Online and Distance Social Work Education

Online and Distance Social Work Education: Current Practice and Future Trends provides a comprehensive presentation of the evolution, current status and future direction of distance learning and online education in the social work profession.

Documenting the current state-of-the-art, this book demonstrates the power of distance learning and online technology and addresses future trends in web-based social work education. Written by widely recognized experts, the chapters represent an authoritative statement of the present state-of-the-art in the application of technology to contemporary social work education. The insights of these experts will be of great interest to students and faculty in the 798 accredited social work programs in the United States. They are creating a revolution in the profession which will forever change the nature of education for professional practice.

Authored by widely recognized educators on the cutting edge of technological innovation, this text will be relevant to social work students and educators in baccalaureate, masters and doctoral programs in the USA and internationally.

The chapters in this book were originally published in the *Journal of Teaching in Social Work*.

Paul A. Kurzman, Ph.D., ACSW, is a Professor of Social Work at Hunter College, USA, and Professor of Social Welfare at The Graduate Center of the City University of New York, USA, where he teaches policy and practice in the MSW and Ph.D. programs. He is an Author/Editor of 10 books and Editor-in-Chief of the *Journal of Teaching in Social Work*.

Melissa B. Littlefield, Ph.D., LGSW, is an Associate Professor and Chair of the Master of Social Work Department at Morgan State University, Baltimore, USA. She is a recognized expert on multiculturalism, race, ethics and computer technology.

Online and Distance Social Work Education

Current Practice and Future Trends

Edited by
Paul A. Kurzman & Melissa B. Littlefield

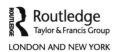

Routledge
Taylor & Francis Group

LONDON AND NEW YORK

First published in paperback 2024

First published 2020
by Routledge
4 Park Square, Milton Park, Abingdon, Oxon OX14 4RN

and by Routledge
605 Third Avenue, New York, NY 10158

Routledge is an imprint of the Taylor & Francis Group, an informa business

© 2020, 2024 Taylor & Francis

Publisher's Note
The publisher has gone to great lengths to ensure the quality of this reprint but points out that some imperfections in the original copies may be apparent.

Disclaimer
Every effort has been made to contact copyright holders for their permission to reprint material in this book. The publishers would be grateful to hear from any copyright holder who is not here acknowledged and will undertake to rectify any errors or omissions in future editions of this book.

British Library Cataloguing-in-Publication Data
A catalogue record for this book is available from the British Library

ISBN: 978-0-367-86036-3 (hbk)
ISBN: 978-1-03-283911-0 (pbk)
ISBN: 978-1-00-301655-7 (ebk)

DOI: 10.4324/9781003016557

Typeset in Minion Pro
by codeMantra

Contents

Citation Information

The chapters in this book were originally published in the *Journal of Teaching in Social Work*. When citing this material, please use the original page numbering for each article, as follows:

Chapter 1
An Introduction: Reimagining Social Work Education for the Digital Age
Melissa B. Littlefield
Journal of Teaching in Social Work, volume 39, issue 4–5 (2019) pp. 278–285

Chapter 2
The Current Status of Social Work Online and Distance Education
Paul A. Kurzman
Journal of Teaching in Social Work, volume 39, issue 4–5 (2019) pp. 286–292

Chapter 3
Community of Inquiry (CoI): A Framework for Social Work Distance Educators
Tami Micsky and Leonora Foels
Journal of Teaching in Social Work, volume 39, issue 4–5 (2019) pp. 293–307

Chapter 4
Beyond the Online Versus On-Campus Debate: Leveraging Technology in a CoI Framework to Enhance Student and Faculty Presence in the MSW Classroom
Jennifer A. Parga, Kathy Bargar, Steve Monte, Ruth A. Supranovich, and Danielle E. Brown
Journal of Teaching in Social Work, volume 39, issue 4–5 (2019) pp. 308–322

Chapter 5
A Synchronous Online Social Work PhD Program: Educational Design and Student/Faculty Response
Dennis Myers, Jon Singletary, Rob Rogers, Jim Ellor, and Sidney Barham
Journal of Teaching in Social Work, volume 39, issue 4–5 (2019) pp. 323–343

Chapter 6
Reflections of an Online Social Work Professor: Illuminating an Alternative Pedagogy
Rachael A. Richter
Journal of Teaching in Social Work, volume 39, issue 4–5 (2019) pp. 344–360

For any permission-related enquiries please visit:
http://www.tandfonline.com/page/help/permissions

Contributors

Eileen Mazur Abel, Ph.D., is a Clinical Professor of Social Work at the Suzanne Dworak-Peck School of Social Work at the University of Southern California, Los Angeles, USA, and can be reached at eabel@usc.edu.

Tanya Nash Andrews, MSW, is a Registered Social Worker at Extendicare Southwood Lakes, Windsor, Canada, and can be reached at tandrews@extendicare.com.

Johanna Creswell Báez, Ph.D., is an Adjunct Assistant Professor and the Manager of Course Development at the Columbia University School of Social Work Online Campus, New York City, USA, and can be reached at jc2515@columbia.edu.

Kathy Bargar, MSW, is an Assistant Professor of Social Work at Brandman University, Irvine, USA, and can be reached at kbargar@brandman.edu.

Sidney Barham, MSW, is a Program Coordinator at St. Alexius Outreach Ministries of Chattanooga, USA, and can be reached at sidneymbarham@gmail.com.

Danielle E. Brown, MSW, is a Clinical Assistant Professor at the Suzanne Dworak-Peck School of Social Work of the University of Southern California, Los Angeles, USA, and can be reached at brownde@usc.edu.

Cynthia Brown Laveist, M.S.E., is the Director of Morgan Online, Division of Academic Outreach & Engagement at Morgan State University, Baltimore, USA, and can be reached at cynthia.brownlaveist@morgan.edu.

Michael Campbell, Ph.D., is an Associate Professor in the Department of Social Work at Saint Leo University, Florida, USA, and can be reached at michael.campbell03@saintleo.edu.

Irene Carter, Ph.D., is a Professor, and MSW Coordinator for Campus Programs at the School of Social Work of the University of Windsor, Canada, and can be reached at icarter@uwindsor.ca.

Rebecca Yae-Eun Chung, MSW, is a Program Manager at the Columbia University School of Social Work Online Campus, New York City, USA, and can be reached at rc2703@columbia.edu.

Laura Curran, Ph.D., is an Associate Professor at the School of Social Work of Rutgers, The State University of New Jersey, USA, and can be reached at lacurran@ssw.rutgers.edu.

Thecla Damianakis, Ph.D., is an Associate Professor at the School of Social Work of the University of Windsor, Canada, and can be reached at damianak@uwindsor.ca.

Beverly Araujo Dawson, Ph.D., is a Professor and the Director of the Online MSW Program at the School of Social Work of Adelphi University, Garden City, USA, and can be reached at baraujo@adelphi.edu.

Jim Ellor, Ph.D., is the Kronzer Endowed Professor at the Diana Garland School of Social Work at Baylor University, Waco, USA, and can be reached at james_ellor@baylor.edu.

Awhina English, Ph.D., is an Honorary Research Associate at the School of Social Work of Massey University, New Zealand, and can be reached at awhinaenglish@gmail.com.

Judy Fenster, Ph.D., is a Professor at the School of Social Work of Adelphi University, Garden City, USA, and can be reached at fenster@adelphi.edu.

Leonora Foels, Ph.D., is an Associate Professor at the School of Social Work of Millersville University, USA, and can be reached at leonora.foels@millersville.edu.

Fontaine H. Fulghum, Ph.D., is a Lecturer at the School of Social Work of Rutgers The State University of New Jersey, USA, and can be reached at fulghum@camden.rutgers.edu.

Kristin Garay, MSW, is Manager of Technologies at the Columbia University School of Social Work Online Campus, New York City, USA, and can be reached at keg2143@columbia.edu.

Jeanna Jacobsen, Ph.D., is a Core Faculty Member of the Barbara Solomon School of Social Work in the College of Social and Behavioral Sciences of Walden University, Minneapolis, USA, and can be reached at jeanna.jacobsen@mail.waldenu.edu.

Janet M. Joiner, Ph.D., is an Assistant Professor and a Chair of the Department of Social Work at the University of Detroit Mercy, USA, and can be reached at joinerjm@udmercy.edu.

Paul A. Kurzman, Ph.D., is a Professor of Social Work at the Silberman School of Hunter College, USA, and a Professor of Social Welfare at The Graduate Center of the City University of New York, USA, and can be reached at pkurzman@hunter.cuny.edu.

Melissa B. Littlefield, Ph.D., is an Associate Professor and Chair of the Master of Social Work Department at Morgan State University, Baltimore, USA, and can be reached at Melissa.littlefield@morgan.edu.

Robert Lucio, Ph.D., is an Associate Professor of Social Work at Saint Leo University, Florida, USA, and can be reached at robert.lucio@saintleo.edu.

Benjamin R. Malczyk, Ph.D., is an Assistant Professor and the Online Program Director in the Social Work Department of the University of Nebraska Kearney, USA, and can be reached at malczykbr@unk.edu.

Matthea Marquart, MSW, is an Adjunct Lecturer and the Director of Administration for the Online Campus at the Columbia University School of Social Work, New York City, USA, and can be reached at msm2002@columbia.edu.

Sumaiya Matin, MSW, is a Strategic Communications Advisor for Ontario Public Service in Toronto, Canada, and can be reached at matins@uwindsor.ca.

Raymond Sanchez Mayers, Ph.D., is an Associate Professor at the School of Social Work of Rutgers, The State University of New Jersey, USA, and can be reached at rsmayers@ssw.rutgers.edu.

Jason S. McKinney, Ph.D., is an Associate Professor and Division Chair of Social Work at Keuka College, Keuka Park, USA, and can be reached at jmckinney@keuka.edu.

Tami Micsky, MSSW, is an Assistant Professor in the Department of Applied Sociology and Social Work of Mercyhurst University, Erie, USA, and can be reached at tmicsky@mercyhurst.edu.

Steve Monte, MSW, is an Adjunct Lecturer at the Suzanne Dworak-Peck School of Social Work of the University of Southern California, Los Angeles, USA, and can be reached at monteste@usc.edu.

Sharon Munro, MSW, MLIS, is an Associate Professor and Social Work Librarian at the Leddy Library of the University of Windsor, Canada, and can be reached at smunro@uwindsor.ca.

Dennis Myers, Ph.D., is the Prince Endowed Professor at the Diana Garland School of Social Work of Baylor University, Waco, USA, and can be reached at dennis_myers@baylor.edu.

Ananda Newmark, Ph.D., is an Associate Professor in Teaching at the School of Social Work of Virginia Commonwealth University, Richmond, USA, and can be reached at anewmark@vcu.edu.

Jennifer A. Parga, MSW, is a Clinical Assistant Professor at the Suzanne Dworak-Peck School of Social Work at the University of Southern California, Los Angeles, USA, and can be reached at jparga@usc.edu.

Debra Patterson, Ph.D., is an Associate Professor at the School of Social Work of Wayne State University, Detroit, USA, and can be reached at dt4578@wayne.edu.

Melanie Reyes, MSW, is a Lecturer at the School of Social Work of Arizona State University, Tempe, USA, and can be reached at melanie.reyes@asu.edu.

Rachael A. Richter, DSW, is an Associate Professor at the School of Social Work of Western New Mexico University, Silver City, USA, and can be reached at rachael.richter@wnmu.edu.

Rob Rogers, Ph.D., is an Associate Professor at the Diana Garland School of Social Work at Baylor University, Waco, USA, and can be reached at rob_rogers@baylor.edu.

Karen Rubinstein, M.Ed., is the Director of Academic Technology Services, Division of Information Technology at Morgan State University, Baltimore, USA, and can be reached at karen.rubinstein@morgan.edu.

Delia Ryan, MSW, is the Live Support Specialist at the Columbia University School of Social Work Online Campus, New York City, USA, and can be reached at der2153@columbia.edu.

Rachel Schwartz, MSW, is the Director of Online Education at the School of Social Work of Rutgers, The State University of New Jersey, USA, and can be reached at rschwartz@ssw.rutgers.edu.

Mary Secret, Ph.D., is Associate Professor Emerita at the School of Social Work of Virginia Commonwealth University, Richmond, USA, and can be reached at mcsecret@vcu.edu.

Elizabeth A. Segal, Ph.D., is a Professor at the School of Social Work of Arizona State University, Tempe, USA, and can be reached at esegal@asu.edu.

Jon Singletary, Ph.D., is the Dean and Professor at the Diana Garland School of Social Work of Baylor University, Waco, USA, and can be reached at jon_singletary@baylor.edu.

Hannah Skinner, MSW, is a Housing Stability Worker at the Optimism Place Women's Shelter and Support Services in Stratford, Canada, and can be reached at hskinner7690@outlook.com

Jennifer Spitz, DSW, is an Adjunct Lecturer at the Silver School of Social Work of New York University, USA, and can be reached at jsg2012@nyu.edu.

Nicky Stanley-Clarke, Ph.D., is a Senior Lecturer at the School of Social Work of Massey University, New Zealand, and can be reached at n.stanley-clarke@massey.ac.nz.

Ruth A. Supranovich, MSW, is a Clinical Associate Professor at the Suzanne Dworak-Peck School of Social Work of the University of Southern California, Los Angeles, USA, and can be reached at supranov@usc.edu.

Christopher Jennings Ward, MSW, is the Online Program Coordinator in the Department of Social Work at Winthrop University, Rock Hill, USA, and can be reached at wardc@winthrop.edu.

Polly Yeung, Ph.D., is a Senior Lecturer at the School of Social Work of Massey University, New Zealand, and can be reached at p.yeung@massey.ac.nz.

Acknowledgments

When we issued a Call for Papers for a text on *Online and Distance Social Work Education*, we had not imagined the response it would receive. While we knew this to be a cutting-edge issue, which prompted our interest in taking the initiative, the sheer number of excellent manuscripts we received, many for the journal's special issue and hence the book, certainly did pleasantly surprise us. Our belief that the time had come for a new and authoritative text on the subject had been validated, and we hope the peer-reviewed selection of these 22 superb chapters confirms that conviction to the reader. Representing the ideas of 51 contributing authors, the chapters herein present new information, novel experimentation, fresh conceptualization and creative templates for what surely represents an important thrust for professional social work education for the present and the future.

As Co-editor, Paul A. Kurzman is very grateful for the can-do spirit and steady support of Abigail Carson, Portfolio Manager for Behavioral Science and Social Care, and Caroline Church, Commissioning Editor of Routledge Special Issues as Books. Their patience and flexibility made a difference. And it is clear that this book would not have been possible without the quiet, steady and focused support of Ruth Flaherty, the Assistant Editor of the *Journal of Teaching in Social Work*, who carried out so many of the tasks of assignment and production with an always skillful and steady hand.

As Co-editor, Melissa B. Littlefield wishes to recognize that the idea for what has ultimately resulted in the publication of this volume was conceptualized by members of the Online Social Work Educators' League, a group that has met since 2016 to share information and to support each other in developing and implementing online MSW programs across the country. In the true spirit of the social work profession, League members identified a gap in the literature regarding successful implementation of online social work programs and set in motion an effort to gather the latest ideas and practice wisdom to advance the state-of-the-art. Special thanks go to the following League members: Trish Cox of University of New Hampshire; Stephen Cummings of University of Iowa; Julia Kleinschmit of University of Iowa; Melanie Reyes of Arizona State University; and Rachel Schwartz of Rutgers, The State University of New Jersey. Finally, I would like to acknowledge Halaevalu Vakalahi, former Associate Dean of the Morgan State University School of Social Work, for encouraging and supporting me in taking on editorship, and Dean Anna McPhatter and the MSW Faculty and Staff at Morgan State University, Morgan Online, and Morgan Academic Technology Services for their groundbreaking efforts to establish the first fully online MSW program at an HBCU.

And to the contributors, whose insights and innovations are so articulately expressed here, we give thanks and tribute for their remarkable creativity and perspicacity. In this book, each of them individually and all of them collectively have made an indelible professional contribution to the topic of *Online and Distance Social Work Education* for the social work profession.

Paul A. Kurzman
Melissa B. Littlefield
January 2020

Part I

An Overview and Perspective

An Introduction: Reimagining Social Work Education for the Digital Age

Melissa B. Littlefield

ABSTRACT

Despite the recent publication of a number of articles, along with current presentations at professional conferences, and a scholarly text all on the topic of distance learning and online social work education, many believe that the subject has not received the level of recognition among academics in our profession that it needs and deserves. This Introduction to a special double issue of a prominent peer-reviewed journal serves to welcome the reader to the contents of the seventeen articles that follow, and to provide both an overview and conceptual framework for the special issue as a whole. Underscoring both the opportunities and quandaries, support and resistance, most of the authors would appear to conclude that social work educators must rapidly become more agile in embracing the unique opportunities presented by the technology that we now have at hand.

Many more social work bachelors and masters programs have initiated hybrid and fully online programs in the intervening years since the *Journal of Teaching in Social Work* published its 2013 special issue on distance and online education (Council on Social Work Education [CSWE], 2019). As programs have launched online delivery options, they have discovered that much more is required to offer online courses and programs than digitizing the content they offer in face-to-face classes. Attention also must be focused on engaging students, maintaining faculty and student motivation, and forming effective student-to-instructor and student-to-peer relationships, as well as addressing ethical and diversity considerations. Moreover, there are program implementation and administration issues, as well.

While there is a plethora of literature on online education generally, and even a fair amount speaking to online professional education (such as nursing education), specific literature around distance and online education for social work is still comparatively sparse. However, in recent years there has been a greater response. For example, articles on the use of technology in delivering social work education increasingly are found in a variety of social work journals; books have now been published on the topic; more conference sessions featuring the use of technology in education now are being presented at the Council on Social Work Education Annual Program Meeting and other social work conferences; and specialty publications have appeared (Kurzman, 2013). Additionally, a Social Work Distance Education Conference (SWDE) has been held annually since 2016.

Yet, the state of the literature has not yet reached the point of providing sufficient knowledge to guide social work programs pursuing the online education arena. Social work faculty and academic staff, including advisors, field educators and program administrators, continue to grapple with the everyday realities of navigating the cyberscape of distance and online education. One response has been the formation of informal groups of online program directors and advisors to share information and strategies and to support one another as they develop and implement such programs at their respective institutions. One such group, now known as "The Online Social Work Educators' League," was formed following the second annual SWDE conference. The group has met synchronously on a monthly basis via web-based video conferencing. Initially, the hosting of sessions rotated among members and topics were determined at the start of each session. The format was tweaked in the second year, with a slate of topics being generated at the beginning of each academic year, based on areas of need and interest, with specific members agreeing to facilitate each session. During sessions participants typically share their experiential knowledge and the resources they have found in their own quests to implement their programs. They also seek feedback, support and advice from each other. Participants represent diverse online programs, including rural and urban, those targeting marginalized as well as more privileged populations, those with both large and small student populations, and those with regional versus national student enrollment. Yet the program implementation issues seem to cut across program contexts. Topics have included student orientation, advising, faculty and staff boundary setting and work-life balance, graduation practices, student support and community building, and instructor training and evaluation, among others. Group members found these sessions to be so useful that they were inspired to propose another special issue on distance and online education to capture new knowledge and strategies that have emerged since the publication of the previous special issue (Distance Learning and Online Education in Social Work, 2013). Special thanks are given to League members Julia Kleinschmidt of the University of Iowa, Rachel Schwartz of Rutgers University, Melanie Reyes of Arizona State University, and Trish Cox of the University of New Hampshire for their important contributions to bringing this current special issue to fruition. Judging from the response to the call for papers, which has resulted in the publication of this double issue, the topic of distance and online education continues to be of great interest to social work educators.

Kurzman's lead article provides an overview of the current status and implications of distance and online social work education. Articles in Part II then address *Emergent Paradigms* for online pedagogy. Micsky & Foels discuss the Community of Inquiry (CoI) as a framework for distance social work course design, implementation and evaluation, which is increasingly a standard for distance education. Parga, Bargar, Monte, Supranovich and Brown's article illustrates how the CoI framework was implemented to enhance student learning outcomes in an online MSW program, and Myers, Singletary, Rogers, Ellor & Barham describe the design and evaluation of a CoI-based online doctoral program. Shifting gears, Richter's article presents a "liberatory pedagogical approach" to facilitate critical thinking, awareness, reflection and social action around constructs such as race, gender, and class. Scholarly Personal Narrative is used as a method to explore the opportunities and challenges of implementing liberatory pedagogy within a virtual classroom.

Part III focuses on *Ethical & Diversity Considerations*. Reyes and Segal use the lens of critical theory to examine the juxtaposition of opportunities afforded by distance education for information globalization, consciousness-raising, and social justice, versus being used as an instrument of colonization and oppression and offer recommendations to prevent social work distance education from becoming the latter. The other articles in this section focus on strategies for teaching online students about diversity and ethics. Jacobsen provides specific recommendations for online teaching about diversity and difference, with regard to both the explicit and the implicit curriculum. Joiner's piece explores the importance of preparing social work students for ethical online behavior by teaching digital ethics and professional online conduct. Spitz asserts the need to preserve the learner-teacher relationship in online education given its significance in social work education.

The offerings in Part IV illustrate innovations in engaging online students using a variety of educational technologies. The article by McKinney and the one by Schwartz, Sanchez Mayers, Curran & Fulghum, exemplify the use of simulations that activate student learning for online, face-to-face, or hybrid courses, while Joiner and Patterson's entry demonstrates the use of a multimedia tool, VoiceThread, for collaborative learning in which students are engaged through content creation. Malczyk provides a glimpse of the new trend toward customized learning in his article on the "HyFlex" blended learning model. Ward, Secret and Newmark then outline the transformation of an entire course to an online format which involved aligning new teaching practices, learning activities and specific technologies to achieve the learning outcomes.

Part V tackles difficult administrative issues facing online programs. Baez, Marquart, Ryan, Chung, and Garay describe a five-week faculty training program for distance social work educators based on best practices in online education that other social work programs can use. Littlefield, Rubinstein and

Brown-Laveist provide an overview of research-informed tools, known as quality rubrics or scorecards, which administrators can deploy to guide the development, support and management of quality online courses and programs. Finally, Campbell, Abel and Lucio discuss the use of a brief assessment tool, called the one minute paper, by online instructors to reinforce learning and to tailor the pedagogical experience, to reinforce student-centered learning.

Social work educators will need to take a more proactive approach in responding to technology and related trends in higher education and developing pedagogical applications for the educational technology that is increasingly accessible to faculty, staff and students. Indeed, distance and face-to-face education have converged somewhat, with online education being at the nexus. In particular, distance education has previously been offered via communication technologies such as interactive television and telephone conferencing, and implies that students participate in courses remotely with little if any physical meetings with the instructor. More recently distance education has become almost synonymous with online education. However, distance education may refer to fully online programs in which students do not meet in the same physical classroom; blended or hybrid programs in which students and instructors sometimes meet physically; or programs that primarily meet in a physical location, but which also use online resources for teaching and learning and course administration. Examples include electronic courses reserves. Learning management systems (such as Canvas, Blackboard, Brightspace), incorporation of video and adaptive learning, as well as use of video conferencing for online office hours, advising, admissions applications and interviews. Hence, going forward it would appear that different pedagogical considerations and frameworks may be necessary, depending on the degree of physical presence versus online presence of students and instructors in programs. Moreover, for degree programs offered fully online, more conceptual literature and empirical studies are needed to address the types of "brass tacks" program implementation issues identified by the aforementioned Online Social Work Educators' League, which are likely to be shared by many online social work programs.

Curiously, despite the explosion of growth in online programs, social work faculty have been cautious about embracing online education (Levin, Fulginiti, & Moore, 2018). In a study of faculty in US schools of social work, Levin and colleagues found that respondents perceived online courses to be less effective with respect to every CSWE competency than face-to-face courses – with practice courses perceived as being least effective when taught online. Although their study has limited generalizability, they report that their findings were almost identical to those of a similar, seminal study conducted almost 15 years prior. This perception is alarming, given that a vast number of social work programs have moved to offering hybrid and online courses, as well as programs and certificates. Levin and colleagues cited faculty concerns about modeling the use of self as a barrier for endorsing online practice method courses. Faculty may be concerned here that human development and interaction, including helping relationships and educational outcomes, could be impacted in unknown ways with the shift to online education. Thus, it would appear that the move of social work programs to offer online courses and degrees often has come at the insistence of their institutions, or in response to economic realities, rather than by their own volition.

Other challenges to more fully developing online instructional modalities involve the resistance of social work academic administrators to using new enhanced communication technology. This resistance is reflected in staffing issues such as restricting the number of online courses allowed in faculty workloads, and disallowing flexible work schedules and telework for staff in online programs who need to interact with students and faculty outside of traditional business hours. Discomfort with telework also limits some programs from hiring staff, and even faculty who reside out of the geographic area where the university is located, thereby limiting the talent pool available to those programs. Another challenge is the lack of innovation in field education which should consider better support for online students in field placements, including appropriate training and supervision for field liaisons and field instructors who are supervising students remotely, and providing opportunities for field internships that focus on technology enhanced social work practice, such as telehealth.

The apparent dissonance among social work educators with regard to the role and value of online education, especially as it relates to their belief about the ability to teach practice, has significant implications for the preparation of students for the current and future work force. In fact, apparent faculty and staff reluctance seems to be out of step with the changing demands of the labor market, as well as students' expectations of their learning experiences, especially for "digital natives", (i.e., students under the age of 30) who have never known life otherwise.

Bonk (2016) asserts that we have entered the age of "Education 3.0", characterized by vast resource abundance and learner empowerment. According to Bonk, "There is a revolution underway in education. Today, learning is more visual, blended, game-based, immersive, digital, comfortable, modifiable, and personal" (p. 7). Bonk identifies 30 ways in which education is changing that can be subsumed under three mega trends: (1) learner engagement, (2) pervasive access to learning [aka, anytime/anywhere learning], and (3) customized and personalized learning. Examples of learner engagement include increasing use of mobile devices, visual versus text based learning, and games and simulations in which learners solve problems to gain understanding of concepts and to demonstrate competence. Students are more immersed in the learning experience via technologies including virtual reality, which allows them to experience situations as though they were actually there, and augmented reality, where information is superimposed on objects in the physical environment. Learning also is more cooperative and collaborative, with students working on team projects remotely. Examples of the concept of pervasive access include learning being more online, more global, and more immediate (i.e., new knowledge is being made available to the masses more rapidly). In terms of customization, learning is becoming more blended (i.e. hybrid), self-directed, competency-based (i.e., learners do not repeat content they already know and can test out of courses) and more on demand (i.e., access to tools, resources and experts based on the learner's schedule rather than the institution's). Similarly, futurist James Canton's (2015) list of ten innovations that will reinvent education mirrors much of Bonk's list, and further includes "big data applied to learning how to learn" and "cloud computing for distributed education." Jeffrey Selingo, former editor of the Chronicle of Higher Education (2016), discusses some of these trends in terms of the disconnect between traditional higher education practices and what the labor market and students actually want and need to meet today's realities. He highlights innovations such as "just in time education" in which providers (other than higher education institutions) are offering "shorter chunks" of learning at the time it is needed by recent college graduates in order to hone their skills.

Therefore, the writing is on the wall for social work education which must seriously begin to consider how it will position itself to be responsive to the changing demands of both the workplace and student expectations. The need for reconsideration extends beyond degree programs to include continuing education and certificate programs that social workers need for licensure and credential renewal, and for staying current with evolving practice knowledge and skills. Advances in technology can enable a variety of models of education to be delivered in ways that are more accessible, congruent with a variety of learning styles and preferences, and are more efficient for learners.

Given the pervasiveness of technology in society, perhaps a larger issue looms than whether social work courses and content can be taught using the new methods. Social work education also must be concerned with creating opportunities to expose and engage students in technologies currently being used in practice environments so they can practice competently in these arenas, as required by our professional Code of Ethics. Further, the profession and its educators have a duty to help students develop an understanding of how contemporary technology impacts the social environments and social problems with which clients have to deal and therefore social work is concerned. Indeed, it has been argued that failure to engage social work students in learning how to effectively use current technology risks further marginalizing an already historically marginalized group of professionals (Littlefield & Roberson, 2005). This reality continues to be a concern, considering that the social work profession continues to be largely populated by women and that technology continues to be socially constructed as masculine – although there is a recent trend in primary education toward making technology more appealing to girls. It should be noted as well that some of the educational trends affected by technological advances and features of online learning, such as the move toward cooperative and collaborative learning, are congruent with women's epistemology (Littlefield & Roberson, 2005) and therefore can be seen as opportunities for social work education.

There is no question that technology currently impacts the profession and consequently social work education. Rather, the question seems to be to what extent the profession will embrace technology and use it to advance its mission. Social work educators who have been exploring the use of digital technology in teaching and practice have long been a niche group, connecting with one another via interest groups at domestic social work conferences as well as via international communities of interest such as the Human Services Information Technology Association (HUSITA). This loose and informal manner can no longer be the case, given the pervasiveness of the Internet, and since the integration of technology into every aspect of life has implications for the *what* as well as the *how* of social work education. The report of the Envisioning the Future of Social Work Task Force (CSWE, 2018) identifies technology as a major trend affecting the future of the profession and poses the question of whether social work will experience technology at an evolutionary pace, incorporating technology to improve existing ways of practice, or whether it will embrace technology to create new forms of practice. Consequently, the relevance of the profession in the digital age is in question, since there is a current gap between the real world and social work classes at many institutions. Anecdotally, in the past 5 years that this author has been conducting a campus technology workshop as part of MSW student orientation, students have indicated a much higher use of technology in their human services workplace, particularly as tools for managing client information and reporting. They also have expressed high use of the Internet and social media for their personal affairs, as social work students increasingly have become "digital natives." Hence, we are likely to see a shifting focus of developing online social work education from not only making it more accessible but responding to customer (that is, student) expectations. Therefore, basic technology-related competencies for social workers might include the following:

- New ways of communicating with client systems (including digital ethics and "netiquette");
- Information literacy (discerning reputable sources of research/information and critiquing it for practice);
- Psychosocial implications of the contemporary technology environment including interpersonal and intrapersonal dynamics;

- New social problems and the impact of technology on current problems social work addresses (e.g. internet addiction, cyber bullying, etc.); and
- Developing skills for distance practice utilizing contemporary technology.

In sum, the impact of contemporary technology has led to changes in all levels and forms of instruction, including graduate and professional education. Social work programs have been, and will continue to be, affected. Social work educators and programs must seriously consider how to become more agile and how to embrace new opportunities brought forward by technological advances while being mindful of technology's challenges and limitations. When so doing, we must determine what is essential about social work practice and social work education, and how the essence can be preserved while updated to meet contemporary needs.

Disclosure statement

No potential conflict of interest was reported by the author.

References

Bonk, C. J. (2016). Keynote: What is the state of e-learning? Reflections on 30 ways learning is changing. *Journal of Open, Flexible and Distance Learning, 20*(2), 6–20.

Canton, J. (2015). *Future smart: Managing the game changing trends that will transform your world.* Boston, MA: DaCapo Press.

Council on Social Work Education [CSWE]. (2018). *Envisioning the future of social work: Report of the social work futures task force.* Alexandria, VA, Council on Social Work Education. Retrieved from https://www.cswe.org/About-CSWE/Governance/Board-of-Directors/2018-19-Strategic-Planning-Process/CSWE-FTF-Four-Futures-for-Social-Work-FINAL-2.aspx

Council on Social Work Education [CSWE]. (2019, August). *Online and distance education offerings by accredited programs.* Retrieved from https://cswe.org/Accreditation/Directory-of-Accredited-Programs/Online-and-Distance-Education

Distance Learning and Online Education in Social Work. (2013). P. A. Kurzman & R. P. Maiden (Eds.). *Journal of Teaching in Social Work, 33*(4/5).

Kurzman, P. (2013). The evolution of distance learning and online education. *Journal of Teaching in Social Work, 33*:(4–5), 331–338. doi:10.1080/08841233.2013.843346

Levin, S., Fulginiti, A., & Moore, B. (2018). The perceived effectiveness of online social work education: Insights from a national survey of social work educators. *Social Work Education, 37*(6), 775–789. doi:10.1080/02615479.2018.1482864

Littlefield, M. B., & Roberson, K. C. (2005). Computer technology for the feminist classroom. *Affilia, 20*(2), 186–202. doi:10.1177/0886109905274676

Selingo, J. (2016). *There is life after college: What parents and students should know about navigating school to prepare for the jobs of tomorrow.* New York, NY: HarperCollins.

The Current Status of Social Work Online and Distance Education

Paul A. Kurzman

ABSTRACT

Over the past three decades, social work education gradually has begun to embrace distance education as a viable alternative (and supplement) to traditional face-to-face education. While some feel that social work's response has been slow, compared to sister professions, it has been explicit, extensive and sure. This paper looks at the current status of social work's response to emerging online and digital options, and concludes with a look to the future.

The electronic revolution

Over the past 35 years, a revolution has taken place, but no troops took to the battlefield, and no shots were fired. This revolution has been electronic and has had a profound impact on citizens of all nations in ways that often were unexpected. The arena of higher education has not been exempt, and most of us would consider this reality to essentially be good news. It is now possible to offer college and university education to more people, at a greater convenience, and often at a lower cost. The advent of distance learning and online education has been heralded by many as a creator of new opportunities, especially in the area of higher and continuing education; and opportunity in a democracy is the coin of the realm.

Lawrence K. Grossman, the original vice-chair of Digital Promise, notes that in this digital age it would be shortsighted "to ignore the great potential that digital technologies have to improve, extend and transform teaching, learning and skills training" at all levels of education (Grossman, 2012, p. 2). In recognition of this reality, in 2008 the U.S. Congress established and appropriated modest start-up funds for a nonprofit and independent national research center. What the National Science Foundation did for science and the National Institutes of Health did for health care, the new National Center for Research in Advanced Information and Digital Technologies is now

NOTE: This manuscript was adapted in part from an article by the author titled, "The Evolution of Distance Learning and Online Education," published in the *Journal of Teaching in Social Work*, 33(4/5), 2013, pp. 331–338.

beginning to do for teaching and education "in order to provide Americans with the knowledge and skills needed to compete in the global economy" (p. 2).

The social work response

In the current issue of the *Encyclopedia of Social Work*, Ouellette and Westhuis (2008, p. 118) presciently observe that "The integration of technology for teaching the social work curriculum has the potential to make social work education, and ultimately direct practice, more effective, more widespread, and less expensive." With the advent of broadband availability, more powerful processors, secure interactive video transmission, simulcast broadcasting with ITV, versatile web conferencing software, high-end graphics, avatar assisted animation, and sophisticated web-based platforms, the options for online education (and therefore distance learning) today are extensive, and are likely to further expand with the development of 5G networks, the next generation of wireless technology. Even field work education, sometimes considered to be the pedagogical exception to the rule, can be secured using a 3D virtual world where clients and students interact with one another visually via digitally generated avatars (Reamer, 2013; Wilson, Brown, Wood, & Farkas, 2013).

Recent reviews of social work education tend to support the early embrace of technology in the delivery of baccalaureate and graduate education. A survey conducted by the Council on Social Work Education (CSWE) Commission on Accreditation in 2005 found that 41% of the respondents from BSW programs and 52% from MSW programs were delivering courses using some form of technology (Vernon, 2006). Vernon, Vakalahi, Pierce, Pittman-Munke, and Adkins (2009) also found that "More than one-third of BSW programs and one-quarter of MSW programs did not require a face-to-face experience as an integral component of course work" (p. 269). Instead, these programs offered courses that were <u>entirely online</u>, without direct human contact.

Along with the two key national sister organizations, the National Association of Social Workers (NASW) and the Association of Social Work Boards (ASWB), CSWE has been supportive of efforts by the programs it accredits to move toward increasing online and distance education options. For example, in 2007, CSWE hosted a Distance Education Summit; has published many articles on the topic in its quarterly *Journal of Social Work Education*; offers many presentations on the topic at its Annual Program Meeting; and has made provisions for this educational innovation in its current Educational Policy and Accreditation Standards (EPAS) document. Moreover, the new 2015 EPAS focus on "core competencies" is supportive, since online education is less interested in how students acquire a competency (i.e., the process) than in offering evidence that the competency was mastered. The NASW has provided support for this new pedagogy as well through an extensive focus on technology, distance learning, and online education in the most recent edition of its frequently cited *Encyclopedia of Social Work* publication; coverage in its widely read journal, *Social Work*; and through co-development (with the ASWB) of *Standards for Technology in Social Work Practice* (2017), an authoritative guidepost for professional education and practice. Finally, the Group for the Advancement of Doctoral Education (GADE), which sets standards for social work doctoral programs, notes that many of the current 79 PhD and 10 DSW offerings are now being provided (primarily or entirely) online (GADE, 2019).

Books and journals also have emerged on the subject during the past decade. In 2005, Professor Paul Abels at California State University-Long Beach issued *Distance Education in Social Work* (Abels, 2005); Professors Richard Beaulaurier (Florida International University) and Martha Haffey (Hunter College) assembled the text titled *Technology in Social Work Education* (Beaulaurier & Haffey, 2005); and in 2014 Professors Paul Kurzman (Hunter College) and Paul Maiden (USC) published *Distance Learning and Online Education in Social Work* (Kurzman & Maiden, 2014). Over the course of the decade, new peer-reviewed social work journals have appeared, such as the *Electronic Journal of Social Work*, and *Technology in Social Work Education and Curriculum*, as well as the *Journal of Technology in the Human Services, American Journal of Distance Education, Journal of Computers in the Human Services, Online Learning Journal, Quarterly Review of Distance Education*, and many more. In addition, ASWB and NASW are approving continuing education units, required for licensure renewal and credential endorsement, that are being offered entirely online by distance education firms such as CEUNITS.com and NetCE.com. Moreover, display advertisements, from CSWE-accredited programs, have begun to appear regularly in *Social Work Advocates* and in *Social Work Today*, promoting their online distance learning educational offerings. By 2019, it became clear that widespread recognition of this alternative pedagogical option had been achieved (CSWE, 2019).

The pros and cons

It is difficult to compare classroom-based social work education with that delivered largely (or entirely) online via the medium of distance education. To some extent, it is an "apples and oranges" comparison, since both modalities meet a need, and both lead to the award of an accredited professional degree and full eligibility for state licensure and professional employment. The latter simply offers an alternate route, and alternatives generally are honored and valued. One faculty member, with MSW and

DSW degrees, stated her opinion quite clearly. She opined, "Well-designed online courses taught by professors at local universities can cultivate autonomous learning strategies and create opportunities for student-to-student engagement as well as student-to-professor engagement". She concluded, "This can provide the student who is juggling school, work and family responsibilities the means to complete college" (Rose, 2013, p. A-27). Providing that online faculty agree to eschew the "sage on the stage" orientation to teaching and are comfortable with a more modern "guide on the side" approach, many would argue that distance learning is an entirely viable framework for professional education. As the Pulitzer Prize–winning columnist and author Thomas L. Friedman (2013, p. A-18) observes, "There is one big thing happening that leaves me incredibly hopeful about the future, and that is the budding revolution in global online higher education." Indeed, there is a quintessentially democratic spirit embedded in the proposition that a potential student's remote location, limited transportation options, family commitments, or work obligations will not be a barrier to the pursuit of higher education and to the opportunities it almost always provides. In fact, these are social work values, articulated in our professional code of ethics. Unless research can uncover a statistically significant difference in student satisfaction, licensing exam pass rates, or post-graduation career achievement, we have no basis to assert that one way of pursuing the BSW, MSW or DSW degree is definitely better than another. Little summative research has been conducted to date, although a small but well-designed study of 183 MSW graduates of the University of Tennessee's distance education and traditional degree pathways found no significant difference in final attainment in EPAS core competency area ratings or in GPA (Cummings & Chaffin, 2012).

Moreover, a recent 2018 research sample survey of more than 1,400 MSW graduates, conducted by the Health Workplace Institute of George Washington University, revealed that currently "almost 80% of accredited baccalaureate and master's social work programs offer part of their program in an online or hybrid format" (George Washington University, 2019, p. 2). This finding would support Allen and Seaman's (2013) earlier observation that the growth in enrollment for online courses is now increasing more rapidly than for traditional on-campus offerings.

Nonetheless, the critics are many and vocal. Some argue that the movement toward online education has primarily been motivated by profitmaking and led by proprietary educational corporations such as Coursera and Udacity, along with for-profit universities like Phoenix, Walden, and American Intercontinental (Cronin & Bachorz, 2006). While there is no question that several proprietary firms and institutions of higher education have taken the lead, it also presently is true that prestigious public and nonprofit colleges and universities have mounted the leading master's and baccalaureate online options. They include such nationally regarded schools of social work as Fordham, Case Western Reserve, Columbia, Rutgers, and the universities of Southern California, Indiana, Alabama, and Tennessee. Although some firms in the emerging industry may primarily be focused on profit, and sometimes accused of fraud, currently such does not seem to be the experience with online and distance education for the social work profession. The quandaries and conundrums for us may be of a different order.

More than 80 years ago, the noted educator John Dewey (1938) stated that learning is based on discovery guided by mentoring, rather than on the transmission of information. Therefore, he argued that students need engagement with their teachers to feel comfortable, confident, and successful. As the provost of a prominent university recently put it, "No PowerPoint presentation or elegant online lecture can make up for the surprise, the frisson, the spontaneous give-and-take of a spirited, open-ended dialogue with another person" (Brooks, 2013, p. A-27). A faculty member and prolific author adds his own concern about the relative "sterility" of the distance learning medium. "A real course," he suggests, "creates intellectual joy, at least in some. I don't think an Internet course ever will. Internet learning promises to make intellectual life more sterile and abstract than it already is – and also, for teachers and students alike, far more lonely" (Edmundson, 2012, p. 11).

The future

Certainly, it is clear that distance learning and online education for the social work profession are here to stay. They are not temporary, passing, or ephemeral phenomena that will dissipate and decline in the coming decades. From a Parsonian structural-functional perspective, they perform a function and, therefore, structures will continue to be put in place to ensure their survival. Indeed, we would expect that these educational modalities will expand in the future and become far more common in the preparation for professional practice than they are today. We have begun to discuss and witness their evolution in this paper, and the reader will see a great deal of further evidence in the superb papers that follow. As one social work authority in this arena has commented, "There is no doubt that new developments in technology will continue at a rapid pace that will make teaching with technology even more effective and widespread." She therefore wisely adds that there is a pressing need "to develop a coherent body of knowledge to support the delivery of teaching in technology-enhanced learning environments for future social work education" (Coe Regan, 2008, p. 218).

We must recognize the medium has limitations, including a higher general rate of attrition and the frequently unstated expectation of a very well-organized, disciplined, and motivated student. Field practicum, sometimes referred to as the signature pedagogy of the profession, often may be more difficult to execute well at a distance. Yet the online revolution offers intriguing opportunities for broadening and extending access to social work education. Whenever possible, perhaps use of a hybrid format, with online education complemented and supplemented by faculty mentoring and personal contact, would lead toward an optimal protocol (Dawson & Fenster, 2015). But as the noted political sage Douglas Schoen (2010, p. 198) reminds us:

> Our society and all of its institutions are in continuous processes of transformation. We cannot expect new stable states that will endure for our own lifetimes … We [reflective practitioners] must learn to understand, guide, influence and manage these transformations.

It is our hope that the articles that follow will help us to continue this journey of understanding together.

Disclosure statement

No potential conflict of interest was reported by the author.

References

Abels, P. (Ed.). (2005). *Distance education in social work*. New York, NY: Springer.

Allen, I. E., & Seaman, J. (2013). *Changing course: Ten years of tracking online education in the United States*. Newburyport, MA: The Sloan Consortium.

Beaulaurier, R., & Haffey, M. (Eds.). (2005). *Technology in social work education*. Binghamton, NY: Haworth.

Brooks, A. C. (2013, February 1). My valuable, cheap college degree. *The New York Times*, p. A–27.

Coe Regan, J. A. (2008). Technology in social work education. In T. Mizrahi & L. Davis (Eds.), *Encyclopedia of social work* (Vol. 4, 20th ed., pp. 217–218). Washington, DC: NASW Press.

Council on Social Work Education. [CSWE]. (2019). *Distance education*. Retrieved from www.cswe.org/accreditation/directory-of-accredited-programs/online-and-distance-education

Cronin, J. M., & Bachorz, P. M. (2006). The rising phoenix and what it means for higher education. *Journal of Education*, *186*(1), 11–21. doi:10.1177/002205740618600103

Cummings, S. M., & Chaffin, K. (2012, November 11). *Comparison of outcomes of a distance education and a traditional MSW program*. Paper presented at the 58th Annual Program Meeting of the Council on Social Work Education, Washington, DC. doi:10.1094/PDIS-11-11-0999-PDN

Dawson, B. A., & Fenster, J. (2015). Web-based social work courses: Guidelines for developing and implementing an online environment. *Journal of Teaching in Social Work*, *35*(4), 365–377. doi:10.1080/08841233.2015.1068905

Dewey, J. (1938). *Logic: The theory of inquiry*. New York, NY: Henry Holt.

Edmundson, M. (2012, January 18). The trouble with online education. *The International Herald Tribune*, p. 11. doi:10.1094/PDIS-11-11-0999-PDN

Friedman, T. L. (2013, January 27). Revolution hits the universities. *The New York Times*, p. A–18.

George Washington University. (2019). A comparison of in person and online master's of social work graduates: Findings from a 2018 survey of social work graduates. Washington, DC: Health Workforce Institute.

Grossman, L. K. (2012, February 6). Reading, 'riting, 'rithmetic, and R & D. Letter to the editor. *The Nation*, p. 2. doi:10.1094/PDIS-11-11-0999-PDN

Group for the Advancement of Doctoral Education. [GADE]. (2019). Retrieved from www. gadephd.org/About-Us.

Kurzman, P. A., & Maiden, R. P. (Eds.). (2014). *Distance learning and online education in social work*. New York, NY: Routledge.

National Association of Social Workers, Council on Social Work Education, and Clinical Social Work Association. (2017). *Standards for technology in social work practice*. Washington, DC: NASW Press.

Ouellette, P. M., & Westhuis, D. (2008). Social work education: Electronic technologies. In T. Mizrahi & L. Davis (Eds.), *Encyclopedia of social work* (Vol. 4, 20th ed., pp. 118–120). Washington, DC: NASW Press.

Reamer, F. G. (2013). Social work in a digital age: Ethical and risk management challenges. *Social Work*, 58(2), 163–172. doi:10.1093/sw/swt003

Rose, L. H. (2013, April 29). Letter to the editor. *The New York Times*, p. A–27.

Schoen, D. E. (2010). *The political fix*. New York, NY: Time Books.

Vernon, R. (2006). *CSWE commission on accreditation distance education survey* (Unpublished manuscript). CSWE, Alexandria, VA.

Vernon, R., Vakalahi, H., Pierce, D., Pittman-Munke, P., & Adkins, L. F. (2009). Distance education in social work: Current and emerging trends. *Journal of Social Work Education*, 45(2), 263–276. doi:10.5175/JSWE.2009.200700081

Wilson, A. B., Brown, S., Wood, Z. B., & Farkas, K. J. (2013). Teaching direct practice skills using web-based simulations: Home visiting in the virtual world. *Journal of Teaching in Social Work*, 33(4–5), 421–437. doi:10.1080/08841233.2013.833578

Part II

Emergent Paradigms

Community of Inquiry (Col): A Framework for Social Work Distance Educators

Tami Micsky and Leonora Foels

ABSTRACT

The Community of Inquiry (Col) framework, a research-based seminal work, provides a structure for integrating a collaborative constructivist approach in course design, implementation, and evaluation. The Col framework suggests that by fostering three essential elements – social presence, cognitive presence, and teaching presence – a community of inquiry can be created to promote student engagement and learning. This paper will present the concepts of the Col framework for social work educators to consider for distance education course design, implementation, and evaluation.

Introduction

Social work education is facing an increased use of distance education formats, including fully online and blended/hybrid/mixed-mode models (Cummings, Chaffin, & Cockerham, 2015; Hill-Jones, 2015; Zidan, 2015). However, many social work educators remain skeptical about the effectiveness of distance education formats (Moore, 2005; Vernon, Vakalahi, Pierce, Pittman-Munke, & Adkins, 2009) and research remains focused on that issue (Bentley, Secret, & Cummings, 2015; Cummings et al., 2015; Hill-Jones, 2015; Zidan, 2015). Moreover, the field of social work education has yet to fully examine or adopt a consistent model for course design, implementation, and evaluation that supports the values and goals of the social work profession (Blackmon, 2013; Reamer, 2013).

Existing research into social work distance education primarily focuses on effectiveness and appropriateness for the field of social work (Bentley et al., 2015; Cummings et al., 2015; Hill-Jones, 2015; Kurzman, 2013; Zidan, 2015) Blackmon (2013) posits that the field of social work education is not addressing the movement toward online education with the same haste as other applied disciplines, such as business and nursing, and recommends that social work educators identify teaching strategies that will thoughtfully integrate technology into courses as part of the learning process, not just as a mechanism for

---

Color versions of one or more of the figures in the article can be found online at www.tandfonline.com/wtsw.

communication. Cummings et al. (2015) concur and suggest identifying "specific pedagogical approaches and instrumental mechanisms" (p. 119) in this regard. Zidan (2015) suggests that future research should focus on formats that provide a high level of interaction between educators and students and the development of curricula that will fit with student needs while maintaining social work pedagogy.

The Community of Inquiry (CoI) Framework provides a model that suits the needs of social work education and provides techniques and insights that will help educators to maintain high-quality social work programs in the online format. The CoI framework can assist in course design and guide a social work educators' instructional approach by focusing on concepts of human presence, inquiry, and community building.

The community of inquiry

The Community of Inquiry (CoI) framework encompasses features and characteristics that create community and encourage student satisfaction and success in learning environments (Garrison, 2016; Vaughan, Cleveland-Innes, & Garrison, 2013). The CoI framework was originally developed to provide a structure to understand the mechanisms of computer-mediated distance education, as well as a methodology to practice and evaluate online learning (Garrison, Anderson, & Archer, 2000). However, Garrison (2016) observed that the framework could have an application to any form of thinking and learning in a collaborative environment. The CoI concept helps educators to understand the process of using presence to create a community of deep learning, critical thinking, and serious inquiry (Garrison, 2017).

Garrison et al. (2000) proposed the three elements that comprise the Community of Inquiry (CoI) Framework: social presence, cognitive presence, and teaching presence. Social presence is defined as "the ability of participants in the Community of Inquiry to project their personal characteristics into the community, thereby presenting themselves to the other participants as real people." Cognitive presence centers on supporting the development of skills, knowledge, and understanding, which would include exploring and examining content, integrating material into assignments, and resolving dilemmas. Teaching presence focuses on course design and organization, instructor preparation, course materials, course facilitation, direct instruction, and learning experiences (Garrison et al., 2000, p. 89). The Community of Inquiry (CoI) model, at its core, submits that the formation of a collaborative constructivist community of learners is reliant on the interface of these three core elements (Garrison, 2017).

The process of group inquiry is stimulated when students are provided with opportunities to share ideas and express diverse opinions. Cognitive presence is the primary stimulus for students to engage in a learning community. Essentially, students are enrolled in courses to engage in content, learn skills, and process new knowledge. Garrison and Arbaugh (2007) described the four phases of the Practical Inquiry Model as a primary progression of cognitive presence: 1) Triggering Event – identification of a problem that requires inquiry; 2) Exploration of the problem through critical reflection and discourse; 3) Integration – construction of meaning and ideas; and 4) Resolution – application of new knowledge in multiple settings. Prior to engaging in "practical inquiry," students must be provided with opportunities to build relationships and safety in the classroom (online or traditional). Students will need this sense of community in order to safely challenge one another, engage in critical thinking, and develop problem-solving skills. Furthermore, teaching presence provides a foundation for the presentation and development of the process of inquiry. Instructors provide assignments, activities, and guidance to help students move through the phases of practical inquiry, which leads in turn to the cognitive presence (Lambert & Fisher, 2013).

History of the community of inquiry (CoI)

The Community of Inquiry (CoI) framework provides a context to understand the formation of a collaborative learning environment in the online and blended/hybrid/mixed-mode classroom (Garrison, 2016, 2017). Such formal distance learning is based on communication for the purposes of learning through networked computer systems (Bangert, 2009). In the educational environment, communication is often focused on asynchronous written communication; however, current formats frequently incorporate synchronous verbal and text communications. A blended/hybrid/mixed-mode format is described as "the organic interaction of thoughtfully selected complementary face-to-face and online technologies" (Garrison & Vaughan, 2008, p. 148). The convergence of the traditional classroom and online environment presents a model of education that takes advantage of the benefits of both formats (Ayala, 2009; Garrison, 2017).

Garrison (2016) reported that Matthew Lipman began using the term "community of inquiry" in the 1980s "when he and his colleagues began to rethink educational practice from the perspective of a reflective paradigm" (p. 53). Lipman (2003) described the reflective paradigm and stated that education should be focused on inquiry. The dominant assumptions of the reflective paradigm include: education is the outcome of participation in a teacher-guided community of inquiry; students are stirred to think when knowledge is ambiguous, equivocal, and mysterious; relationships between and among disciplines are properly recognized; teachers are prepared to concede error; students are expected to be thoughtful, reflective, reasonable, and judicious; and "the focus of the educational process is not on the acquisition of information but on the grasp of relationships within and among the subject matters under investigation " (p. 19).

Lipman's (2003) reflective paradigm is grounded in the work of John Dewey and his concept of inquiry. Dewey (1959) highlighted the value of an emphasis on activity versus passivity, the importance of communication, and social relations. He described the process of inquiry in the classroom as follows:

> The problem is to find what conditions must be fulfilled in order that study and learning will naturally and necessarily take place, what conditions must be present so that pupils will make the responses which cannot help having learning in their consequence. The pupil's mind is no longer to be on study or learning. It is given to doing the things that the situation calls for, while learning is the result (p. 125).

Dewey (1959) reminds educators of the importance of the environment in learning, placing much of the responsibility of the educator to create and foster conditions that lead to inquiry and learning. Furthermore, he suggests that education is conceived as a reconstruction of experience, making the process of inquiry and education also the end goal. Dewey (1938) advanced that the foundation of instruction should begin with the experience that learners already possess; growth and expansion of content will follow from the attention to prior experience and inquiry.

Theoretical underpinnings of the community of inquiry (CoI)

Constructivism acknowledges the influence of experience and environment and provides a lens which views learning as the construction of knowledge, meaning, and identity. According to Garrison (2016), "The constructivist approach focuses on individuals constructing meaning and making sense of new experiences by integrating them with prior knowledge" (p. 16). Grossman-Dean (1993) further suggest that constructivism promotes the idea that "we cannot know an objective reality apart from our views of it" (p. 58). Thus, knowledge is, essentially, created through interaction with the environment.

The creation of a community of inquiry involves collaboration, learning through active participation and the construction of a social context. At the core of the Community of Inquiry is a collaborative learning theory, which highlights the need for shared activities that motivate students to participate and to use critical thinking skills (Garrison, 2016, 2017; Vaughan et al., 2013). Collaborative activities encourage a shift from independent learning, which is a common approach to distance learning, toward interdependence among the students and instructor. Garrison (2017) postulates that learning in isolation is an illusion and that learners, in reality, are influenced by their environment, experiences, and communication with others. Thinking and learning are often dependent upon the social environment and communication, encouraging exposure to alternative perspectives, ideas, and solutions. Collaboration with others in a safe, established community of learning allows learners to explore, examine, and express new ideas (Fox, 2013; Garrison & Arbaugh, 2007; Palloff & Pratt, 2007).

The philosophical and theoretical assumptions associated with the Community of Inquiry theoretical framework are grounded in collaborative constructivism (Garrison, 2016, 2017; Vaughan et al., 2013). A collaborative constructivist community of learners requires a balance between individual needs and the needs of the collective learning community. Garrison highlights a focus on shared interests in a learning community, indicating that people have the propensity to join with others who have common interests, forsaking personal predilections to join a community where the central dynamic is collaborative thinking. In the online classroom, the common interest typically is focused on learning content, increasing knowledge, and improving skills. However, a learning community, no matter the setting, has multiple purposes. Beyond the focus on academic endeavors, learners are concerned with social aspects and find value in the interpersonal interaction of a classroom (Kim, Kwon, & Cho, 2011; Picciano, 2002; Richardson, Maeda, Lv, & Caskurlu, 2017; Richardson & Swan, 2003).

The premise of the Community of Inquiry (CoI) framework is that the classroom incorporates a collaborative experience that is also individually constructivist, a seemingly contradictory, but essential combination. The sense of community in a learning environment is essential to the sharing of divergent ideas, open communication, and the formation of relationships.

Interdependence of the elements

Garrison et al. (2000) theorized that the CoI model assumes that collaborative learning is constructed within the community through the interaction of three core elements. [Figure 1 depicts them as social presence, cognitive presence, and teaching presence.] The coming together of the three mutually reinforcing elements creates a community through communication, shared teaching responsibilities, and collective learning activities (Garrison, 2017).

Vaughan and colleagues indicate that the presences and corresponding indicators are progressive or developmental in nature, gradually building throughout the course. However, Garrison notes that the process of building a community is not linear; rather, it is fluid and will shift as the learning experience evolves. Garrison (2016) goes on describing the goal of the Community of Inquiry as the attempt to unify the elements of an educational experience (social, cognitive, and teaching presences) in a theoretical framework that highlights the balance between thinking and learning, personal reflection and peer discussion, and self and co-regulation. The process of collaborative inquiry here requires a balance and movement between individual and collective environments.

Community of Inquiry

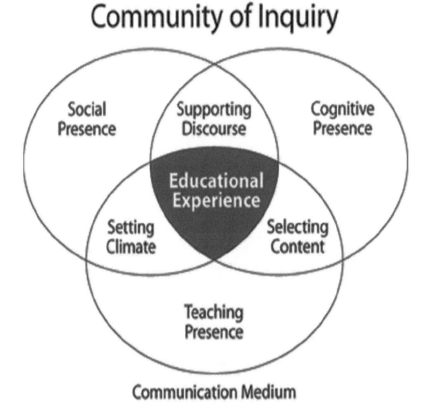

Communication Medium

Figure 1. The community of inquiry model. Reprinted from "Critical inquiry in a text-based environment: Computer conferencing in higher education." Garrison et al. (2000). *The Internet and Higher Education, 2*, p. 88.

Social presence

Hackman and Walker (1990) provide a description of social presence as "teacher immediacy" and describe behaviors that create nearness as "encouragement, praising and self-disclosure, and nonverbal behaviors that reduce the psychological distance between interactants such as smiling, gesturing, and movement" (p. 198). Others have expanded the definition by including the students' contribution to social presence and have focused on mutuality and interaction not only between the instructor and student, but also between and among students (McClellan, 1999; Rourke, Anderson, Garrison, & Archer, 1999). Garrison (2009) described social presence as "the ability of participants to identify with the community (e.g., course of study), communicate purposefully in a trusting environment, and develop inter-personal relationships by way of projecting their individual personalities" (p. 352). Prior to the significant growth of online and distance education formats, the definition of social presence was limited to the actions of the educator and suggested that physical proximity and in-person interaction were necessary for its development. Recent definitions of social presence, however, offer a broader perspective of the element, defined as "the extent to which persons are perceived to be real and are able to be authentically known and connected to others in mediated communication" (Bentley et al., 2015, p. 494).

Social presence is no longer restricted by the physicality of the educator (LaMendola, 2010). However, creating presence in the online education environment presents a distinct challenge. Generating social presence at a distance differs greatly from the traditional classroom setting. Interactions are time delayed, lack the additional information provided by body language and other non-verbal cues, and can be altered by one's interpretation of text alone (Fox, 2013). Hackman and Walker (1990) have suggested that social presence can be measured in terms of gesturing, smiling, and using vocal variety. Because these types of actions and interactions require a physical interface, they are difficult, if not impossible, to incorporate into the fully online classroom. The blended/hybrid/mixed-mode model of online instruction may offer opportunities for instructors to incorporate gestures, facial expression, and emotional interaction in synchronous sessions. Some actions that increase social presence are achievable in the blended/hybrid/mixed-model format and include addressing students by name, using "get to know you" postings/activities and self-disclosure activities (Sung & Mayer, 2012), questioning (Vaughan et al., 2013), praising (Hackman & Walker, 1990), encouraging online discussion (Barnett-Queen, Blair, & Merrick, 2005), allowing expression of emotion (Garrison, 2017), and providing individualized feedback (Sung & Mayer, 2012).

Cognitive presence

Cognitive presence is a fundamental element in critical thinking, a process, and outcome that most see as a primary goal of higher education. (Garrison et al., 2000).

Cognitive presence has been defined as the extent to which learners are able to construct and confirm meaning through sustained reflection and discourse in a critical community of inquiry (Garrison, 2016; Garrison et al., 2000). The concept has a foundation in the work of Lipman and Dewey, who both highlighted the importance of constructing learning from experience and reflective thinking. Hence, cognitive presence involves critical thinking and rational judgment within purposeful relationships.

In order to achieve "deep learning," students must develop the cognitive capacity for metacognition (Garrison & Akyol, 2013). Garrison (2017) described metacognition as "an awareness and ability to individually and collaboratively assume responsibility to regulate the thinking and learning process" (p. 60). Such awareness leads to the ability to assess the learning process and to self-regulate. The application of metacognition to the CoI framework necessitates consideration beyond the individual. Shared meta-cognition further allows the learner to monitor and actively regulate the inquiry process of self and others, and in doing so, develop cognitive presence.

Teaching presence

Anderson, Rourke, Garrison, and Archer (2001) define teaching presence as "the design, facilitation, and direction of cognitive and social processes for the purpose of realizing personally meaningful and educationally worthwhile learning outcomes" (p. 50). Teaching presence, which establishes the structure of the course, is conceptualized by Garrison et al. (2000) as having three dimensions – instructional design and organization; facilitating discussion and activity; and direct instruction. Teaching presence often is viewed as the most challenging responsibility for educators as the element provides the curriculum, approaches, methods, guidance, and focus for the course (Garrison & Vaughan, 2008; Vaughan et al., 2013).

It is important to understand the shared responsibility embedded in the concept of teaching presence. Researchers point out that the element is titled "teaching presence" versus "teacher presence" because the responsibility for this (and all) elements is shared between and among the instructor and students. Participants (instructor and students) in a constructivist community of inquiry hold responsibility for teaching presence. Both students and instructor clarify expectations and requirements, engage in discussion, process misconceptions, and evaluate understanding (Vaughan et al., 2013). Garrison (2017) stressed that while the participants must have open communication and shared responsibility for learning, there is a need for a facilitator or leader to design and direct the interactions. While student to student interaction is highly important, direction and feedback from an instructor are always valued, motivating, and effective.

Community of inquiry (CoI) survey instruments

The research has determined that the Community of Inquiry Survey instrument is a valid, reliable measure of the CoI and its essential elements. While a considerable number of studies have focused on the individual components of the CoI framework (Picciano, 2002; Richardson et al., 2017; Richardson & Swan, 2003; Sung & Mayer, 2012; Wisneski, Ozogul, & Bichelmeyer, 2015), research regarding the dynamic relationships between and among the presences has increased recently, primarily as a result of the validation of the Community of Inquiry Survey instrument. The CoI Survey consists of 34 items derived from the presences that allow researchers to study the contextual dynamics.

Arbaugh et al. (2008) reported on the development and validation of the CoI survey instrument and their findings suggest that it is a valid, reliable, and efficient measure of the dimensions of the CoI. It has been further modified and is now utilized as a tool to examine instructor perceptions. The 40 item educator version of the survey was developed by Cleveland-Innes and is being tested via workshops at Mid-Sweden University and the Open University of China. Research is being conducted at the School of Nursing at Oregon Health and Science University (OHSU), which is expected soon to be published (Cleveland-Innes, 2017).

Evidence and insights

Garrison et al. (2000) have provided the foundation for empirical research with respect to the Community of Inquiry (CoI) framework across multiple disciplines and in varied educational settings which has received wide-ranging empirical support in the literature (Akyol, Garrison, & Ozden, 2009; Akyol, Ice, Garrison, & Mitchell, 2010; Garrison, Cleveland-Innes, & Fung, 2010). In fact, descriptive analysis (of distance and online learning) publications during the period of 2009 to 2013 has revealed the most frequently used theoretical perspective was the community of inquiry framework (Bozkurt et al., 2015). The same study reported a CoI seminal article (by Garrison et al., 2000) as the most cited in the studies of this period (Bozkurt et al., 2015). Researchers have investigated areas of the CoI framework including, but not limited to, the Community of Inquiry Survey Instrument, the individual elements, the relationship among the elements, student perceptions, satisfaction, and performance among varied disciplines, and course format and design.

Research regarding the Community of Inquiry (CoI) design has been primarily focused in the realm of technology and education but has expanded into the applied, skill-based fields of business (Arbaugh & Rau, 2007) and nursing (Mills et al., 2016). Garrison and Arbaugh (2007) indicated that the framework "has resonated with the online learning community and provided insights and methodology for studying online learning" (p. 157). The Community of Inquiry Survey Instrument presents a tool to examine conceptual refinement of the relationships and interactions between/among the essential elements (Garrison & Arbaugh, 2007). In addition, Garrison (2017) recommends the use of qualitative methods to fully explore and gather insights into student and faculty perceptions of the presences.

Research regarding the applicability of the Community of Inquiry to social work education is sparse. The social work profession has continued to focus much of its research on the effectiveness of online and blended/hybrid/mixed-mode formats, while essentially overlooking an already validated, effective model for successful distance course design, implementation, and evaluation. Ferrara, Ostrander, and Crabtree-Nelson (2013) used the CoI to conduct a qualitative examination of two hybrid clinical social work courses taught in an MSW Program and found value in the application of the CoI approach and its collaborative learning environment. Bentley et al. (2015) provided a conceptual review of social presence in online social work courses and highlighted the importance of such social presence stating that the "professional demands of our discipline, which are centered in connective capabilities, interpersonal exchange, shared problem-solving, and collaboration with peers and other providers are addressed through the concept of social presence and the larger Community of Inquiry (CoI) framework" (p. 503). The authors recommend that future research address the use of social presence to inform the development of practice skills, peer collaboration, and decision-making. LaMendola's (2010) conceptual paper examined social presence in online social work courses and opines that social work "needs to confront the changes in culture that are taking place" (p. 113). The author advocates for a broadened vision of creating human associations to include online interactions, encouraging social work educators to consider technological forms of communication.

Importance to social work education

Social work educators seek to socialize and acculturate future social workers to the profession (Anastas, 2010). Whether delivered in-person or in an online format, the process of social work education involves the transmission of the knowledge, skills, and values of the profession and takes place both inside and outside the classroom. A considerable amount of social work practice is grounded in face-to-face interaction, leading to understandable concerns about the ability to effectively impart and assess these skills in a distance education format (Ferrara et al., 2013). Generalist social work practice is grounded in rapport building, empathetic communication, and the importance of human relationships (Hepworth, Rooney, Dewberry-Rooney, & Strom-Gottfried, 2016; Howe, 2008; Walsh, 2014). Similarly, social work educators use a sense of community, relationships, and presence with and among students to encourage learning and to provide a model for future professional practice. Fox (2011) suggests that educators' relationships with students establish meaning beyond the instruction and parallel that of social worker and client. Hill-Jones (2015) asserts that through classroom interaction, educators mentor students and model professional behavior and clinical skills. Therefore, interpersonal interaction and presence clearly are central to social work education. Moreover, effective use of interaction and presence in the classroom may increase students' learning outcomes specific to the course and may be of further benefit as students gain generalist practice skills that are applied later in field placements and professional practice upon graduation.

In November 2016, the Council on Social Work Education (CSWE) Commission on Research Priorities for Improving Social Work Education published results of a survey of members highlighting eight research priorities including "supporting inquiry around the outcomes of online and hybrid education and the consistency of online programs with accepted standards of 'quality' in online learning" (CSWE Education Commission on Research, 2017, p. 4). CSWE also collaborated with sister organizations – the National Association of Social Workers (NASW), the Association of Social Work Boards (ASWB), and the Clinical Social Work Association (CSWA) – to develop the Standards for Technology in Social Work Practice. The document details the need for social work educators to remain current with emerging knowledge and techniques in technology-enhanced and technology-based education formats. Standard 4.01 specifically addresses the use of technology in social work education stating, "Social workers who use technology to design and deliver education and training shall develop competence in the ethical use of the technology in a manner appropriate for the particular context" (National Association of Social Workers (NASW), Association of Social Work Boards (ASWB), Council on Social Work Education (CSWE), & Clinical Social Work Association (CSWA), 2017, p. 44). Furthermore, Standards 4.11 and 4.12 outline criteria for the use of technology in field instruction and supervision, including adherence to organizational policy and to the NASW Code of Ethics (NASW et al., 2017).

The NASW Code of Ethics (2017) was very recently updated to include extensive technology-related revisions pertaining to informed consent, competent practice, conflicts of interest, confidentiality, intimate relationships, sexual harassment, interruption of services, unethical conduct of colleagues, supervision and consultation, education and training, client records, and evaluation and research. The increased use of technology in social work practice necessitates increased experience with technological platforms and an understanding of the ethical challenges presented by technology. Social work students who are exposed to online formats and communication will likely learn from those experiences, transferring those skills to later practice.

Discussion and implications

Social work programs can use the Community of Inquiry (CoI) framework to evaluate overall curriculum delivery, including the distance delivery of field education components. The signature pedagogy of undergraduate and graduate social work curriculums, the field practicum frequently is being supervised by social work faculty from a distance. In conjunction with their field placement, students are often engaged in the final senior seminar course via online or blended delivery. Although some research has examined distance format field education and its inherent challenges (Dillingham, 2018), research regarding the applicability of the CoI framework to the field placement and supporting seminar course has not yet been carried out. Research into the signature pedagogy of social work education, however, would usefully provide a robust understanding of the CoI framework's applicability to the full breadth of social work education.

Further, the Community of Inquiry (CoI) paradigm could provide a rich resource for assessment of the Council on Social Work Education (CSWE) competencies. The essential elements of the CoI (social presence, teaching presence, and cognitive presence) directly align with the competencies outlined by CSWE (knowledge, skills, values, and cognitive and affective processes). Consequently, the CoI could be used to evaluate an entire social work curriculum plan, including traditional and distance format courses.

Social work educators can utilize the Community of Inquiry (CoI) framework and the associated CoI Survey Instruments also for student, peer, or self-assessment. As noted, the survey tools provide a valid and reliable instrument that could be included in annual evaluations, as well as tenure and promotion considerations. Educators could implement the CoI survey instruments in multiple courses, examining themes and relationships over time, and then implementing changes and improvements to distance format social work courses. Further examination and use of the Community of Inquiry (CoI) framework in social work education have the potential to advance distance education format course delivery, thereby improving the distance education experience for both social work students and educators.

Disclosure statement

No potential conflict of interest was reported by the authors.

References

Akyol, Z., Garrison, D. R., & Ozden, M. Y. (2009). Online and blended communities of inquiry: Exploring the developmental and perceptual differences. *International Review of Research in Open and Distance Education, 23*(2), 123–136.

Akyol, Z., Ice, P., Garrison, D. R., & Mitchell, R. (2010). The relationship between course socio-epistemological orientations and student perceptions of community of inquiry. *The Internet and Higher Education, 13*(1–2), 66–68. doi:10.1016/j.iheduc.2009.12.002

Anastas, J. W. (2010). *Teaching in social work: An educators' guide to theory and practice.* New York, NY: Columbia University Press.

Anderson, T., Rourke, L., Garrison, D. R., & Archer, W. (2001). Assessing teacher presence in a computer conferencing context. *Journal of Asynchronous Learning Networks, 5*(2), 1–17.

Arbaugh, J. B., Cleveland-Innes, M., Diaz, S. R., Garrison, D. R., Ice, P., Richardson, J. C., & Swan, K. P. (2008). Developing a community of inquiry instrument: Testing a measure of the community of inquiry framework using a multi-dimensional sample. *Internet and Higher Education, 11*(3), 133–136. doi:10.1016/j.iheduc.2008.06.003

Arbaugh, J. B., & Rau, B. I. (2007). A study of disciplinary, structural, and behavioral effects on course outcomes in online MBA courses. *Decision Sciences Journal of Innovative Education, 5*(1), 65–95. doi:10.1111/j.1540-4609.2007.00128.x

Ayala, J. (2009). Blended learning as a new approach to social work education. *Journal of Social Work Education, 45*(2), 277–288. doi:10.5175/JSWE.2009.200700112

Bangert, A. W. (2009). Building a validity argument for the community of inquiry survey instrument. *Internet and Higher Education, 12,* 104–111. doi:10.1016/j.iheduc.2009.06.001

Barnett-Queen, T., Blair, R., & Merrick, M. (2005). Student perspectives of online discussions: Strengths and weaknesses. *Journal of Technology in Human Services, 23*(3–4), 229–244. doi:10.1300/J017v23n03_05

Bentley, K. J., Secret, M. C., & Cummings, C. R. (2015). The centrality of social presence in online teaching and learning in social work. *Journal of Social Work Education, 51,* 494–504. doi:10.1080/10437797.2015.1043199

Blackmon, B. (2013). Social work and online education with all deliberate speed. *Journal of Evidence-Based Social Work, 10,* 509–521. doi:10.1080/15433714.2012.663672

Bozkurt, A., Akgun-Ozbeck, E., Yilmazel, S., Erdogde, E., Ucar, H., Guler, E., ... Aydin, C. H. (2015). Trends in distance education research: A content analysis of journals 2009–2013. *International Review of Research in Open and Distance Learning, 16*(1), 330–363. doi:10.19173/irrodl.v16i1.1953

Cleveland-Innes, M. (2017, July 2). *Faculty development and the community of inquiry at Oregon health and science university school of nursing.* [web log comment]. Retrieved from http://www.thecommunityofinquiry.org/project4

Council on Social Work Education Commission on Research. (2017). *Annual report to the CSWE board.* Retrieved from https://cswe.org/getattachment/About-CSWE/Governance/Commissions-and-Councils/Commission-on-Research/Commission-on-Reseach-Report-of-Board-of-Directors.pdf.aspx

Cummings, S. M., Chaffin, K. M., & Cockerham, C. (2015). Comparative analysis of an online and a traditional MSW program: Educational outcomes. *Journal of Social Work Education, 51,* 109–120. doi:10.1080/10437797.2015.977170

Dewey, J. (1938). *Experience and education.* New York, NY: Free Press.

Dewey, J. (1959). *Dewey on education.* New York, NY: Teachers College Press.

Dillingham, J. L. (2018). Developing community among social work field seminar students: Lessons learned from the online classroom. *The Field Educator, 8*(2). Retrieved from http://fieldeducator.simmons.edu/article/developing-community-amongsocial-work-field-seminar-students-lessons-learned-from-the-onlineclassroom/

Ferrara, M., Ostrander, N., & Crabtree-Nelson, S. (2013). Establishing a community of inquiry through hybrid courses in clinical social work education. *Journal of Teaching in Social Work, 33,* 438–448. doi:10.1080/08841233.2013.835765

Fox, R. (2011). *The use of self: The essence of professional education.* Chicago, IL: Lyceum Books.

Fox, R. (2013). *The call to teach: Philosophy, process, and pragmatics of social work education.* Alexandria, VA: CSWE Press.

Garrison, D. R. (2009). Communities of inquiry in online learning: Social, teaching and cognitive presence. In C. Howard, P. Rogers, G. Berg, J. Boettcher, L. Justice & K. Shenk (Eds.,), *Encyclopedia of distance and online learning* (2nd, pp. 352–355). Hershey, PA: IGI Global.

Garrison, D. R. (2016). *Thinking collaboratively: Learning in a community of inquiry.* New York, NY: Routledge.

Garrison, D. R. (2017). *E-Learning in the 21st century: A community inquiry framework for research and practice.* New York, NY: Routledge.

Garrison, D. R., & Akyol, Z. (2013). Toward the development of a metacognition construct for communities of inquiry. *The Internet and Higher Education, 17,* 84–89. doi:10.1016/j.iheduc.2012.11.005

Garrison, D. R., Anderson, T., & Archer, W. (2000). Critical inquiry in a text-based environment: Computer conferencing in higher education. *The Internet and Higher Education, 2*, 87–105. doi:10.1016/S1096-7516(00)00016-6

Garrison, D. R., & Arbaugh, J. B. (2007). Researching the community of inquiry framework: Review, issues, and future directions. *The Internet and Higher Education, 10*, 157–172. doi:10.1016/j.iheduc.2007.04.001

Garrison, D. R., Cleveland-Innes, M., & Fung, T. S. (2010). Exploring causal relationship among teaching, cognitive and social presence: A holistic view of the community of inquiry framework. *The Internet and Higher Education, 12*(1–2), 31–36. doi:10.1016/j.iheduc.2009.10.002

Garrison, D. R., & Vaughan, N. (2008). *Blended learning in higher education: Framework, principles, and guidelines.* San Francisco, CA: Jossey-Bass.

Grossman-Dean, R. (1993). Teaching a constructivist approach to clinical practice. *Journal of Teaching in Social Work, 8*(1/2), 55–75. doi:10.1300/J067v08n01_04

Hackman, M. Z., & Walker, K. B. (1990). Instructional communication in the televised classroom: The effects of system design and teacher immediacy on student learning and satisfaction. *Communication Education, 39*(3), 196–209. doi:10.1080/03634529009378802

Hepworth, D. H., Rooney, R. H., Dewberry-Rooney, D., & Strom-Gottfried, K. (2016). *Direct social work practice: Theory and skills.* Boston, MA: Cengage Learning.

Hill-Jones, S. (2015). Benefits and challenges of online education for clinical social work: Three examples. *Clinical Social Work Journal, 43*, 225–235. doi:10.1007/s10615-014-0508-z

Howe, D. (2008). Relationship-based thinking in social work practice. *Journal of Social Work Practice, 12*, 45–56. doi:10.1080/02650539808415131

Kim, J., Kwon, Y., & Cho, D. (2011). Investigating factors that influence social presence and learning outcomes in distance education. *Computers & Education, 57*, 1512–1520. doi:10.1016/j.compedu.2011.02.005

Kurzman, P. A. (2013). The evolution of distance learning and online education. *Journal of Teaching in Social Work, 33*(4/5), 331–338. doi:10.1080/08841233.2013.843346

Lambert, J. L., & Fisher, J. L. (2013). Community of inquiry framework: Establishing community in an online course. *Journal of Interactive Online Learning, 12*(1), 1–12.

LaMendola, W. (2010). Social work and social presence in an online world. *Journal of Technology in Human Services, 28*, 108–119. doi:10.1080/15228831003759562

Lipman, M. (2003). *Thinking in education* (2nd ed.). Cambridge, UK: Cambridge University Press.

McClellan, H. (1999, *September-October*). Online education as interactive experience: Some guiding models. *Educational Technology, 39*(5), 36–42.

Mills, J., Yates, K., Harrison, H., Woods, C., Chamberlain-Salaun, J., Trueman, S., & Hitchins, M. (2016). Using a community of inquiry framework to teach a nursing and midwifery research subject: An evaluative study. *Nurse Education Today, 43*, 34–39. doi:10.1016/j.nedt.2016.04.016

Moore, B. (2005). Faculty perceptions of the effectiveness of web-based instruction in social work education: A national study. *Journal of Technology in Human Services, 23*(1/2), 53–66. doi:10.1300/J017v23n01_04

National Association of Social Workers (NASW). (2017). *Code of Ethics.* Retrieved from https://www.socialworkers.org/about/ethics/code-of-ethics

National Association of Social Workers (NASW), Association of Social Work Boards (ASWB), Council on Social Work Education (CSWE), & Clinical Social Work Association (CSWA). (2017). *Standards for technology in social work practice.* Retrieved from https://www.socialworkers.org/includes/newIncludes/homepage/PRA-BRO-33617.TechStandards_FINAL_POSTING.pdf

Palloff, R. M., & Pratt, K. (2007). *Building online learning communities*. San Francisco, CA: Jossey-Bass.

Picciano, A. G. (2002). Beyond student perceptions: Issues of interaction, presence and performance in an online course. *Journal of Asynchronous Learning Networks*, 6(1), 21–40.

Reamer, F. G. (2013). Distance and online social work education: Novel ethical challenges. *Journal of Teaching in Social Work*, 33(4/5), 369–384. doi:10.1080/08841233.2013.828669

Richardson, J. C., & Swan, K. (2003). Examining social presence in online courses in relation to students' perceived learning and satisfaction. *Journal of Asynchronous Learning Networks*, 7(1), 68–88.

Richardson, J. J., Maeda, Y., Lv, J., & Caskurlu, S. (2017). Social presence in relation to students' satisfaction and learning in the online environment: A meta-analysis. *Computers in Human Behavior*, 71, 402–417. doi:10.1016/j.chb.2017.02.001

Rourke, L., Anderson, T., Garrison, D. R., & Archer, W. (1999). Assessing social presence in asynchronous text-based computer conferencing. *Journal of Distance Education*, 12(2), 50–71.

Sung, E., & Mayer, R. E. (2012). Five facets of social presence in online distance education. *Computers in Human Behavior*, 28, 1738–1747. doi:10.1016/j.chb.2012.04.014

Vaughan, N. D., Cleveland-Innes, M., & Garrison, D. R. (2013). *Teaching in blended learning environments: Creating and sustaining communities of inquiry*. Edmonton, AB: Athabasca University, AU Press.

Vernon, R., Vakalahi, H., Pierce, D., Pittman-Munke, P., & Adkins, L. F. (2009). Distance education programs in social work: Current and emerging trends. *Journal of Social Work Education*, 45(2), 263–275. doi:10.5175/JSWE.2009.200700081

Walsh, J. (2014). *Theories for direct social work practice*. Belmont, CA: Brooks Cole.

Wisneski, J. E., Ozogul, G., & Bichelmeyer, B. (2015). Does teaching presence transfer between MBA teaching environments? A comparative investigation of instructional design practices associated with teaching presence. *The Internet and Higher Education*, 25, 18–27. doi:10.1016/j.iheduc.2014.11.001

Zidan, T. (2015). Teaching social work in an online environment. *Journal of Human Behavior in the Social Environment*, 25, 228–235. doi:10.1080/10911359.2014.1003733

Beyond the Online versus On-campus Debate: Leveraging Technology in a CoI Framework to Enhance Student and Faculty Presence in the MSW Classroom

Jennifer A. Parga, Kathy Bargar, Steve Monte, Ruth A. Supranovich, and Danielle E. Brown

ABSTRACT

While research typically utilizes Student Learning Outcomes (SLO) to evaluate online education programs (OEP) compared to on-campus programs (OCP), little attention is given to other qualitative elements which enhance student social presence or faculty teaching presence. The authors examine the Community of Inquiry (CoI) framework and demonstrate how MSW programs with an OEP can incorporate elements to enhance student learning. Research and data included will attempt to move the discussion beyond the OEP versus OCP debate and include more pertinent ideas regarding the importance and impact of leveraging technology in MSW social work education.

Introduction

Eight years after the launch of the first national online MSW program, the Council on Social Work Education (CSWE) lists 26 bachelor and 77 master degree programs that offer some portion of their graduate curriculum online (Council on Social Work Education [CSWE], 2018; Flynn, Maiden, Smith, Wiley, & Wood, 2013). Yet, extant research continues to debate the value of online education programs (OEP) when compared to on-campus programs (OCP) (Arkorful & Abaidoo, 2015; Daymont, Blau, & Campbell, 2011; Sun, Tsai, Finger, Chen, & Yeh, 2008; Wyatt, 2005). The authors believe the debate is fueled by (a) the belief that the two educational delivery methods cannot be adequately compared, (b) the argument that social work practice cannot be conveyed online (c) faculty resistance to technology and to learning a new teaching methodology, (d) the inability of institutions to support rapid expansion required to create online platforms, and (e) ideological conflicts between nonprofit program partnerships with for-profit educational technology companies. Yet, as Kurzman (2013) aptly points out, unless there are statistically significant differences found in the post-graduation career outcomes, licensing exam pass rates or student satisfaction reports, the argument of comparison between modalities of MSW educational delivery is insignificant, or unknown.

The authors assert that the future of social work education should build on the equivalent student learning outcomes, identified in OEP and OCP research, and elevate student engagement, teaching presence, and the broader use of technology, using a Community of Inquiry (CoI) framework.

Online education: utilization, perception, and definition

Since 2006, the Online Report Card (ORC) has been able to document enrollment, online perceptions, and types of online delivery in the United States (Allen, Seaman, Poulin, & Straut, 2016). Recently, their enrollment tracking found that the number of students not taking any online courses continues to drop (Allen et al., 2016). With students consistently selecting OEP over OCP, the ORC now considers OEP a mainstream option. Nevertheless, their latest report stated that 28.6% of academic leaders still believe that OEP is inferior to OCP methods (Allen et al., 2016). However, this perception is not supported by other research which shows 92% of all studies (comparing OEP and OCP) found OEP learning outcomes are at least equivalent, if not better than, OCP learning outcomes (Nguyen, 2015).

Perceptions have been slow to change despite the following quality research demonstrating equivalent SLOs. Cavanaugh and Jacquemin (2015) examined 5,000 undergraduate courses, which included over 100 faculty, covering 10 academic terms. They found a negligible difference between grade-based performance in both formats when the course was taught by the same faculty member. (The significant factor in this study was the same faculty member taught the same course both online and on campus.) Cummings, Chaffin and Cockerham's (2015) research also found no significant difference between 345 online versus on-campus students for the "majority of educational outcomes" (p.117). This study included knowledge and skill-related variables reflected in exams and field placement performance, respectively. A significant factor noted in this article is that the online curricula was identical to that offered on-campus and taught by the same faculty in real time (Cummings et al., 2015). Even with the aforementioned research, the authors cannot help but think those persistent in the opinion that "in person is better" may be unaware of such research, or are not teaching online.

Just a few decades ago, OEP meant e-learning, where all content was delivered through a static website. With advancing technologies, the current components of e-learning are much more complex (Weller, 2018). OEPs can now encompass multiple formats and a variety of delivery models; however, there is still not a universal definition of what constitutes an OEP among educational institutions. Terms like online, virtual, synchronous, hybrid, distance education, and distance learning are often used interchangeably, and using one particular term may or may not mean the same type of programming at any two schools. Academics, instructional designers, and educational institutions seem to prefer to define for themselves what constitutes their own particular version of an OEP. For the purposes of this article, however, the authors will refer to OEP as defined by Phillips et al. (2018), and focus on the content delivery method as either (a) synchronous (live class with real-time audio and visual), and/or (b) asynchronous (self-paced work).

OEP and OCP student learning outcomes

The explicit curriculum

In 2015, CSWE changed accreditation standards to require social work programs to systematically collect, review, and act on student learning outcome measures. This new focus on accountability for what students learn (rather than what is taught) meant that programs had to develop evaluation tools and respond accordingly to adjust their programs. Although the SLOs primarily focused on cognitive outcomes, they are inherently tied to knowledge, skills, and values that are measured by a student's ability to demonstrate proficiency in nine areas of competency in both their field placement and their academic courses (CSWE, 2015). To examine these standards, the University of Southern California – providing both OEP and OCP instruction – began tracking student learning outcomes in 2016. Their evaluation data was gathered from surveys completed at the end of each semester by faculty, based upon student behavior observed in the classroom, and then combined with field evaluation scores to produce an overall measure on each competency. Data for the past 2 years (2016–2017 and 2017–2018) indicate that both the OEP and OCP have comparable SLO scores and both met or exceeded the school's internal threshold of 90%. This outcome means that in order to consider the program successful in preparing students to be proficient in the nine competencies, 90% of students must meet or exceed expectations on this aggregated measure.

The implicit curriculum

While the explicit curriculum has garnered greatest attention in the literature in terms of comparing student learning outcomes for OEPs versus OCPs, CSWE also emphasizes the importance of the implicit curriculum as it "promotes an educational culture that is congruent with the values of the profession and the mission, goals, and context of the program" (CSWE, 2015,

p. 14). Described as "the learning environment in which the explicit curriculum is presented" (p.14), the implicit curriculum refers to program elements such as the school's commitment to diversity, its policies and procedures, faculty composition and experience, administrative structure, and student engagement in governance. While some studies have begun to explore ways to conceptualize and measure the implicit curriculum both in OCPs (Grady, Swick, & Powers, 2018; Peterson, Farmer, Donnelly, & Forenza, 2014) and OEPs (Quinn & Barth, 2014), this aspect of the curriculum warrants more attention.

Quinn and Barth (2014) describe the engagement of OEP students to the same extent as OCP students as the biggest challenge for OEP faculty. The same authors note that there appear to be opportunities to foster this engagement and recommend the creative use of technologies, and a combination of synchronous and asynchronous media not currently being used by the programs they studied. While aspects of the implicit curriculum, such as "the culture of human interchange" and the "spirit of inquiry" (CSWE, 2015, p. 14) can present particular challenges to OEP faculty, the authors of this article propose that the Community of Inquiry (CoI) framework provides a helpful way to think about this particular aspect of OEPs. Furthermore, they present a number of examples which leverage technology to provide enhanced student experience in OEPs, and attempt to dispel lingering doubts about an OEP's ability to educate and produce, well-rounded, competent social workers.

Community of inquiry: a framework supporting current and future innovation

The CoI framework provides a useful lens to examine the MSW student and faculty experience. The CoI framework, derived from John Dewey's (1938) examination of the nature of knowledge formation, has been advanced by Garrison, Anderson, and Archer (2000) as a basis for understanding the transactional nature of online learning. This framework specifically highlights the interactive composition of social, teaching, and cognitive presence in online courses of instruction and provides structure for the examination of successful learning experiences. [See Figure 1].

The CoI framework illustrates three elements which together constitute an optimal educational experience: (a) teaching presence, (b) cognitive presence, and (c) social presence. Teaching presence refers to the design, facilitation and direct delivery of content with the goal of maximizing learning outcomes (Garrison et al., 2000). This process relies on the provision of expertise and implementation of forward thinking modalities of content delivery in an online environment. Cognitive presence is conceptualized as the extent to which students develop and demonstrate critical thinking while integrating

Community of Inquiry

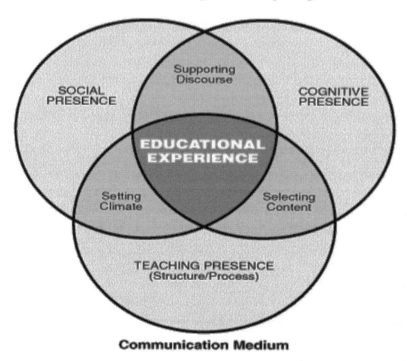

Figure 1. The community of inquiry model. *Source*: Garrison et al. (2000). Reprinted with permission.

meaning from concepts and ideas learned. The cognitive presence of the student develops through a cycle of progressive examination, which includes understanding and exploring a problem, and then integrating it into the learning experience through the application of the knowledge learned (Garrison & Arbaugh, 2007). Social presence in OEPs refers to the student's ability to socially and emotionally connect in the online learning community through self-expression, communication and group cohesion (Garrison et al., 2000).

Student learning outcome measures in social work tend to focus primarily on the cognitive process of the student as demonstrated via behavioral examples of competency, yet they are implicitly tied to the values and the knowledge base of social work, as well as the skills put forth in the CSWE Educational Policy and Accreditation Standards. The CoI framework establishes that these three elements of the learning experience are interconnected, with the cognitive presence of the student cultivated through the teaching presence of faculty and the social presence of the student. The CoI lens suggests that examining the overall effectiveness of OEPs in social work needs to look deeper within SLO measures and focus on the enhancement of the social presence of the student and the teaching presence of faculty.

Garrison and Arbaugh (2007) posit that social presence is an essential element in facilitating higher-order learning. Engagement in a positive social climate of online learning cultivates positive overall regard for online learning and increased emotional investment by students (Arbaugh & Benbunan-Fich, 2006). Thus, social work OEPs would benefit from intentionally enhancing the ways in which students are connected to their educational cohort and intentional social experiences in the program. The recommendation for social work OEPs is to incorporate specific goals for cultivating student social presence in OEPs. Interactions which closely mirror the exchanges occurring in an OCP environment allow OEPs to engage and develop the social presence of the online student and include (a) student-to-student interactions, (b) faculty-to-student interactions, and (c) group work.

Informal student-to-student exchanges increase student satisfaction and investment in the learning environment, leading to enhanced knowledge retention (Taylor, 2016). These informal exchanges could involve creating online spaces for students to interact with one another socially prior to the commencing of synchronous class time. Functionally, this is comparable to opening the classroom door early and allowing students to engage with one another while class preparation is undertaken. Alternatively, in the asynchronous environment, the instructor can request students create an introduction video they then share online with their cohort just prior to or during the first week of the term. For example, students could be encouraged to share a picture depicting their self-care activities and post this via the program's learning management system. Student-led water-cooler discussions, using online meeting room technologies and not tied to the specific course objectives, can be hosted by any student and allow opportunities for the larger student body to socially connect even though not physically in the same space. Online student caucuses are an additional format for the larger student body to associate with one another and identify with the larger educational institution. Even the simple act of encouraging students to exchange phone numbers or emails communicates the importance of student social connection. When faculty encourages informal student-to-student social interactions, the result is more effective student investment in the course, and in each other (Ma, Han, Yang, & Cheng, 2015).

Faculty-to-student interaction can enhance topical integration of the coursework while leveraging student social presence. Encouraging opportunities for students to connect with one another and to faculty around course themes and assignments do not have to be complex. If the OEP consists primarily of asynchronous text, video, discussion boards, and student submissions, this too can facilitate students' engagement with one another and the instructor. Online video discussion programs (like Flipgrid) can be leveraged to encourage recorded video discussion of various topics related to coursework. The instructor provides a sample video, with a topical introduction, and then students record responses via short video clips, expressing their unique perspectives, connecting with their instructor, and exchanging ideas with their class cohort (Flipgrid Inc., 2018). For hybrid models, students can use real time/synchronous breakout interactions to discuss how course material relates to their personal and professional lives, and how they might use information from the course in their current or future professional activity. Faculty members can provide students with examples from their own professional practice to create even deeper faculty-to-student connections. These practices depend on faculty embracing the importance of student connection as core to achieving teaching presence. When student social interactions are delivered through innovative practices by faculty, the results are valued as a direct component of teaching presence within the CoI framework.

Student group activities also can be encouraged and incorporated through-out the curriculum to further enhance the social presence of the student (Garrison et al., 2000). Goldingay and Land's (2014) study on social presence in online social work education affirms a positive impact on student motiva-tion when a strong relationship among peers is established. The use of group work to encourage student-to-student contact in online social work educa-tion can lead to greater student investment and cohesion, especially if structured around themes that support the coursework. One such example is a group assignment to create a word cloud reflecting the group discussion on a course topic. Another illustration would be the use of problem-based learning as a group experience for students during synchronous class, in order to examine a fictional client and address the biopsychosocial aspects of service delivery. These group activities are most effective when monitored by instructors through online comments, feedback, and encouragement (Carter et al., 2018). In this sense, group projects focused on the exploration of specific educational objectives, help tie students to the curriculum and to one another.

Individual or group digital storytelling is an additional example of an activity that engages the social presence of students. As humans, we naturally connect through the use of stories, and storytelling is acknowledged as a powerful strategy for learning that allows students to build connections via sharing unique experiences around a common theme (Lowenthal & Dunlap, 2009). Digital storytelling is operationalized when a student is able to demonstrate a point of view or experience through pictures or graphics, with the student voice usually shown in a video along with music, vocal narration or subtitles (Storycenter.org, 2018). Storytelling is personal narra-tive and allows students in OEPs to present themselves as authentic to their cohort while exploring their connection to an educational topic and to a larger group (Lowenthal & Dunlap, 2009). Programs like WeVideo permit online learners to co-create and edit individual or group video storytelling presentations (WeVideo, 2017). The Center for Digital Storytelling (currently referred to as "Story Center") has led efforts to incorporate this narrative approach in online education (Storycenter.org, 2018). Analogous to current pedagogical practice of small group discussion, using personal narrative and the practice of starting where the client is, digital storytelling can be explored during synchronous instruction when the class is placed in virtual breakout rooms with general oversight of the instructor to educate and support around the use of narrative within social work practice (Reissman & Quinney, 2005). The Shoah Foundation is another free resource, which houses curated, visual testimonies of survivors from the European Holocaust and Rwandan Genocide, among other world-altering events (USC Shoah Foundation, 2019). The testimony is a valuable visual history, which not only educates students about the past but allows for deep and meaningful conversation related to the value of storytelling at any level: faculty to student, student to student, in groups.

Cultivating the student's sense of identification with the larger university is yet another simple way to engage the social presence of the student. For example, one of the authors allocated just 4 minutes at the start of the first three synchronous class meetings to take students through a video photo tour of the physical space of the campus-based institution. Students were shown images of the University administration offices, the bookstore, and even the mascot while they were encouraged to embrace identification with the campus as part of their university experience. Informal student feedback via electronic poll response demonstrated a strong positive objective response to this approach and a subjective sense of greater investment in the educational program.

These examples demonstrate several ways to engage the social presence of the student through the innovative teaching presence of faculty. Best practices and research into student engagement online are just beginning to form in the literature (Farrell et al., 2018). Ultimately, we believe that studies will demonstrate that students participating in courses with attention to building a strong social presence experience a significant sense of community, support of peers, and connection to others and their program of participation (Taylor, 2016).

Implications for future research

Cavanaugh and Jacquemin (2015) and Cummings et al. (2015) suggest that SLOs in OEPs compare well with OCPs. Those who seek to advance OEPs can use the concepts from the ORC report (Allen et al., 2016), the CoI framework (Garrison et al., 2000), and additional research referenced in this article as guidelines and models. As MSW programs accept such evidence, questions about the overall efficacy of OEPs likely will become less germane; however new questions will emerge, calling for further reflection and research. The following questions we suggest are critical for future research:

- What specific technologies (e.g., use of synchronous (real time) and asynchronous (self-paced) material, live web chat, online discussion forums, social media, mobile apps, telepresence robots (described more in case example 1), augmented reality (AR), virtual reality (VR) simulations, artificial intelligence (AI) chatbots, etc.) will have the largest positive impact on cognitive, social, and teaching presence, as described above?
- What specific technologies will be used specifically in social work practice settings five or 10 years from now?
- How will faculty and staff within schools of social work be trained and encouraged to incorporate technology into the classroom?
- What training and education will MSW students need in order to be competent and ethical practitioners when using these technologies?
- What other disciplines (e.g., computer and data science, business management, etc.) need to be involved as future technology is built, tested, evaluated, and scaled for social work practice?
- How do we address the legal and ethical questions, such as those highlighted by Reamer (2013), which can arise as we incorporate technology into social work education?

As research seeks to answer these questions, along with others that will inevitably arise, it may be helpful to consider the current wave of innovation in education. The following examples highlight how educators are beginning to pioneer around the themes of social, cognitive, and teaching presence utilizing new technology. Not all of these innovations have been formally evaluated and few publications are available to document their efficacy in increasing SLOs. As such, references to both peer-reviewed journals and popular media appear here.

Case example 1: Telepresence robots in the classroom to expand social presence

Students at a large, east coast university participated in a clinical nursing simulation as part of a course requirement. This simulation occurred in a mock hospital room and involved collaboration with other nursing students who used a telepresence robot. The robot was a wheeled, remote-controlled device with a display screen, and was able to stream real-time audio and video, which enabled others who were not physically present to participate remotely (Shaw et al., 2018). The experience of using this technology mirrors that of other health-care practitioners, including social workers in behavioral health roles, who collaborate via video conferencing systems as a regular part of their work. Researchers here used standardized measures to assess the feasibility and acceptability of using technology in this manner. Students reported high mean scores on both elements of the simulation. In another example, a large public university-integrated robot-mediated communication (RMC) into their synchronous hybrid doctoral course and evaluated the social presence, compared to Zoom, a video conference platform. RMC is a technology which allows participants in different locations to utilize a screen (like a TV or computer monitor), web camera, microphone and speakers (thus enabling real-time audio and visual) – plus the ability to move to the camera in different directions between remote and local participants. The results indicated that working with a robot (such as Kubi or Double) allows students to experience a more genuine interaction, authentic communication, and an increased sense of belonging when compared to traditional video conferencing (Gleason & Greenhow, 2017).

Case example 2: clickers and engagement reports to enhance cognitive presence

Canadian researchers from a large, publicly funded university gathered data from 5,459 students regarding the use of clicker technology in physical classrooms (Han & Finkelstein, 2013). As discussed in that study, clicker technology functions much like a remote control, except instead of changing the channel, one can respond to a prompt or question (generally from the course instructor) through the click of a button. The prompt or question, as well as aggregated student responses, are then displayed by a video projector at the front of the classroom for all to see. Using this technology allows students to provide anonymous, real-time feedback to instructors about any topic related to course material, which then could be covered in more detail to improve comprehension and learning outcomes. In the study, students consistently reported that clicker technology allowed them to have a deeper understanding of the content covered and their ability to be attentive to the class (Han & Finkelstein, 2013). Comparable technology is also available without the physical components of a clicker in online education. For example, polling and engagement tracking features in AdobeConnect web applications used for synchronous video connection between faculty and students help with class attention (Phillips et al., 2018). Additionally, clicker technology has since evolved to use as a web-based application or website, utilizing the individual student's cell phone instead of a physical clicker to collect their responses to a prompt (e.g., Poll Everywhere, MicroPoll, Flisti, and PollDaddy).

Case example 3: virtual reality simulations as a novel approach in teaching presence

At one small, public university in the southeastern United States, social work students now have the opportunity to learn about therapeutic group dynamics by using virtual reality (VR) headsets (Beal, n.d.). The immersive environment allows students to engage with four virtual clients, hear the pre-recorded dialogue, and choose how to respond when given a series of options. (The work was funded in part by a grant and represents a unique, collaborative effort with the theater department, where the voice recordings were produced.) Similarly, Koetting and Freed (2017) have used a virtual patient simulation to teach nursing students how to screen for drug and alcohol use. Their research showed that "students felt significantly more confident about their ability to screen, assess patients' readiness to change their behavior, discuss patient's substance use, advise them to change their behavior, and to refer patients with alcohol problems" (p. 245) as a result of the virtual simulation. As an increasing number of universities open virtual reality labs, social work educators can create VR content and continue assessing the value of this new medium for pedagogical purposes related to practicing interventions with minimal risk.

In addition to these illustrations from higher education, other examples could be given in a world where innovation quickly makes its way into practice at the micro (Sage & Sage, 2016) and macro levels (Folayan, Hitchcock, & Zgoda, 2018). Consider the following: the use of virtual reality has demonstrated efficacy in the treatment of anxiety disorders (Rothbaum et al., 2014); researchers have deployed social media data to predict depressive symptoms among users (De Choudhury, Counts, Horvitz, & Hoff, 2014); machine learning algorithms can often accurately predict psychosis (Corcoran et al., 2018); and use of particular smartphone applications can reduce symptoms of anxiety and depression (Campbell & McColgan, 2016) consistently for clients from many demographic backgrounds (Mohr et al., 2017).

Concluding remarks

It is curious that despite good data and evidence to the contrary, social work educators continue to doubt the reliability, efficacy, and validity of online social work education. It is beyond the scope of this article to investigate the reasons behind such skepticism, but it is a topic well worth exploring in the future. As long as online MSW programs continue to offer the equivalent programs and SLOs as their OCPs, students will likely continue to choose to open their laptops rather than a classroom door to access their education. Hence, moving forward, dialogue will benefit from embracing a broader perspective to technology, innovation, and learning. CSWE accreditation standards require that faculty in both OEPs and OCPs intentionally engage with both implicit and explicit curricula. Therefore, evaluation design that is holistic, and includes measures of teaching, cognitive, and social presence, will not only serve to maximize student learning experiences but acknowledge and validate the shifts both in contemporary social work education and professional practice.

In 2017, the National Association of Social Workers (NASW), Association of Social Work Boards (ASWB), Council on Social Work Education (CSWE), and Clinical Social Work Association (CSWA) created the "Standards for Technology in Social Work Practice." CSWE also added the "appropriate use of technology" to competency number one: Demonstrate Professional and Ethical Behavior (CSWE, 2015). The NASW updated its Code of Ethics to include use of technology, and presently one of the twelve Grand Challenges developed by the American Academy of Social Work and Social Welfare is "Harnessing Technology for Social Good" (Berzin, Singer, & Chan, 2015). Digital literacy is now seen as a cultural competency; failure to grapple with this fact ignores the reality and needs of many of our clients and their communities and the explicit future expectations of the profession. It is time for faculty and accredited programs to do the same, refining the use of technology in OEPs and expanding its use in OCPs, to support positive learning outcomes for all students.

Disclosure statement

No potential conflict of interest was reported by the authors.

References

Allen, I. E., Seaman, J., Poulin, R., & Straut, T. (2016). *Online report card: Tracking online education in the United States*. [online] Babson Survey Research Group and Quahog Research Group, LLC. Retrieved from http://onlinelearningsurvey.com/reports/onlinere portcard.pdf

Arbaugh, J. B., & Benbunan-Fich, R. (2006). An investigation of epistemological and social dimensions of teaching in online learning environments. *Academy of Management Learning & Education, 5*, 435–447. doi:10.5465/amle.2006.23473204

Arkorful, V., & Abaidoo, N. (2015). The role of e-learning, advantages and disadvantages of its adoption in higher education. *International Journal of Instructional Technology and Distance Learning, 12*(1), 29–42.

Beal, B. (n.d.). *Teaching group dynamics using virtual reality*. Retrieved from https://social worker.com/feature-articles/technology-articles/teaching-group-dynamics-using-virtual-reality/

Berzin, S. C., Singer, J., & Chan, C. (2015). *Practice innovation through technology in the digital age: A grand challenge for social work* (Grand Challenges for Social Work Initiative. Working Paper No. 12). Cleveland, OH: American Academy of Social Work and Social

Welfare. Retrieved from http://grandchallengesforsocialwork.org/wp-content/uploads/2015/12/180604-GC-technology.pdf

Campbell, A., & McColgan, M. (2016). Making social work education App'ier: The process of developing information-based apps for social work education and practice. *Social Work Education*, *35*(3), 297–309. doi:10.1080/02615479.2015.1130805

Carter, I., Damianakis, T., Munro, S., Skinner, H., Matin, S., & Andrews, T. N. (2018). Exploring online and blended course delivery in social group work. *Journal of Teaching in Social Work*, *38*(5), 486–503. doi:10.1080/08841233.2018.1523824

Cavanaugh, J. K., & Jacquemin, S. J. (2015). A large sample comparison of grade based student learning outcomes in online vs. face-to-face courses. *Online Learning*, *19*(2), 8. doi:10.24059/olj.v19i2.454

Corcoran, C. M., Carrillo, F., Fernández-Slezak, D., Bedi, G., Klim, C., Javitt, D. C., … Cecchi, G. A. (2018). Prediction of psychosis across protocols and risk cohorts using automated language analysis. *World Psychiatry*, *17*(1), 67–75. doi:10.1002/wps.20491

Council on Social Work Education [CSWE]. (2015). *Educational policy and accreditation standards*. Retrieved from https://www.cswe.org/getattachment/Accreditation/Standards-and-Policies/2015-EPAS/2015EPASandGlossary.pdf.aspx

Council on Social Work Education [CSWE]. (2018). *Online and distance education offerings by accredited programs*. Retrieved from https://cswe.org/Accreditation/Directory-of-Accredited-Programs/Online-and-Distance-Education

Cummings, S. M., Chaffin, K. M., & Cockerham, C. (2015). Comparative analysis of an online and a traditional MSW program: Educational outcomes. *Journal of Social Work Education*, *51*(1), 109–120. doi:10.1080/10437797.2015.977170

Daymont, T., Blau, G., & Campbell, D. (2011). Deciding between traditional and online formats: Exploring the role of learning advantages, flexibility, and compensatory adaptation. *Journal of Behavioral and Applied Management*, *12*(2), 156.

De Choudhury, M., Counts, S., Horvitz, E., & Hoff, A. (2014). *Characterizing and predicting postpartum depression from shared facebook data*. Proceedings of the 17th ACM conference on computer supported cooperative work & social computing (pp. 626–638). ACM. Retrieved from https://dl.acm.org/citation.cfm?id=2531675&dl=ACM&coll=DL

Dewey, J. (1938). *Experience and education*. New York, NY: Collier Books.

Farrell, D., Ray, K., Rich, T., Suarez, Z., Christenson, B., & Jennigs, L. (2018). A meta-analysis of approaches to engage social work students online. *Journal of Teaching in Social Work*, *38*(2), 183–197. doi:10.1080/08841233.2018.1431351

Flipgrid Inc. (2018) *Flipgrid (version 7.1.5)* [Mobile application Software]. Retrieved from http://itunes.apple.com

Flynn, M., Maiden, R. P., Smith, W., Wiley, J., & Wood, G. (2013). Launching the virtual academic center: Issues and challenges in innovation. *Journal of Teaching in Social Work*, *33*(4–5), 339–356. doi:10.1080/08841233.2013.843364

Folayan, S. W., Hitchcock, L. I., & Zgoda, K. (2018). Using twitter in reclaiming macro practice, and affirming our social work roots. *Reflections: Narratives of Professional Helping*, *24*(1), 56–64.

Garrison, D. R., Anderson, T., & Archer, W. (2000). Critical inquiry in a text-based environment: Computer conferencing in higher education. *Internet and Higher Education*, *11*(2), 87–105.

Garrison, D. R., & Arbaugh, J. B. (2007). Researching the community of inquiry framework: Review, issues and future directions. *The Internet and Higher Education*, *10*, 157–172. doi:10.1016/j.iheduc.2007.04.001

Gleason, B., & Greenhow, C. (2017). Hybrid education: The potential of teaching and learning with robot-mediated communication. *Online Learning Journal*, *21*(4), 87–105.

Goldingay, S., & Land, C. (2014). Emotion: The 'e' in engagement in online distance education in social work. *Journal of Open, Flexible and Distance Learning, 18*(1), 58–72.

Grady, M., Swick, D., & Powers, J. (2018). The Implicit curriculum survey: An examination of the psychometric properties. *Journal of Social Work Education, 54*(2), 261–269. doi:10.1080/10437797.2017.1404527

Han, J., & Finkelstein, A. (2013). Understanding the effects of professors' pedagogical development with clicker assessment and feedback technologies and the impact on students' engagement and learning in higher education. *Computers & Education, 65*(C), 64–76. doi:10.1016/j.compedu.2013.02.002

Koetting, C., & Freed, P. (2017). Educating undergraduate psychiatric mental health nursing students in screening, brief intervention, referral to treatment (SBIRT) using an online, interactive simulation. *Archives of Psychiatric Nursing, 31*(3), 241–247. doi:10.1016/j.apnu.2016.11.004

Kurzman, P. A. (2013). The evolution of distance learning and online education. *Journal of Teaching in Social Work, 33*(4–5), 331–338. doi:10.1080/08841233.2013.843346

Lowenthal, P. R., & Dunlap, J. C. (2009). From pixel on a screen to real person in your students' lives: Establishing social presence using digital storytelling. *The Internet and Higher Education, 13*(1–2), 70–72. doi:10.1016/j.iheduc.2009.10.004

Ma, J., Han, X., Yang, J., & Cheng, J. (2015). Examining the necessary condition for engagement in an online learning environment based on learning analytics approach: The role of the instructor. *The Internet and Higher Education, 24*, 26–34. doi:10.1016/j.iheduc.2014.09.005

Mohr, D. C., Tomasino, K. N., Lattie, E. G., Palac, H. L., Kwasny, M. J., Weingardt, K., … Caccamo, L. (2017). IntelliCare: An eclectic, skills-based app suite for the treatment of depression and anxiety. *Journal of Medical Internet Research, 19*(1), e10. doi:10.2196/jmir.6645

NASW, ASWB, CSWE, & CSWA Standards for Technology in Social Work Practice. (2017). Retrieved from https://www.socialworkers.org/includes/newIncludes/homepage/PRA-BRO-33617.TechStandards_FINAL_POSTING.pdf

Nguyen, T. (2015). The effectiveness of online learning: Beyond no significant difference and future horizons. *MERLOT Journal of Online Learning and Teaching, 11*(2), 309–319.

Peterson, N., Farmer, A., Donnelly, L., & Forenza, B. (2014). Assessing the implicit curriculum in social work education: Heterogeneity of students' experiences and impact on professional empowerment. *Journal of Teaching in Social Work, 34*(5), 460–479. doi:10.1080/08841233.2014.955943

Phillips, E., Wood, G., Yoo, J., Ward, K., Hsiao, S., Singh, M., & Morris, B. (2018). A virtual field practicum: Building core competencies prior to agency placement. *Journal of Social Work Education, 54*(4), 620–640. doi:10.1080/10437797.2018.1486651

Quinn, A., & Barth, A. (2014). Operationalizing the implicit curriculum in MSW distance education programs. *Journal of Social Work Education, 50*(1), 34–47. doi:10.1080/10437797.2014.856229

Reamer, F. (2013). Social work in a digital age: Ethical and risk management challenges. *Social Work, 58*(2), 163–172. doi:10.1093/sw/swt003

Reissman, C. K., & Quinney, L. (2005). Narrative in social work: A critical review. *Qualitative Social Work, 4*, 391–412. doi:10.1177/1473325005058643

Rothbaum, B., Price, M., Jovanovic, T., Norrholm, S., Gerardi, M., Dunlop, B., … Ressler, K. (2014). A randomized, double-blind evaluation of d-cycloserine or alprazolam combined with virtual reality exposure therapy for posttraumatic stress disorder in Iraq and Afghanistan war veterans. *American Journal of Psychiatry, 171*(6), 640–648. doi:10.1176/appi.ajp.2014.13121625

Sage, T. E., & Sage, M. (2016). Social media use in child welfare practice. *Advances in Social Work, 17*(1), 93–112. doi:10.18060/20880

Shaw, R., Molloy, M., Vaughn, J., Crego, N., Kuszajewski, M., Brisson, R., & Hueckel, R. (2018). Telepresence robots for pediatric clinical simulations: Feasibility and acceptability. *Pediatric Nursing, 44*(1), 39–43.

Storycenter. (2018). Retrieved from www.storycenter.org

Sun, P. C., Tsai, R. J., Finger, G., Chen, Y. Y., & Yeh, D. (2008). What drives a successful e-Learning? An empirical investigation of the critical factors influencing learner satisfaction. *Computers & Education, 50*(4), 1183–1202. doi:10.1016/j.compedu.2006.11.007

Taylor, B. L. (2016). *The Struggle is real: Student perceptions of quality in online courses using the community of inquiry (CoI) framework* (unpublished doctoral dissertation). University of California, Department of Education Studies, San Diego.

USC Shoah Foundation. (2019). *The institute for visual history and education.* Retrieved from https://sfi.usc.edu/

Weller, M. (2018). Twenty years of edtech. *Educause Review Online, 53*(4), 34–48.

WeVideo. (2017). *WeVideo (version 4.3.7)* [Mobile Software]. Retrieved from http://itunes.apple.com

Wyatt, G. (2005). Satisfaction, academic rigor and interaction: Perceptions of online instruction. *Education, 125*(3), 460–468.

A Synchronous Online Social Work PhD Program: Educational Design and Student/Faculty Response

Dennis Myers, Jon Singletary, Rob Rogers, Jim Ellor, and Sidney Barham

ABSTRACT
Faculty and students evaluate the curriculum design and delivery of a synchronous online PhD program in social work that prepares scholar-practitioners in social work research, education, and organizational practice. The designers envision a collaborative community of scholars and leaders nurtured by a cohort-based, sequenced curriculum, and intentional faculty mentoring. This teaching and learning platform provides an opportunity to engage with a globally diverse population of doctoral students while fostering both relationships and quality learning outcomes. Educational design and pedagogical features of the program are described and analyzed through the collaborative thinking and learning platform of the Community of Inquiry (CoI) model's interdependent elements–teaching, cognitive, and social presence. Eighteen students and ten faculty evaluated the strengths and limitations of the online program across each dimension of the model through student course evaluations, focus-group reflections, and qualitative faculty survey data. Student and faculty respondents specified the benefits of synchronous presence across all three dimensions. They also identified significant barriers, particularly in the areas of teaching and social presence. Implications and recommendations are based on a review of findings that inform pedagogical decisions and design options for online PhD education in social work.

The authors report here on student and faculty evaluations of the design and delivery of the PhD program in Social Work at Baylor University, a private Christian university in Texas. The program launched in 2013 utilizing synchronous, web-based pedagogy commonly described as a virtual classroom. Like many other social work doctoral education programs, Baylor adopted distance education technologies as a response to one of the challenges impacting the profession and the academy–access to doctoral social work programs for graduates working full-time (Kurzman, 2015). This pedagogical shift to distance education is occurring in the context of a remarkable increase in web-based instruction across all sectors of higher education. According to the most recent data on social work PhD programs, there are two completely online programs, and four that combine online and physical presence hybrid instruction (Lightfoot & Beltran, 2016). Each of them benefit from wider broadband availability, more nimble information processors, and increasingly sophisticated learning management software (Kurzman, 2015). Online platforms vary in the utilization of asynchronous and/or synchronous capabilities, applied exclusively or in combination (blended format). Synchronous (or virtual) online classroom engagements are frequently complemented by opportunities for physical presence in a traditional (non-virtual) setting. Whether a program is considered to be synchronous or asynchronous, it is also possible that schools can employ asynchronous classroom management tools such as Blackboard and Canvas.

Social work educators who are willing to share their research findings and lessons learned from online programs are a vital resource for addressing design, technology, and learner issues, thereby improving student satisfaction and program outcomes. As Golde (2007) observes, careful assessment of new doctoral programs is especially important so that effective pedagogies are shared and "ineffective pedagogies can be avoided" (p. 350).

Consistent with the call for lessons learned and informed observations, the authors provide a program-level description and analysis of Baylor University Garland School of Social Work's PhD program that focuses on two aspects of synchronous program delivery–development and design decisions and student and faculty impact. The importance of attention to program-level evaluation (rather than course-level assessment of online curricula) is supported by the observation of Merisotis and Phipps (1999) that "a major gap in the research is the lack of studies dedicated to measuring the effectiveness of total academic programs taught using distance learning" (p. 15). More recently, Kumar (2014) observed that studies of online program design and development is important because a majority of the research published on distance education continues to focus on teaching and learning within individual courses.

The program under discussion is a traditional Doctor of Philosophy in that it is a research degree that teaches not only research methods but also the philosophy of science which undergirds social science research. Rather than writing a traditional dissertation, students produce three publishable articles, a requirement directly related to establishing the doctoral student as a participant and future leader in an area of substantive inquiry. Qualitative as well as quantitative methodologies are central to the research curriculum that also includes courses in measurement and program evaluation. Since preparation of social work educators is also a goal of the PhD program, the curriculum includes courses on academic leadership, administration, and higher education instruction, as well as a teaching practicum.

The object of this inquiry is the pursuit of higher quality design and delivery of online PhD programs and, ultimately, more effective social work practice and knowledge development.

The authors analyzed the responses of students and faculty to program design and delivery inquiries utilizing data from three primary sources: student course evaluations, focus-group reflections of the most recent cohort, and qualitative survey feedback from faculty about their online teaching experience. Before reporting student and faculty responses about the program, we will examine historical developments and current design features as well as the conceptual frames and research that inform the structure and pedagogy of the cohort-based, virtual classroom approach.

Program development and design features

As background and context for the discussion of program design and student/faculty responses, the authors here will provide a brief overview of the development of the program and a glimpse into the synchronous classroom experience. Prior to developing the PhD program, the School of Social Work began experimenting with distance education in 2003 when the university installed teleconference technology in one of the social work classrooms. The installation enabled a maximum of four MSW students engaged in distant field internships to participate in seminars conducted on campus. This delivery system soon was replaced by Collaborate, a more robust teleconferencing mechanism within the Blackboard learning management system, and the university purchased licenses for a high definition Cisco videoconferencing system in 2011. Baylor University's experience with this higher quality network provided the technology platform and confidence needed to complete the development of the PhD program. One year later, the university switched to Canvas, a learning management system that allows faculty and students to interact online through submitting and posting documents, discussion threads, videoconferencing, and more. Canvas also includes the Big Blue Button (BBB) videoconferencing system which students and faculty quickly developed a preference for using for their virtual classroom experiences.

Since 2013, three doctoral cohorts (one cohort every other year) have been admitted for a total of 18 students. Throughout the program, students connect for class via videoconference each week at a set time. Using the BBB platform, all students and faculty can see and speak with one another. In this virtual classroom, the instructor can post documents, share desktop materials, or walk through presentation slides. In addition to talking, students and the instructor can use a text chat box to further facilitate communication. The BBB platform also supports the creation of multiple "rooms" where students can meet in small groups while the instructor rotates among them.

Online educational design and best practices

Research related to online doctoral education provides a rich resource for guiding program design, learning methodologies, and relational strategies. The Carnegie Mellon Open Learning Initiative in fact found that students in online classes perform as well as or better than students in traditional classes (Bowen, Chingos, Lack, & Nygren, 2013). When strategically placed and rigorously developed, online courses are comparable to those which are face-to-face in activities, assignments, outcomes, student quality, and methods of addressing academic honesty (Jones, 2015). In addition, online field seminars have been shown to be effective for distance placements. For example, in one study, it was found that students experienced equivalent educational outcomes and were able to report the value of online collegial relationships with other seminar participants (Harris & Myers, 2013).

While these and other studies report that student perceptions of online course quality and learning are comparable to traditional in-person courses (Topper, 2007; Tucker, 2000), agreement here is not unanimous. For example, Castle and McGuire (2010) concluded that students in face-to-face classes generally agreed with the statement, "I gained significant knowledge about this subject" (p. 37) more frequently than students in (asynchronous) online classes. However, they reported that student satisfaction with courses tended to be higher with online courses where synchronous learning opportunities were offered.

Even though empirical and anecdotal evidence in general support the efficacy of online social work education, and synchronicity as a preferred pedagogy (Flynn, Maiden, Smith, Wiley, & Wood, 2013), significant questions remain concerning how to enrich student outcomes as well as student and faculty engagement and satisfaction with the design and delivery of social work doctoral education at a distance. In the literature, potential barriers to a satisfactory learning experience include unreliable Internet connection (Bolliger & Martindale, 2004), Internet and virtual classroom anxiety (Simonson, Smaldino, Albright, & Zvacek, 2009), virtual versus physical presence comparisons (Bowen et al., 2013), responsiveness of the faculty (Herbert, 2006), and social integration (Moore, 2014).

Overcoming social isolation and creating a collaborative and viable learning community are challenges often associated with online education, particularly in asynchronous learning contexts. Community, connectedness, and social presence are all terms often used in the literature synonymously with social integration and are associated with doctoral candidates' reported intent to persist in their course of study (Cockrell & Shelley, 2011; Terrell, Snyder, & Dringus, 2009). Rovai, Wighting, and Lucking (2004) explain that social community, "represents the feelings of the community of students regarding their spirit, cohesion, trust, safety, trade, interdependence, and sense of belonging" (p. 269). This definition highlights the importance of creating a thinking and learning context that nurtures the interdependence among social, cognitive, and teaching presence as is seen in the Community of Inquiry (CoI) model, especially in the context of the virtual, synchronous environment where passive learning approaches may become the default option.

Some of the online technological and collaborative challenges were addressed at Baylor University by using a learning management system (LMS) with a reputation for excellent responsiveness and reliability. In online courses, when student-to-student collaboration is properly facilitated, students have expressed feelings similar to those of being together physically (Chang, 2012); therefore, the authors provide examples of how Baylor's doctoral education program sought to create this level of relationality through design features focusing on social integration and cohort solidarity, including a one week in-person experience in tandem with the synchronous, virtual classroom.

Conceptual lens

The opportunities and challenges of technology-mediated teaching and learning elevate collaboration with one another (and with the learning) as essential components in building and sustaining the academic community. Casey and Kroth (2013) observe that presence may be experienced differently in an online classroom, stating that "online environment interactions are mediated through technology which changes the character of the interactions and can change the ways in which they are perceived" (p.104). The Community of Inquiry (CoI) model, developed by Garrison, Anderson, and Archer (2000), is a frequently applied framework for several important educational ends. The authors of the model recognize the active learning opportunities available in classrooms mediated by technologically connected, synchronous learning environments. Seemingly outdated yet valued educational characteristics, such as smaller classes, now reemerge in this space. Traditional passive learning approaches and written communication can make important contributions to asynchronous content delivery but they are insufficient within programs aspiring to create a community-based environment for doctoral level collaborative thinking and learning. The CoI approach provides "a coherent, heuristic, and proven theoretical framework for studying and designing a community of thinkers and learners" (Garrison, 2016, p. 9). In this transactional space, doctoral students' questions activate a collaborative exchange with real potential for challenging bias and providing participants with a window into their unexamined patterns of thinking. The CoI design, if successful in inspiring collaborative inquiry, prescribes three forms of presence (termed core elements) within the learning environment–cognitive, social, and teaching.

Cognitive presence

The nature of inquiry and discourse within the model invites students to trust the thinking and learning ethos enough to offer their private deliberations and questions to colleagues who care enough to engage in critical molding of incomplete notions, biases, and new ideas, yielding a shared, recursive, and mutually beneficial educational resolution. Ideally, the additional benefit of this process is that students develop the habit of metacognitive awareness (Garrison, 2016), particularly when the doctoral seminars provide opportunities to lead discussions and engage in peer facilitation.

From the perspective of the CoI framework, Baylor University's curriculum creates conceptual contexts to develop collaborative intellectual intentionality and to value the life of the mind. Several courses address the intersection among teaching, practice, and research. Students review conceptual analyses and research as well as facilitate peer discussions around the ethical integration of religious faith and social work practice in seminars devoted to religious and cultural diversity, as well as social policy and religion, with an emphasis on the Christian worldview. Related to the program's academic leadership emphasis, students critically engage theoretical scholarship, faculty and curriculum issues, and research related to the higher education administration of social work educational programs.

Consistent with Costa and Kallick's (2008) observation of doctoral education as a process for developing scholarly habits of mind, students translate their assessments of theoretical paradigms and current research into proposals for knowledge development, innovative interventions, and/or teaching and learning strategies. Whenever possible, scholarship in the context of promoting collegial and collaborative teams is encouraged. Furthermore, students are expected to immediately develop a program of work that clearly identifies a coherent and bounded area of inquiry consistent with social work values and research excellence.

Social presence

The CoI design also includes provision for social integration and virtual community building among students. Considered the backbone of the CoI process, social presence is the ability of students to experience a sense of belonging and trust with their doctoral colleagues so that open communication can become the norm, peer relationships can grow, and collaborative learning can flourish. Garrison (2016) identifies three deliverables: purpose of the inquiry (identity), conditions for free and open communication (cohesion), and personal relationships (natural growth).

Sense of community, which is developed through interaction (Rovai, 2002) and is closely related to student engagement (Young & Bruce, 2011), is a crucial element to ensuring online student success (Moore, 2014). These phenomena play a major role in social and academic integration, which affect student decision-making and outcomes (Tinto, 1997). In addition, Fletcher, Comer, and Dunlap (2014) suggest that technology can facilitate a virtual holding environment that nurtures doctoral students' investment in their learning, to include the dissertation process.

To this end, Baylor University's online doctoral program adopted a cohort model for admission and matriculation, which is reported to be an important factor in promoting online doctoral student morale and retention (Kumar, Johnson, & Hardemon, 2013). As observed by Kumar (2014), "online programs have to provide structures for peer interactions but also communicate the value of such interactions, especially at the doctoral level where research and writing are often individual and isolating endeavors" (p. 66). The program requires a one-week in-person, on-campus orientation with two face-to-face class sessions to foster a social presence at the start of the program. The small size of the cohort (n = 5–7) further increases the likelihood of relationship development.

One caveat to an overemphasis on social presence is offered by Arbaugh and Rau (2007) who reported that intense engagement in peer relationships among graduate students is correlated with course dissatisfaction, particularly in the dissertation phase. In this case, attention to where students are along the matriculation path may need to be considered when encouraging higher levels of social presence. The findings of this study provide examples of how students and faculty responded to Baylor University's intention to elevate social presence through attention to social integration and cohort solidarity.

Teaching presence

The teaching presence element of the CoI framework addresses the leadership function in nurturing social presence and in designing, facilitating, and directing cognitive presence. In fact, Garrison's (2016, p. 88) seven principles of social and cognitive presence are ordered according to the three categories of teaching presence (design, facilitation, and direct instruction). In this model, faculty have a defined instructional leadership role that is balanced with the relational needs of the seminar participants.

Numerous studies document the adverse effects on the learning and the learner when this dimension of presence is compromised. Challenges to effective delivery of teaching presence (including synchronous classrooms) are faculty's lack of responsiveness to student needs (Herbert, 2006); unreliable technology and interactivity (Bolliger & Martindale, 2004; Dennen, Darabi, & Smith, 2007); and anxiety associated with technology (Simonson et al., 2009; Sun, Tsai, Finger, Chen, & Yeh, 2008).

As currently constituted, the architecture of the synchronous, online social work PhD program design includes facets associated with promoting collaborative thinking and learning grounded in cognitive, social, and teaching presence. Examples of these program components include synchronous delivery, cohort admission and matriculation (Kumar & Dawson, 2014), initial orientation requiring physical presence (Byrd, 2016), reliable LMS (Dennen et al., 2007), opportunities for continued full-time employment (Castle & McGuire, 2010), the integration of faith and practice (Byrd, 2016), and faculty responsiveness (Herbert, 2006). After reviewing the methods applied in this study, the researchers report the extent to which students and faculty perceive that the educational design delivered the dimensions and levels of collaboration and presence associated with responsive online doctoral education.

Methods

Research questions and design

The following questions guided this evaluation of the PhD program: To what extent do PhD students and faculty experience cognitive, social, and teaching presence in this program, and what is the role of technology in their learning and teaching? The authors used a mixed-methods, primarily qualitative approach with archival data of student course evaluations, a focus group with students, and a brief survey of the students, and of the faculty who had taught courses in the program.

Sample selection

The sampling frame consisted of all of the 18 students from three cohorts (starting in 2013, 2015, and 2017) and all of the 10 faculty who taught courses in the program. (This research, conducted between May and July 2017, was deemed exempt from review by the university's Institutional Review Board.) The identity of the students who contributed to the course evaluations was confidential. Students from Cohort Three, who participated in the focus group, signed consent forms; both students and faculty who responded to the confidential email surveys did so voluntarily; and there were no incentives offered for participation.

When the survey was sent, faculty were told that their data would be deidentified by the graduate associate before being sent to the investigators. Students completed a survey asking for non-sensitive data, such as how many online courses they had taken prior to entering the PhD program. Data from these surveys were compiled by the PhD program manager before being sent anonymously to the investigators. Qualitative student data were obtained from the University's confidential course evaluation system which is an IRB approved protocol for program evaluations such as this one.

Instrumentation and data collection

The archival data sources were 12 course evaluations completed by students in Cohorts One and Two (n = 12) and demographic data in the students' files. The authors focused on seven questions related to the role of technology. Three were Likert-type questions with a four point *agree* scale (Not at All, Very Little, Somewhat, and Very Much): How prepared were you for online learning? To what extent did the technology itself help your learning? To what extent did the technology itself hinder your learning? Four questions were open-ended: What do you think are the benefits of being in this class online? What do you think you have lost by being in this class online? How did the technology itself affect your relationship with other students in the class and with the professor? From this experience, how do you think that your learning outcomes in a virtual classroom compare to a face-to-face classroom?

Cohort One did not have the opportunity to answer these seven additional course evaluation questions until the end of the second year of their coursework in Summer 2015 when Cohort Two began. Cohort Two had the opportunity to answer these questions in every course. Further, faculty who teach in the PhD program were sent an email survey with questions similar to those in the course evaluations.

Cohort Three began with six students in Summer 2017. Since this cohort started as this manuscript was being written, the authors conducted a focus group with the six students asking about their expectations regarding the program, including the role of technology in their learning.

To provide additional context for interpreting the data from the course evaluations, students were sent an email survey asking the number of courses they had taken online prior to entering the Ph.D. program, the number of semesters they had taught a course (adjunctively, full-time), and the number of courses they had taught online. All students in the program (n = 18) and seven out of a possible 10 faculty members responded to the survey. At the time the survey was sent in June, two PhD faculty had left the university at the end of the academic year and several others were out of the office, which most likely accounts for the 70 percent response rate.

Data analysis

A five-member research team consisting of the co-directors of the doctoral program, two faculty teaching in the program, and a graduate associate analyzed the quantitative course evaluation data from the first two cohorts by reporting the percentage of student responses to the three Likert-type questions by course and cohort. An analysis of the significance of differences over time could not be conducted due to the small numbers of respondents for each course evaluation. The team members also analyzed the qualitative data in an inductive manner, using constant comparison (Strauss & Corbin, 1998), which involves looking for key issues, themes, or experiences in the data that can then become categories for focus (Glaser & Strauss, 1967).

This process of qualitative analysis is inherently subjective, and so, rather than looking for objective meaning in the data, researchers sought to develop higher order meaning in their interpretation of the data sources. To do so, each team member read through all of the data and offered highlights of the phenomena related to the role of technology in teaching and learning. Additional team members read iterative drafts of the interpretations. Through a peer review process, the team achieved consensus and had confidence in the narrative report.

Each of these steps in analysis contributes to what qualitative researchers discuss as the trustworthiness of analysis methods in an effort to promote the rigor of their research (Guba, 1990). According to Rodwell (1998), trustworthiness "demonstrates elements necessary to ensure that there can be confidence in the research findings" (p. 96). Prolonged engagement with the data, persistent observation and interpretations over time, triangulation of the qualitative and quantitative data, dependability in analysis (akin to interrater reliability), and peer review of the analysis by team members all contribute to the trustworthiness and therefore rigor of the analysis.

Results

The sample

The sample of 18 students consisted of 15 (83.33%) females and three (16.67%) males. Their median age at the time of entry into the program was 34.5 years with a range of 26–50 years. The sample included two African American, one Hispanic, and 15 Caucasian students. Seventeen held MSW degrees and one had a degree from a sister profession. Regarding the students' experience with online teaching and learning prior to entering the PhD program, five (27.78%) had taught adjunctively or full-time, six (33.33%) had taken online courses, and two (11.11%) had taught an online course. In addition, three (16.57%) had taught an online course since entering the program.

Student and faculty response themes

The experiences of PhD students and faculty with the pedagogy and technology of the PhD program are presented in four categories. The first focuses on how program design and technology fostered teaching presence and offered flexibility, making their education feasible. The second includes challenges to teaching and social presence, such as technical issues, learning fatigue, and the nature of building relationships in an online learning community. In the third, students and faculty discuss how the synchronous approach in virtual classrooms delivered social and cognitive presence. The final category focuses on the nature of the program's learning outcomes.

The benefits of technology

Students and faculty repeatedly described how technology fosters social and teaching presence. Several highlighted the benefits of a learning community enriched by the intellectual and geographic diversity of their student colleagues, with one stating,"Being able to hear the stories and to appreciate the experiences of students across America was extremely motivational as well as educational."

Preparation for online education in the program occurs because of prior student experience with technology used in in-person courses (online videos, virtual labs, and demonstrations), taking online courses, and/or teaching online. The quantitative evaluation findings indicate that more online experiences result in greater comfort with this format. By their seventh semester, all students in the first cohort felt "very prepared" for online courses. One student noted, "Our entire program is pretty much online, so two years in, I feel like a pro." Students in the second cohort felt "somewhat" or "very much prepared" during their first semester, and all felt "very prepared" by the sixth. As one student from this cohort noted, "I have been doing this for two years now. I am very comfortable in the virtual classroom. Our cohort feels as if we are together in class even though we are across the country. Our instructors have been well prepared to use technology effectively." As for the third cohort in the focus group, none of the students reported having substantial online experience, and none had a clear understanding of how interactions among students occurs online. In addition, the quantitative findings suggested a positive link between prior online experience and perceiving benefits of technology. For example, over time (first to sixth semester), students in the second cohort reported technology being slightly more helpful and slightly less of a hindrance.

Whether students were beginning the program or were close to completion of the program, they shared ways that technology provided highly valued flexibility and teaching presence. Half of the incoming third cohort reported that an attraction of the program was that they could keep working and did not have to move their families, and that it works with their schedule–a theme echoed across all cohorts. In addition to convenience benefits, economies of time also were mentioned, to wit, "When I attended my master's program at a local university, I clearly recall lamenting how much time I wasted commuting to/from class rather than actually being productive. With the additional rigor of a doctoral program, any time I can save is to my benefit!"

Faculty reported similar benefits related to teaching presence for the online courses they taught. Providing access to doctoral education within the students' locality was also of paramount importance to them. In addition, the online venue increased the diversity of student identities and viewpoints. Scheduling flexibility also was favorably mentioned by all the faculty, including the convenience of being able to lead the class from a variety of spaces.

Struggles with technology

Despite the benefits of technology, there are challenges in a synchronous model of online learning, particularly in the areas of teaching and social presence. Third cohort students (new to the program) expressed discomfort regarding how they would talk with each other and how group dynamics would work when mediated by computers. They also expressed a hope that the faculty would be flexible with their learning so that, if they fail to understand something, they can continue to address it until all are comfortable. One student provided this helpful observation:

> Trust between students and instructors comes with a sense of community, the same for cohort members. Baylor University needs to create a sense of community and intentionality about implementation. It is challenging when instructors are new to the online format and/or do not get a sense of cohort dynamics and navigate them effectively.

This reservation was addressed in part by having each cohort meet in person on campus for one week prior to the start of their online experience. Fostering the development of relationships among students and with faculty is a priority during this week, and a process that continues after online classes begin.

Relationship building for online students, even in a synchronous setting and with a week-long in-person orientation, was a significant concern related to the virtual nature of the learning community. Specifically, one student remarked that she missed the collegiality and the informal conversations that happen in the hallways, saying "Occasionally I find it distracting being in my own house taking coursework. Some emotional/relational information gets missed." A fellow student echoed this concern, "I always feel somewhat disconnected from both my classmates and my professor in this format. It is often difficult for me to speak up and contribute to class discussions in this format." Another acknowledged this challenge but added, "I have to listen harder, so I give them fuller attention, and that enhances my relationships." Others observed that, without the intimacy of physical presence, they felt less impetus to be vulnerable when discussing divisive or difficult topics.

The most significant technology struggle for both students and faculty was with teaching presence caused by connectivity issues, but almost always with the caveat, "they were minimal."

A common theme across all student cohorts was, "There were glitches at times when the instructor could not hear or students were kicked off. Time spent rebooting was frustrating at times. Being able to join just with audio would be useful when there are connectivity issues." Each of the faculty respondents mentioned the negative effect of losing connection, whether due to a student's computer or bandwidth capacity. One faculty respondent noted, "It is cumbersome and challenging to maintain focus and engage with students when either the instructor or students continue dropping off throughout class."

Other struggles were also related to teaching presence. For example, students mentioned fatigue related to the online learning context, "the length of time spent online contributes to eye and physical fatigue that an in-person class that meets for four hours each session does not"; "lecture is hard to listen to when you're in a virtual classroom. It's easy to get distracted–it was sometimes hard to stay focused during a lecture that lasted longer than 30 minutes"; and "Face-to-face is more effective for an intense, twice-weekly class. An online class should be limited in time due to the ways we learn and our human limits such as eye fatigue."

Faculty also mentioned social presence concerns related to the student-faculty relationship when compared to traditional, in-person classes. One professor commented, "It was clear my online students experienced me very differently than my in-person students, which I think in some ways hindered my teaching. I need to be much more intentional in building relationships with my students in subsequent online courses which requires a different set of skills I didn't anticipate, or initially know how or where to acquire." Another reported, "I can't even identify most of my students when I have finally seen them in the flesh. A 2-D dimension of a person just isn't the same as being in the room as them." On a collective level, a student noted that "some instructors do not get a sense of a cohort's dynamics and navigate them effectively."

Several faculty respondents mentioned a loss in capacity to discern how the student is engaging in the learning process. For example, interpretation of eye contact is compromised in the distance learning environment, complicated by an inability to discern to what the students are giving their attention (e.g., email, social media, etc.), whereas students in an in-person setting can be asked to keep their computers closed and remain attentive. Another faculty member opined, "though we can see one another and engage in the virtual classrooms easily, there's something about physically being in the same space together that cannot be captured in an online class." A different perspective was offered by a respondent who encouraged faculty to not frame the online experience as a "less-than" experience but to see the challenges as opportunities to further develop and perfect this pedagogical method. The same respondent credited an intentional one-on-one virtual meeting twice during the semester as an approach to developing an effective teacher-student relationship.

Strengths of synchronous learning

While challenges exist in any learning environment, and while some are unique to online learning, there are also strengths in various approaches to online learning. The synchronous model (the virtual classroom) is seen as an asset to the program by many students and faculty who described the technology as "fostering relationships," "enhancing the learning experience," and "making the program what it is." The strengths identified primarily tended to be related to social presence. For example, students reported, "we have built our relationships with primarily technology. In fact, not being able to all talk at the same time has really helped our class and our relationships!" and "I grow closer to my classmates and professors with each class. My cohort is full of amazing, talented, and inspiring individuals who help me to grow as a person and a scholar."

Collaboration benefits extended to the creation of learning communities supported by technology. This statement reflects this advantage: "Being able to also conference online (speaking one-on-one with fellow students) outside the classroom more than made up for any short-fall (in technology)." One faculty respondent noted that the capacity of the learning management system to create small group settings mirrored well this positive aspect of an in-person class taught in the traditional manner.

Social presence advantages extended to presence in the student-faculty relationship. Two students addressed this benefit, "I can't just wander into the professor's office during office hours, but I can log in and meet with her anytime, anywhere" and "our professor made it a point that all students were required to meet with her at least once throughout the semester outside of class, to have a personal conversation, which helped develop some rapport."

Synchronous learning outcomes

Students and faculty compared their perceptions of outcomes in the synchronous online program with probable learning outcomes of the in-person setting. Remarkably, students reported, "sometimes getting distracted during lectures, [but] don't feel that my learning outcomes were compromised at all in this virtual classroom experience" and "this model of synchronous, and cohort-based, works just like a face-to-face classroom."

However, when discussing learning outcomes, students do point out some challenges. One weighed the costs and benefits, "I believe I would be learning more in a face-to-face classroom setting. However, the other conveniences of the online model win out." Another provided a more in-depth reflection:

> I believe that an in-person environment, for this class, would have allowed for there to be more of a personal touch and tone between students. Vulnerability and willingness to challenge ideas is extremely important for learning. While there were honest conversations, I don't know that these discussions went as deep as they could have in an in-person environment.

One student described the value of community as a mediating variable in her learning outcomes, "Online is preferable because of the flexibility of options to study while staying in my hometown and keep my current employment. Face-to-face is more interactive and builds a closer sense of community that does get a little lost in an online environment."

Students also shared how effective teaching presence in the design of synchronous learning contributed to their accountability and improved outcomes, "Synchronous learning systems also provide more accountability than face-to-face because of the camera always being on faces ... instead of being in a classroom where you are only looking forward at the instructor." They also described in detail how faculty supported their learning, one saying, "The professors are also adapting and finding a way to encourage thoughtful conversation in this medium." Another added, "Professors have been prepared to deliver their content in engaging ways."

Two students identified additional ways that a well-designed virtual class contributed to learning outcomes in unanticipated fashion. One observed, "On this level of education, and given my maturity, this virtual experience definitely outweighed by far the classroom. There is nothing like having theory translated into practice each week ... by those who were actually in the practice arena in other cities."

Like their students, most faculty offered observations that the learning outcomes appeared to be the same when comparing online synchronous and in-person delivery. Some faculty distinguished between content outcomes, which were positive, and student-faculty relationship outcomes, which were lower. One faculty member made this observation:

> In-person provides easier relationship building, fully present without as many distractions, and less dependent on technology working. Online, particularly synchronous delivery, offers learning to participate and communicate in real-time virtual meetings (which will serve them well after graduating), flexibility with addressing technology issues, and cultivation of an informal community.

In summary, overall satisfaction was the majority response of students and faculty to the current program design and delivery. Teaching presence offered in the context of the students' home and professional practice appears to be a significant factor that energized their decision to enroll in a synchronous online program. Connectivity, both in terms of technology performance and social presence, was an additional factor that appeared to play an important role in mediating the quality and impact of the virtual classroom experience.

Discussion

The CoI framework (Garrison et al., 2000) for online pedagogy provided a heuristic framework for communicating and analyzing collaboration across three elements of presence–teaching, social, and cognitive–that are central to the experience Baylor University seeks to provide in its PhD program. The analysis of student and faculty evaluations yielded an informed conclusion that the synchronous online model not only fosters learning comparable to the in-person experience but also provides greater flexibility, making doctoral education feasible for a new generation of working students. Social presence (Hostetter, 2013) in a learning community is key to the success of this model, and students and faculty affirm the capacity of virtual classrooms to deliver at least an acceptable level of this essential element of effective online learning.

Deepening student support

Literature about online doctoral learning identifies a primary challenge of finding ways to deepen social presence to the extent that students will feel supported in their educational program. While not every student significantly engages faculty and colleagues in on-campus programs, it is more difficult to maintain relationships online that will allow students to feel like they can just walk into a virtual office and chat with the instructor. Hence, faculty teaching in online programs need to learn new ways to foster and sustain supportive educational relationships with students within and outside of the classroom. As noted, Winnicott's (2018) holding environment and Bowlby's (1988) attachment theory, as applied by Fletcher et al. (2014), inform this effort to enrich faculty-student relationality and educational support. Therefore, the program will benefit significantly from an in-depth review that applies the CoI concept of teaching presence.

The findings of this study support several practices that need continuing reinforcement and can be adapted rather easily. Foremost is to insist that students as well as faculty, generally working from home, have Internet service with the capacity to sustain audio and video connectivity throughout class sessions. Negative consequences for poor connectivity need to be included in the course attendance policy and enforced. In addition, faculty can record lengthy lectures for students to view asynchronously prior to class. Then shorter synchronous sessions, focused on discussion, can reduce eye fatigue and stimulate attentiveness. Furthermore, faculty can be more intentional about sharing with colleagues their observations about the dynamics of relationships and interactivity within each cohort. Recognizing that these dynamics vary somewhat here with each instructor can guard against stereotyping and enable faculty to consistently reinforce strengths and address negative patterns. Students can contribute to this effort by proactively sharing collective preferences which they feel will enhance their learning experience. Finally, faculty and students need to inform administrators and technical staff about deficiencies in the videoconferencing platform and LMS and advocate for upgrades or for new systems. Rapidly evolving technologies (and a competitive marketplace) are making educational outcomes, as well as costs, a driving force for systems changes.

A *value-added signature pedagogy*

The Carnegie Foundation for the Advancement of Teaching (Shulman, Golde, Bueschel, & Garabedian, 2006) identified signature pedagogy as one of the four areas for the professional doctorate in education. Shulman (2005) defines signature pedagogy as "the characteristic forms of teaching and learning ... that organize the fundamental ways in which future practitioners are educated for their new professions" (p. 52). Current research centers on the comparability of online and in-person delivery (Arbaugh & Rau, 2007; Kumar et al., 2013; Topper, 2007), with synchronous delivery rated over asynchronous in approximating the in-person experience. However, Kurzman (2015) points out that comparisons of in-person versus online educational programs are difficult to make because they employ very different mediums but both result in quality learning outcomes. Some also argue that online programs are focused on profit and, while some may be, one cannot ignore the practicality of these programs that allow students to complete degrees at a distance while engaged in a variety of other work and family responsibilities.

The findings of this research may contribute to understanding the benefits and limitations of collaborative synchronous learning as a key component in the signature pedagogy of online social work doctoral education. Numerous observations of students and faculty in this study provide insight into the synchronous vs. in-person comparison. Critics of the online environment express concern that online learning is significantly more sterile than the in-person, which may make it ill-suited for social work education (Kurzman, 2015). Nevertheless, the reality is that there are differences that matter, and improvement of the technology and deeper adoption of the CoI collaboration model, can move beyond the defined expectations set by the in-person experience.

In fact, there are unique features and potential contributions which are often overlooked. Students and faculty provided several examples of substantive educational assets not available within the in-person context. The videoconferencing tool (BBB) of the LMS used by the program has a chat box feature that provides a venue for students to simultaneously respond as classroom content is being delivered. This supplemental channel offers another mode of student engagement that students and faculty can use to share information such as website links and commentary that enriches teaching presence and learning opportunities. Another asset is the capacity to record classroom content for review after the initial presentation. Moreoever, topic experts, such as authors of the students' texts, can be more conveniently invited to a virtual classroom, regardless of their location. Both Kurzman (2015) and Ferrera, Ostrander, and Crabtree-Nelson (2013) acknowledge the practicality of the virtual classroom and Ferrera et al. (2013)

point to the diversity of ways in which students can engage with the material and with one another in the online environment.

Indeed, videoconferencing is an increasingly common part of the social fabric, from Skype to Google Hangouts to Facetime. Bringing these social technologies into the classroom makes sense, and both the academic literature and student experience point to the value of this methodology for teaching and learning. While these examples of educational assets are not exhaustive, they highlight the value of a shift from viewing the virtual classroom as a margin of approximation of optimization to a stand-alone, signature pedagogy with unrealized potential for revolutionizing social work doctoral education.

Study limitations

The research design deployed had inherent limitations often associated with cross-sectional, small and unrepresentative samples. Clearly, future research initiatives will need to overcome such limitations to definitively examine the impact of online, synchronous approaches to doctoral social work education. Nevertheless, the strengths of this study are its focus on program-level analysis and design-based research utilizing the CoI model, along with program evaluation based on the observations of respondents most affected by the educational design.

While this study represented a limited application of the CoI model, the framework yielded insight into the strengths and limitations of virtual social work doctoral education. Further attention to the seven principles proposed by Garrison (2016) should provide a more comprehensive view of how social work educators are preparing scholars for knowledge development, teaching, and organizational leadership.

Impact on future social work doctoral education

Online education will continue to develop in new ways and transform instruction in Baylor University's programs irrespective of the mode of communication (asynchronous or synchronous) or venue (online or in-person). In the program addressed in this study, the shift was largely from a synchronous in-person classroom to a synchronous online one. A truly hybrid or blended model may evolve where more and more classes will include both synchronous and asynchronous elements, in-person and online.

Conclusion

The decision of faculty to develop a synchronous online PhD program that can simultaneously deliver teaching, social, and cognitive presence has been supported by the responses of students and faculty. The continuing challenges are primarily in the arena of social presence, particularly with respect to faculty and student relationships. Students, however, are able to learn in place while completing the program, which means less disruption for their careers and families.

While Berzoff and Drisko (2015) provocatively suggest that "PhD programs in social work may be abdicating their responsibility as stewards of the profession in favor of stewarding only an academic discipline" (p. 84), we feel this pilot program did just the opposite. By maintaining a full-time job in the field while completing a rigorous course of study, students in this doctoral program should graduate not only with skills in research and teaching but also as more seasoned and collaborative social work practitioners.

Disclosure statement

No potential conflict of interest was reported by the authors.

References

Arbaugh, J. B., & Rau, B. L. (2007). A study of disciplinary, structural, and behavioral effects on course outcomes in online MBA courses. *Decision Sciences Journal of Innovative Education*, 5(1), 65–95. doi:10.1111/j.1540-4609.2007.00128.x

Berzoff, J., & Drisko, J. (2015). Preparing PhD-level clinical social work practitioners for the 21st century. *Journal of Teaching in Social Work*, 35(1–2), 82–100. doi:10.1080/08841233.2014.993107

Bolliger, D. U., & Martindale, T. (2004). Key factors for determining student satisfaction in online courses. *International Journal on E-Learning*, 3(1), 61.

Bowen, W. G., Chingos, M. M., Lack, K. A., & Nygren, T. I. (2013). Online learning in higher education: Randomized trial compares hybrid learning to traditional course. *Education Next*, 13(2), 58.

Bowlby, J. (1988). *A secure base: Parent-child attachment and healthy human development.* New York, NY: Basic Books.

Byrd, J. C. (2016). Understanding the online doctoral learning experience: Factors that contribute to students' sense of community. *Journal of Educators Online*, 13(2), 102–135. doi:10.9743/JEO.2016.2.3

Casey, R. L., & Kroth, M. (2013). Learning to develop presence online: Experienced faculty perspectives. *Journal of Adult Education*, 42(2), 104–110.

Castle, S. R., & McGuire, C. (2010). An analysis of student self-assessment of online, blended, and face-to-face learning environments: Implications for sustainable education delivery. *International Education Studies*, 3(3). doi:10.5539/ies.v3n3p36

Chang, H. (2012). The development of a learning community in an e-learning environment. *International Journal of Pedagogies & Learning*, 7(2), 154–161. doi:10.5172/ijpl.2012.7.2.154

Cockrell, C. N., & Shelley, K. (2011; 2010). The relationship between academic support systems and intended persistence in doctoral education. *Journal of College Student Retention*, 12(4), 469–484. doi:10.2190/CS.12.4.e

Costa, A. L., & Kallick, B. (2008). *Learning and leading with habits of mind: 16 essential characteristics for success.* Alexandria, VA: Association for Supervision and Curriculum Development.

Dennen, V. P., Darabi, A., & Smith, L. J. (2007). Instructor-learner interaction in online courses: The relative perceived importance of particular instructor actions on performance and satisfaction. *Distance Education, 28*(1), 65–79. doi:10.1080/01587910701305319

Ferrera, M., Ostrander, N., & Crabtree-Nelson, S. (2013). Establishing a community of inquiry through hybrid courses in clinical social work education. *Journal of Teaching in Social Work, 33*(4–5), 438–448. doi:10.1080/08841233.2013.835765

Fletcher, K. L., Comer, S. D., & Dunlap, A. (2014). Getting connected: The virtual holding environment. *Psychoanalytic Social Work, 21*(1–2), 90–106. doi:10.1080/15228878.2013.865246

Flynn, M., Maiden, R. P., Smith, W., Wiley, J., & Wood, G. (2013). Launching the virtual academic center: Issues and challenges in innovation. *Journal of Teaching in Social Work, 33*(4–5), 339–356. doi:10.1080/08841233.2013.843364

Garrison, D. R. (2016). *Thinking collaboratively: Learning in a community of inquiry.* New York: Routledge.

Garrison, D. R., Anderson, T., & Archer, W. (2000). Critical inquiry in a text-based environment: Computer conferencing in higher education. *The Internet and Higher Education, 2* (2–3), 87–105. doi:10.1016/S1096-7516(00)00016-6

Glaser, B. G., & Strauss, A. L. (1967). *The discovery of grounded theory: Strategies for qualitative research.* Chicago, IL: Aldine Publishing Company.

Golde, C. M. (2007). Signature pedagogies in doctoral education: Are they adaptable for the preparation of education researchers? *Educational Researcher, 36*(6), 344–351. doi:10.3102/0013189X07308301

Guba, E. G. (1990). *The Paradigm dialog.* Newbury Park, CA: Sage.

Harris, H., & Myers, D. (2013). Student perceptions of integrative field seminar: A comparison of three models. *Administrative Issues Journal: Education, Practice, and Research, 3*(2), 2–16. doi:10.5929/2013.3.2.3

Herbert, M. H. (2006). *Predicting retention in online courses utilizing the noel-levitz priorities survey™ for online learners* (Doctoral dissertation). California State University, San Bernardino. Retrieved from ProQuest. (3241669).

Hostetter, C. (2013). Community matters: Social presence and learning outcomes. *Journal of the Scholarship of Teaching and Learning, 13*(1), 77–86.

Jones, S. H. (2015). Benefits and challenges of online education for clinical social work: Three examples. *Clinical Social Work Journal, 43*(2), 225–235. doi:10.1007/s10615-014-0508-z

Kumar, S. (2014). Signature pedagogy, implementation and evaluation of an online program that impacts educational practice. *The Internet and Higher Education, 21,* 60–67. doi:10.1016/j.iheduc.2013.11.001

Kumar, S., & Dawson, K. (2014). *The impact factor: Measuring student professional growth in an online doctoral program.* Boston, MA: Springer US. doi:10.1007/s11528-014-0773-2

Kumar, S., Johnson, M., & Hardemon, T. (2013). Dissertations at a distance: Students' perceptions of online mentoring in a doctoral program. *Journal of Distance Education, 27*(1), 1.

Kurzman, P. A. (2015). The evolution of doctoral social work education. *Journal of Teaching in Social Work, 35*(1–2), 1–13. doi:10.1080/08841233.2015.1007832

Lightfoot, E., & Beltran, R. (2016). *The GADE Guide: A program guide to doctoral study in social work.* St. Paul, MN: The Group for the Advancement of Doctoral Education in Social Work. Retrieved from http://www.gadephd.org/GADE-GUIDE

Merisotis, J. P., & Phipps, R. A. (1999). What's the difference?: Outcomes of distance vs. traditional classroom-based learning. *Change: the Magazine of Higher Learning, 31*(3), 12–17. doi:10.1080/00091389909602685

Moore, J. (2014). Effects of online interaction and instructor presence on students' satisfaction and success with online undergraduate public relations courses. *Journalism & Mass Communication Educator, 69*(3), 271–288. doi:10.1177/1077695814536398

Rodwell, M. K. (1998). *Social work constructivist research.* New York, NY: Garland Publishing, Inc.

Rovai, A. P. (2002). Development of an instrument to measure classroom community. *The Internet and Higher Education, 5*(3), 197–211. doi:10.1016/S1096-7516(02)00102-1

Rovai, A. P., Wighting, M. J., & Lucking, R. (2004). The classroom and school community inventory: Development, refinement, and validation of a self-report measure for educational research. *The Internet and Higher Education, 7*(4), 263–280. doi:10.1016/j.iheduc.2004.09.001

Shulman, L. S. (2005). Signature pedagogies in the professions. *Daedalus, 134*(3), 52–59. doi:10.1162/0011526054622015

Shulman, L. S., Golde, C. M., Bueschel, A. C., & Garabedian, K. J. (2006). Reclaiming education's doctorates: A critique and a proposal. *Educational Researcher, 35*(3), 25–32. doi:10.3102/0013189X035003025

Simonson, M., Smaldino, S., Albright, M., & Zvacek, S. (2009). *Teaching and learning at a distance: Foundations of distance education* (4th ed.). Boston, MA: Allyn & Bacon.

Strauss, A. L., & Corbin, J. (1998). *Basics of qualitative research: Procedures and techniques for developing grounded theory.* Thousand Oaks, CA: Sage.

Sun, P., Tsai, R. J., Finger, G., Chen, Y., & Yeh, D. (2008). What drives a successful e-learning? an empirical investigation of the critical factors influencing learner satisfaction. *Computers & Education, 50*(4), 1183–1202. doi:10.1016/j.compedu.2006.11.007

Terrell, S. R., Snyder, M. M., & Dringus, L. P. (2009). The development, validation, and application of the doctoral student connectedness scale. *The Internet and Higher Education, 12*(2), 112–116. doi:10.1016/j.iheduc.2009.06.004

Tinto, V. (1997). Classrooms as communities: Exploring the educational character of student persistence. *The Journal of Higher Education, 68*(6), 599–623.

Topper, A. (2007). Are they the same? Comparing the instructional quality of online and face-to-face graduate education courses. *Assessment & Evaluation in Higher Education, 32* (6), 681–691. doi:10.1080/02602930601117233

Tucker, S. Y. (2000). *Assessing the effectiveness of distance education versus traditional on-campus education.* Paper presented on April 24- 28at the Annual Meeting of the American Educational Research Association, New Orleans, LA.

Winnicott, D. W. (2018). *The maturational processes and the facilitating environment: Studies in the theory of emotional development.* New York, NY: Routledge.

Young, S., & Bruce, M. A. (2011). Classroom community and student engagement in online courses. *Journal of Online Learning and Teaching, 7*(2), 219.

Reflections of an Online Social Work Professor: Illuminating an Alternative Pedagogy

Rachael A. Richter ⓘ

ABSTRACT

Research in distance education has investigated student satisfaction and learning outcomes, comparing face-to-face with online delivery formats, and tested various technological tools, but has yet to consider alternative pedagogies. Liberatory pedagogy facilitates critical thinking, awareness, reflection and social action around constructs such as race, gender, and class. This paper uses Scholarly Personal Narrative to explore opportunities and challenges of implementing liberatory pedagogy within a virtual classroom. Themes include identity, body, mind, spirit, voice, authenticity, and self-actualization. Liberatory pedagogy emphasizes critical consciousness of oppression, aligns with professional values and ethics, encourages societal well-being, and would appear to enhance online social work education.

Urging all of us to open our minds and hearts so that we can know beyond the boundaries of what is acceptable, so that we can think and rethink, so that we can create new visions, I celebrate teaching that enables transgressions–a movement against and beyond boundaries. It is that movement which makes education the practice of freedom.

–bell hooks (1994, p. 12)

The moment I read these words, I was hooked. I felt alive and energized about teaching in a way I had never experienced. I also felt intimidated. bell hooks' conceptualization of a liberatory pedagogy – as detailed in her book, *Teaching to Transgress* – resonated with every fiber of my being but the idea of trying to implement this approach in my own teaching practice in an online Master of Social Work (MSW) program seemed daunting. Was it even possible?

As I discerned my own teaching philosophy in the weeks that followed, I could not stop thinking about the concepts within this critical paradigm. I literally could not find the "off switch"; thoughts about body, mind, and spirit in virtual spaces raced through my sleep-deprived brain. Finally, I came

Author Note

The author is an Associate Professor at Western New Mexico University. She received her DSW from St. Catherine University and the University of St. Thomas School of Social Work.

to the conclusion that an exploration of liberatory pedagogy *must* form the basis of my doctoral research.

Excited, but more than a bit anxious about the prospect, I began reading and re-reading the volumes in bell hooks' Teaching Series (1994, 2003, 2010). I became aware that I had never read anything written by radical Brazilian educator, Paulo Freire; what kind of professor was I!? hooks' work on liberatory pedagogy was inspired by Freire's ideas about "conscientization" which hooks understood to mean a critically aware and engaged pedagogy (hooks, 1994). So, I read some Freire and wrote question after question in my little brown "I Am a Scholar" notebook, a gift from our doctoral orientation session, "Developing a Scholarship Agenda." I searched for current literature that examined online education. Exhausted (in that good, I am a doctoral student in every sense of the word, kind of way), I developed my dissertation proposal. To fully implement a liberatory pedagogical approach in the asynchronous online classroom I needed an understanding of how students experienced key concepts, such as body, mind, and spirit, during their online educational experience. So, I proposed a qualitative study to explore the student experience. Then I realized what I needed first was a better understanding of my *own* experience of body, mind, and spirit as an online instructor to provide some context for this exploration. Sigh. More discernment, reflection, and sleepless nights followed as I wrestled with issues of lack of confidence and vulnerability. True, I had been involved in online higher education since I taught my first online course in 2002. Yes, I have been teaching full-time in an online MSW program since 2013. Okay, maybe I did have something to offer others by sharing my thoughts.

In the pages that follow, I will use a Scholarly Personal Narrative (SPN) methodology to present my argument for using a liberatory pedagogy to enhance online social work education; explore my personal and professional development as an online educator; and reflect on my experience with liberatory pedagogical concepts. This type of scholarship integrates the writer's personal stories and knowledge of theory and practice with other relevant scholarly works in a format that explores the larger implications of identified themes. Although the structure of SPN may vary, the process developed by Robert Nash contains four specific elements: (a) identifying topics and themes, (b) telling the stories, (c) connecting the personal to the scholarly, and (d) commenting on universal aspects (Nash & Bradley, 2012). Other authors have used SPN and autoethnography to examine their experiences in social work education (Jensen-Hart & Williams, 2010; McGranahan, 2008; Sy, 2013; Tinucci, 2017). SPN felt like an appropriate method here for my exploration because it honors my qualitative experience and allows for alternative ways of thinking and knowing.

Distance education is one way to achieve social justice regarding access to higher education. Additionally, the use of liberatory pedagogy enhances social work education because this paradigm is aligned with professional values and ethics, emphasizes critical awareness of injustices, and encourages social change. A liberatory approach improves on the "banking system" of education – a phrase coined by Freire (1970) – which describes a scenario where deposits of knowledge are made from the wise professor to the passive student. Unlike this model, liberatory pedagogy produces engaged, critically aware, empowered, and self-actualized individuals capable of achieving the mission of social work: to enhance well-being for all human beings.

However, implementing liberatory pedagogy in the online environment presents unique challenges. To successfully overcome such challenges, educators must understand how online participants experience philosophical concepts central to a liberatory pedagogical framework. The purpose of this narrative is to explore my development as an online educator and to illuminate my experiences of key concepts, relevant opportunities, and realistic constraints within this educational approach. I may raise more questions than answers, but hopefully sharing my evolution as both learner and teacher will be useful to others who desire to expand their educational praxis. First, I will provide a brief overview of liberatory pedagogy and its value for social work education. Next, I will reflect on my identity and path to becoming an online social work instructor. Finally, I will highlight my online teaching experiences around the themes of body, mind, spirit, voice, authenticity, and self-actualization.

Liberatory pedagogy in social work education

The classroom remains the most radical space of possibility in the academy.
                                                                – bell hooks (1994, p. 12)

Education is an act of love, and thus an act of courage. It cannot fear the analysis of reality or, under pain of revealing itself as afarce, avoid creative discussion.
                                                                – Freire (1973, p. 38)

Taking a radical path requires bravery regardless of the context. In my experience, this is definitely the case in higher education. When my doctoral cohort was getting to know one another, we completed an exercise where we identified strengths we brought to the group and supports we needed from the group. Out of this process came our defining mantra: Be Brave. So, here goes.

As the quotations above suggest, academia presents many opportunities for growth, but only if we are willing to be creative and courageous as we consider all the possibilities. (Allowing our fear of what we might discover to blind us, would do just that.) Liberatory pedagogy is an alternative approach to education that emphasizes the shared responsibility of teachers and students to think critically, challenge the status quo, and connect classroom learning with life experience. The goal of developing a critical consciousness – through reflection about oppression and privilege based on cultural differences – and the integration of this reflection with practice contributes to the mission of social work: social justice, social change, and well-being for all. In addition, this framework is holistic and aligns with social work values and ethical principles; an "engaged pedagogy" facilitates self-actualization of the instructor, empowerment of students, and attention to well-being (hooks, 1994). To hooks, who was inspired by Freire and Buddhist monk Thich Nhat Hanh, engaged pedagogy incorporates praxis and wholeness, "a union of mind, body, and spirit" (1994, p. 14).

Similarly, social justice as a core social work value is an integral part of social workers' ethical responsibility to society at large (National Association of Social Workers [NASW], 2017). Offering professional social work education in an online delivery format is consistent with this perspective: As Abels (2005) suggests, distance education is not about technology, it is about access and opportunities that help students overcome economic or geographic barriers. Historically, social work education has evolved to meet ever-changing training needs; distance education is one more example of this appropriate and necessary evolution (Abels, 2005; Kurzman, 2013). Therefore, from a social justice perspective, social work education is enhanced by both a liberatory pedagogy and online access.

However, this method of teaching and learning has traditionally incorporated dialogue within a community of learners who are physically present to clearly see and hear one another, who are encouraged to negotiate the conflicts that arise as individuals from various social locations and confront differences of privilege and power. In fact, hooks (1994) challenges the academic notion of a mind/body split by explicitly acknowledging the value of the physical body, voice, and emotion within the transformative learning process. Hence, my significant dilemma in the asynchronous classroom. hooks might disagree with how I understand liberatory pedagogy, and my insistence in the potential for its online application, but for myself as an educator, and for my students, this exploration appears both timely and worthwhile.

A look in the mirror

...good teaching cannot be reduced to technique; good teaching comes from the identity and the integrity of the teacher.

– Palmer (1997b, p. 16)

As I began to review my identity development as an educator, I realized September has always been my favorite month. Some people thought this was because it is the month of my birthday, but the real reason is because, to me, September represents the start of a new school year. I have always loved reading and learning; I wanted to be a teacher when I grew up so that I could always be "in school." When my younger sisters and I played school together, I insisted on being the teacher. My father, who started his career as a high school English teacher and then became a guidance counselor, was an early role model.

As a high school student, I developed an interest in psychology, and by the time I was ready to graduate with a bachelor's degree, the practical aspects of achieving social justice through social work had caught my attention. After completing my MSW in 1991, I enjoyed a meaningful career practicing medical social work. As the universe would have it, in 1997, while working as the Coordinator of Client Services for the AIDS Foundation Miami Valley in Dayton, Ohio, I was contacted by Dr. Robin Johnson from Capital University about supervising a Bachelor of Social Work intern. Within a year I began teaching Human Behavior as an adjunct for Capital. Robin became a mentor and dear friend, and his ongoing support has afforded me opportunities to share my social work expertise as a full-time assistant professor at two institutions.

Remembering my youthful desire to be a teacher, I realized I had many teaching roles (including peer education and teaching Sunday School) which paved the way to my first formal teaching experience in the face-to-face college classroom. I loved everything about it! Well, I didn't love grading papers late at night after I came home from my full-time job, and my preschooler and six-month old were finally in bed, who does? But I loved interacting with students, the energy we created together in the classroom, learning new things, the smell of new textbooks, and the feel of the highlighter gliding across the page. I loved the privilege of witnessing lightbulb moments when just the right idea pops into your mind, you share it with the students, and you can actually see the wheels turning as cognitive connections emerge. I will never forget the day students in my Diversity class realized their service-learning experiences – facilitating educational groups in a residential facility for previously incarcerated women – mirrored research they had just read about regarding the gender differences of group development. Most especially, I loved being able to blend my identity as a social worker (this is who I am, not just what I do) with my newly developing identity as a professor.

I have always appreciated the importance of integrity. My parents taught me to always tell the truth and obey laws; my father never drove over the speed limit (which was maddening during family vacations but made a lifelong impression). The social work professional Code of Ethics (NASW, 2017) has much to say about integrity and competence and has guided my professional life for many years. So, despite what educator Parker Palmer (1997b) says about technique and good teaching in the quote above, the perfectionist in me was desperate to do it "right." I felt uncomfortable and inexperienced. To compensate, I searched for direction, worried I might negatively impact my students' future careers – and more horrifically, their vulnerable clients – if I didn't cover all the required content or give comprehensive feedback on assignments. Clearly, I was an imposter; where's the integrity in that?

The truth is, I am always asking questions and rarely satisfied with the answers. Although this can be overwhelming at times, it also means that I will never run out of research topics. So, I have muddled through over the years, learning from my mistakes and the wisdom of my mentors, but most of all from interacting with students. I am incredibly grateful for those opportunities to develop new skills and experiment with different ways of knowing, being and doing social work education. I have come full circle, a student again, in a doctoral program where education is honored as a form of social work practice.

These developmental steps I have recounted are only part of the identity to which Palmer is referring. On a more personal level, I care deeply about equality, equity, justice, and people who are vulnerable and marginalized in our racist, patriarchal, capitalist society. I am a middle-aged woman, a mother of two adult sons, a daughter, a divorcee, a lesbian who came out later in life, a partner in a committed relationship, an intellectual, an activist, an extrovert who occasionally needs quiet time. I am passionate and spiritual. I believe in the power of love and peace and the potential of both/and (as opposed to either/or). I am also – sometimes overly – responsible, and I pride myself on producing quality in all that I do. I acknowledge my white and class privilege but have personally experienced the pain of discrimination based on my gender and sexual orientation.

When contemplating Palmer's assertion that "we teach who we are" (1997b, p. 15) perhaps the more important question is not who am I, but rather, how do my students' perceive who I am? Can they determine my social location from how I teach? The comments I make? The personal information I choose to share? According to Palmer, "Good teachers join self, subject and students in the fabric of life because they teach from an integral and undivided self; they can manifest in their own lives, and evoke in their students, a 'capacity for connectedness'" (1997b, p. 16). From hooks' (1994) perspective being whole requires a willingness to be vulnerable with ones' students and an active commitment toward self-actualization. Am I teaching from a place of integrity and wholeness? How does all of this occur in the online environment?

From face-to-face to virtual space

The next logical stop (on this personal and professional development part of the journey) was to review how I became involved in distance education. In 2002 and 2003, I had the opportunity to participate in a series of online training modules about how to teach online. The training required a significant amount of time spent reading and posting to an asynchronous discussion board. I will fully admit I did not initially embrace this gift with open arms; I was working one full-time job, one part-time job, and had two young children at the time, so how could I possibly add homework to my already overloaded schedule? In addition, I was very skeptical about teaching social work – a profession that places a very high value on human relationships – in an online format. Could aspiring social workers learn anything about how to work with *real* people over the internet? Thankfully, I decided to dive into this pool of enormous possibilities. While completing the training, I developed hybrid and online courses and subsequently facilitated faculty workshops at my institution. At the time, I did not feel worthy of the "resident online expert" designation I was given, but in hindsight, what I was doing *was* cutting edge and provided a solid foundation for my academic career.

Reflecting on the last 15 years of teaching online, I realize that my approach to developing effective learning communities in the virtual classroom is not representative of a specific technique, although there are many suggested tools and techniques documented in the distance education literature (Dietz-Uhler & Hurn, 2013; Garrison, Anderson, & Archer, 1999; Gibson, 2013; Kirby & Hulan, 2016) and I certainly use some of them. Rather, it is evidence of my commitment to social work values and ethics in action. My dedication to a timely response to student emails, and the energy I invest providing constructive feedback on discussion posts and assignments illustrates my belief in the dignity and worth of all human beings, the importance of relationships, and my obligation to competent practice. My unwavering support for an online delivery format is consistent with my opinion that all students deserve opportunities for access to higher education.

Nevertheless, there is always room for improvement. In my doctoral studies, I have been exposed to a variety of teaching and learning paradigms and required to formally determine my own teaching philosophy. I have examined social work literature that investigates online education. Overall, this literature compares face-to-face to online offerings and finds no major differences in educational outcomes (Cummings, Chaffin, & Cockerham, 2015; O'Neill & Jensen, 2014) or student perceptions (Hostetter & Busch, 2006), regardless of delivery format. In addition, Saleebey and Scanlon (2005) consider the possibility of a critical pedagogy in social work education. What I did not find was any research that investigated the exciting and engaging promise of liberatory pedagogy in the virtual social work classroom. I will begin to address this gap in the literature by reflecting on my experiences of the liberatory pedagogical themes of body, mind, spirit, voice, authenticity, and self-actualization embedded in online social work education.

Is distance education dis-embodied education?

Liberatory pedagogy really demands that one work in the classroom, and that one work with the limits of the body, work both with and through and against those limits: teachers may insist that it doesn't matter whether you stand behind the podium or the desk, but it does.

– bell hooks (1994, p. 138)

Although I was captivated from the very first chapter of *Teaching to Transgress*, it was this passage that sparked my interest in exploring liberatory pedagogy within the scholarship of teaching and learning online. Just visualizing hooks at work in the classroom made me tingle all over – this was exactly the kind of teaching and learning I wanted to facilitate. Questions quickly threatened my enthusiasm. How is the body represented and experienced by instructors and students in online education? How can one be *virtually* fully present? I also mused about whether the absence of "real" bodies in the virtual classroom reinforced the mind/body split – a Western philosophical dualism that hooks (1994) argues must be challenged through conversations about power differences and oppression based on gender, race, class, and sexual orientation. From this perspective, ignoring our bodies and emotions in the service of the "Academic Mind," is a betrayal of self; the antidote is to enter the classroom whole. Easier said than done.

When I think about "the body" in the online classroom, my first thought is of profile photos. I think about students as real human beings and what I know about them from their introduction posts (such as partner/kids/pets, work/field experiences, and geographic location). I realized that I feel more connected to students who share both a photo and a rich description of themselves. Should I more actively encourage students to post a profile picture? Or, do profile pictures facilitate implicit racial and gender bias?

As I reflected more deeply, I also concluded that my understanding of the concept of body includes active engagement. As I read students' work, I visualize them posting to the discussion board, interviewing policy experts, and completing their real-world advocacy projects. In lieu of warm bodies in a circle of chairs, attendance is noted by timely posts and submission of assignments. If students are missing deadlines (in other words, not coming to class), I reach out with an email to inquire about their absence and offer my assistance. This is one way I show respect for students as human beings possessing dignity and worth; every voice matters, and I want them to know I am missing them and their contributions to our learning community.

Contemplating hooks' thoughts about the location of the teacher's body in the classroom, I considered what I do in virtual space to "move around rather than stand behind the furniture." I don't like to lecture; when I taught face-to-face I often rearranged the chairs to facilitate dialogue. In my online classes, I make an intentional effort to engage in the discussion as it unfolds, sharing my opinions as appropriate, asking thought-provoking questions, providing affirmation and encouragement. Although my comments are typically brief, this effort reminds the students that I am "present" with them as the conversation is occurring, not just when it is time to evaluate what they said.

Another way I am aware of the body in the asynchronous environment involves students' potentially traumatic physical and emotional responses when exposed to readings and videos about difficult subjects. Currently, this is a controversial topic in higher education (American Association of University Professors [AAUP], 2014). My use of content warnings in my Human Trafficking elective is an exhibition of ethical and professional social work behavior and shows care and concern for my students. As hooks (1994, p. 13) suggests, "to teach in a manner that respects and cares for the souls of our students is essential if we are to provide the necessary conditions where learning can most deeply and intimately begin".

I have also spent some time thinking about students' impressions of me as a person, and how my presence influences them within and beyond the course experience. Do they feel any connection with me? How would I know? This is where the constructs of body, mind, and spirit overlap significantly for me. I post a profile picture and introduce myself to the class on the discussion board. If I am honest though, what I currently choose to share in the asynchronous environment is more guarded than what I think might occur face-to-face. I will explore this more when I address authenticity. Recently, I have begun posting introductory videos to engage another human sense (voice); this allows me to show passion for the topic, and hopefully encourages students to feel excited. It feels like a step in the right direction, but I'm not entirely satisfied.

Mind meld: developing a critical consciousness in the classroom

> Conditions of radical openness exist in any learning situation where students and teachers celebrate their abilities to think critically, to engage in pedagogical praxis.
>
> – bell hooks (1994, p. 202)

In her work, hooks advises that an emphasis on critical thinking is central to an engaged pedagogy that liberates students (1994, 2010). When I examined my experience of mind in online education, the process of critical thinking was prominent. Following this train of thought led me to ideas about conflict, posing questions, playing devil's advocate to get students to think outside the box, group conversations, critical awareness, reflection, and students' different learning styles. As the free association continued, I pondered about the trust required to share one's honest thoughts. To create an environment where all this intense mind activity can occur, it is crucial to develop a welcoming learning community and, as the teacher, it is my responsibility to initiate this process. However, a liberatory pedagogical approach calls for the co-creation of learning opportunities so course design decisions must allow for shared responsibility as well.

In my experience, getting to know one another virtually requires additional intentional effort. Space for introductions and encouragement to share personal information are only the beginning. For some, perhaps not being face-to-face makes it easier to share what they really think about controversial topics. On the other hand, those who express themselves better orally might be intimidated by the need to write everything they want to say. Posting also means there is a permanent record of what has been said. Add to all this an emphasis on interrogating cultural hegemony and learning from conflict, which are inherent in a critical paradigm, and the challenges may seem formidable.

Having a virtual dialogic conversation takes considerably more effort as well. One of the benefits of online learning is the opportunity to carefully think about what you want to say before you say it. Time to ponder theoretically allows for more meaningful learning. But reading everyone's comments can be tedious for both professor and student, and the conversation often feels disjointed even when everyone is responding to the same prompts. To be honest, I find myself disappointed when student posts don't show evidence of higher order thinking, and even though I try to monitor and facilitate the process by commenting and asking follow-up questions, by the time students respond (if they respond) it almost seems beside the point. According to Freire (1973), true dialogue is necessary for developing critical consciousness. He defines dialogue as "a horizontal relationship between persons. A with B = communication [and] inter-communication. Relation of 'empathy' between two 'poles' who are engaged in a joint search." He continues, "when the two 'poles' of the dialogue are thus linked by love, hope and mutual trust, they can join in a critical search for something. Only dialogue truly communicates" (p. 45). Does the kind of conversation that takes place on the discussion board allow for such true dialogic communication?

I believe the answer to this question can be yes, but as I thought about specific examples of true dialogue in action, I realized that more of these instances have occurred in *my* online exchanges with highly engaged and self-motivated students, but far less frequently between the students themselves. What can I do to change this? My gut tells me this goes beyond setting an example and designing discussion prompts to promote critical thinking. Mind, as a construct, is also about students' cognitive abilities and motivation for learning. Still, there must be something I can do to inspire connections that achieve deep, lasting learning. Educational experts Chickering (2006) and Freire (1970) both suggest a holistic approach which includes students solving personally relevant problems. Chickering also argues that deep learning requires learners to reflect on the ways new ideas build, connect, and challenge existing understanding and knowledge. "Reflection is the absolutely necessary intervening activity that converts input – whatever the experiences are – into meaningful working knowledge that can then be tested in other settings" (2006, p. 143). My real-world approach in the policy course, with assignments and conversations centered around student identified policy advocacy topics that are meaningful to them, is a start toward shared responsibility for deep learning. This approach is not unique to the online environment, but it can be used to transcend distance. It seems reasonable to expect that students who are encouraged to study and follow their passions will also be motivated to dialogue with one another about their interests irrespective of delivery format.

Moved by the spirit

> The emphasis on rational empiricism, on conceptions of truth as objective and external, and on knowledge as a commodity delegitimizes active, public discussion of issues of purpose and meaning, authenticity and identity, spirituality and spiritual growth.
>
> – Chickering, Dalton, and Auerbach (2006, p. 30)

I was baptized Catholic and attended Mass regularly until I was in my early twenties. For many years and reasons, I did not participate in organized religion, although occasionally I searched for a spiritual home. I also studied Reiki, an energy healing practice. I don't think it is a coincidence that shortly before I started my doctoral endeavors, I discovered Science of Mind (SOM). SOM honors the wisdom of many religious and spiritual traditions and feeds my postmodern soul. Joining this spiritual community of individuals who collectively strive to create a world that works for everyone, and personally committing to daily positive affirmations and meditation, have significantly contributed to my success as a student and my continued growth as a person and an educator. In retrospect, the holistic emphasis on body, mind, and spirit taught in this tradition set me on this very pedagogical path before I even knew where I was headed. I am grateful for the synergy yet reminded by Chickering et al. (2006) that spirituality is not always embraced in the academy.

However, there are models, such as liberatory pedagogy, which insist spirituality can and must be a part of the process. hooks writes, "I can testify to the meaningfulness of spiritual practice and that such a practice sustains and nurtures progressive teaching, progressive politics, and enhances the struggle for liberation" (2003, p. 164). Similarly, Cynthia Dillard comments, "what is spirituality in education? Spirituality in education is education with purpose, education that is liberatory work, education that is emancipation … " (as cited in Dillard, Abdur-Rashid, & Tyson, 2000, p. 447). Both Freire (1970, 1973)) and Palmer (1997a, 1997b)) have written eloquently about the pedagogical importance of spirituality and related concepts of authenticity, love, emotion, purpose, and meaning. In the social work education literature, a qualitative study of Canadian student and professor perspectives on spirituality and religion found that participants identified connections between social work values and spiritual values and believed classroom discussions about spirituality were worthwhile for developing self-awareness and appreciation for diversity (Coholic, 2006).

My passionate commitment to social justice is one way I express my spirituality. I learned values of care and concern for others, generosity, and social justice from my parents and extended family. Our family get-togethers always include people who are not biologically or legally related to us in any way as there is always room for one more at the table. Rooting for the underdog is a family creed. As an educator, I try to share this perspective with my students. The energy I feel when engaging with students is sacred. Each learning community has its own vibe: the collective spirit of *this* unique group of individuals together in *this* time and space. I feel jubilant when students share their passions and the discussion board is alive with connections and activity beyond the required weekly post. But as I critically examined my current pedagogy, I concluded that I am not being as explicit about my perception of spirituality as I want to be, nor am I overtly asking students about theirs.

Can you hear me now?

One of the aspects I appreciate most within liberatory pedagogy is the value of each voice and respect for the diversity represented by those voices. hooks (1994) provides examples of how she teaches students to really listen to one another, and creates intentional opportunities for them to speak freely. She believes awareness of one another as individuals comes from hearing these voices. These opportunities to speak is especially important for students who previously have been marginalized in academia and the larger society. It is here where power differences, based on societally constructed ideas about race, gender, class, sexual orientation, and positions of authority, may be confronted.

Reflecting on my teaching experiences, I thought about all those marginalized voices: students of color, women, first-generation college students, those for whom English is a second language, people with disabilities, and the LGBTQIA community. I thought about students who attend online because they also must work full-time to support their families or because they live in rural communities. Since there is no lurking quietly in the back of an online classroom, thoughts of students, intimidated by the writing intensive nature of asynchronous courses, filled my mind. Reading their posts, I can hear excitement, joy, understanding, and pride, as well as confusion, frustration, irritation, exhaustion, and anger; sometimes I even hear silence. I wonder how they hear my voice in this virtual experience. Do they perceive my frustration when the conversation lags or their comments don't show understanding of connections that seem perfectly obvious to me? Do they sense my irritation when they ask a question before trying to find the answer themselves (did you even *read* the syllabus I painstakingly created?). My insecurities flourish – have I clearly communicated that I value their voices? Do my students feel heard, encouraged, and respected by me? Or is my "professor voice" (as an evaluative authority) the only voice they really hear? To mitigate this power differential, I include my teaching philosophy in my syllabus, post introductory videos, and make myself available by phone and video conference. I try to join in the conversation as it unfolds on the discussion board and start my feedback on assignments with positive comments. But, the lack of verbal interaction available in an asynchronous delivery format remains a definite challenge and limitation.

The real me

Authenticity is about knowing your truest, realest, juiciest self and honoring it.

– Paz-Armor (2014, p. 149)

This quote from Paz-Armor's SPN really struck a nerve. At this point in my life, I am pretty confident I know my "self," but less certain I am honoring that self in my online professorial role. With most of my friends, family members, and colleagues, I am an open book. When I meet new people, while I don't typically lead with "Hi, my name is Rachael and I am a lesbian, social work activist," early on I mention my female significant other and, if the topic of conversation is at all political, my activism and advocacy for LGBTQIA rights and anti-human trafficking efforts. Every interaction is a teachable moment to normalize my reality and transform how others think. This feels authentic to me since honesty is one of my personal values. But somehow in the virtual classroom this hasn't happened yet – for some reason it seems awkward and contrived to post my sexual orientation in my intro-duction, even though when I was married to a man, I occasionally mentioned my husband. There have been a few times when I have referred to my partner in relevant online conversations with individual students, but never the whole class. I am not worried about rejection as I work for a university that is very inclusive, and I definitely do not have internalized homophobia. So, what is this reluctance all about?

One limitation of teaching online is the absence of context. If I were teaching on a campus, students would see a picture of my partner and me in my office, and know that I am involved with and supportive of LGBT campus organiza-tions and events. In addition, temporal constraints in an asynchronous structure can impede the flow of conversation. Appropriate self-disclosure would be more natural in the context of spontaneous synchronous or face-to-face classroom conversations about discrimination where I could model exploration of personal bias as a strategy to develop professional self-awareness. I struggle with students who admit to their own personal discomfort with gays and lesbians, especially when they mention this "choice" or "lifestyle" is against their religious beliefs. I am frustrated by students who comment that I focus too much on such topics in my courses. I am not teaching from a place of integrity and wholeness by keeping this part of my authentic self hidden from students. I am missing an opportunity to help them interrogate heterosexual privilege. I have a personal bias toward the need for social workers to develop cultural competence for this marginalized population to which I belong, and students have a right to know my social location. At the same time, I need to maintain balance, be respectful of different opinions, and include discussion about all vulnerable groups. I realized that reflecting on this theme has been quite an "a-ha" moment for me.

hooks remarks " … no education is politically neutral" (1994, p. 37). As a social work educator, it *is* my job to expose my students to professional values and strongly encourage them to consider how these values fit with their personal beliefs. To truly implement a liberatory pedagogy, I must be willing to be vulnerable, to take risks, and to "make [my] teaching practices a site of resistance" (hooks, 1994, p. 21) regardless of the delivery format.

Journey toward self-actualization

…teachers must be actively committed to a process of self-actualization that promotes their own well-being if they are to teach in a manner that empowers students.

– bell hooks (1994, p. 15)

I remember studying the concept of self-actualization as an undergraduate psychology major. At the time the idea seemed nebulous, like Nirvana; was this something mere mortals could ever hope to achieve? But from my current middle-aged vantage point, self-actualization means acknowledging my best self and bringing that self to every situation. When applying the lens of liberatory pedagogy, it means prioritizing personal well-being, being aware of my intentions, teaching from a place of wholeness – with an integrated body, mind, and spirit – being authentic, and speaking with integrity. It means allowing self-growth, learning, and transformation to occur alongside my students. What a relief to not have to know it all – very liberating indeed!

But, have I achieved self-actualization? As this narrative illustrates, some days yes, some days no. I know I am on the pedagogical path that is right for me. I am committed to the process of self-actualization which hooks recommends in the quote above. I have grown as a person and professor since my first adjunct experience. In addition, I am actively working toward bringing wholeness and authenticity into the online classroom. Reflecting on my successes and failures has empowered me to forge ahead.

As hooks suggests, liberatory pedagogy can lead to student empowerment. She advocates "making the classroom a democratic setting where everyone feels a responsibility to contribute is a central goal of transformative peda-gogy" (1994, p. 39). *I* think my teaching practices have successfully overcome some of the constraints the asynchronous online environment presents for a liberatory pedagogical approach. But do my students feel empowered to share responsibility for their learning? Since I am only one person in this co-creative process, the next step in my professorial journey will be to explore and understand the student experience with a qualitative study to answer the research question: How do students experience body, mind, and spirit in the asynchronous MSW classroom?

Final reflections

As predicted, my reflective process has generated more questions than answers. However, since I am a work in progress, I am okay with this. I have been honest about the unique challenges of using an alternative teaching and learning paradigm such as liberatory pedagogy in online social work education. Some educators (even hooks) might argue these challenges are insurmountable. As a full-time online professor, I recognize that I may be biased, however, I wholeheartedly believe it is possible to apply this holistic approach in the virtual classroom. I have argued that it is imperative to do so because the alignment with professional social work values and ethics enhances social work education, and because online access to education achieves social justice. Indeed, a critically engaged pedagogy produces criti-cally aware social workers.

But, as I have illustrated, to thoroughly explore this application, and expand my educational praxis, required a genuine willingness to discern the larger philosophy behind this pedagogical approach. In this narrative, I have reflected on my identity as a person and a teacher, as well as my understanding of the liberatory pedagogical concepts of body, mind, spirit, and authentic voice, and have connected my findings to thoughts from other educational scholars. In addition, I have ruminated about my experiences in bringing this understanding to life in my online teaching practice. The result has been a very illuminating trip so far, and I can't wait to see what discoveries lie ahead.

Disclosure statement

No potential conflict of interest was reported by the author.

ORCID

Rachael A. Richter ⓘ http://orcid.org/0000-0002-0887-0428

References

Abels, P. (2005). The way to distance education. In P. Abels (Ed.), *Distance education in social work: Planning, teaching, and learning* (pp. 3–22). New York, NY: Springer Publishing Company.

American Association of University Professors [AAUP]. (2014). *Trigger-warnings*. Retrieved from https://www.aaup.org/report/trigger-warnings

Chickering, A. W. (2006). Curricular content and powerful pedagogy. In A. W. Chickering, J. C. Dalton, & L. S. Auerbach. (Eds.), *Encouraging authenticity and spirituality in higher education* (pp. 113–144). San Francisco, CA: Jossey-Bass.

Chickering, A. W., Dalton, J. C., & Auerbach, L. S. (2006). *Encouraging authenticity and spirituality in higher education*. San Francisco, CA: Jossey-Bass.

Coholic, D. (2006). Spirituality in social work pedagogy: A Canadian perspective. *Journal of Teaching in Social Work, 26*(3/4), 197–217. doi:10.1300/J067v26n03_13

Cummings, S. M., Chaffin, K. M., & Cockerham, C. (2015). Comparative analysis of an online and a traditional MSW program: Educational outcomes. *Journal of Social Work Education, 51*, 109–120. doi:10.1080/10437797.2015.977170

Dietz-Uhler, B., & Hurn, J. E. (2013). Strategies for engagement in online courses: Engaging with the content, instructor, and other students. *Journal of Teaching and Learning with Technology, 2*(1), 62–65. Retrieved from https://jotlt.indiana.edu/article/view/3294

Dillard, C. B., Abdur-Rashid, D., & Tyson, C. A. (2000). My soul is a witness: Affirming pedagogies of the spirit. *International Journal of Qualitative Studies in Education (QSE), 13*(5), 447–462. doi:10.1080/09518390050156404

Freire, P. (1970). *Pedagogy of the oppressed*. New York, NY: Seabury Press.

Freire, P. (1973). *Education for critical consciousness*. New York, NY: Seabury Press.

Garrison, D. R., Anderson, T., & Archer, W. (1999). Critical inquiry in a text-based environment: Computer conferencing in higher education. *The Internet and Higher Education, 2*(2–3), 87–105. doi:10.1016/S1096-7516(00)00016-6

Gibson, K. M. (2013). Fostering collaboration and learning in asynchronous online environments. *Journal of Teaching and Learning with Technology, 2*(2), 60–78. Retrieved from https://jotlt.indiana.edu/article/view/4003

hooks, B. (1994). *Teaching to transgress. Education as the practice of freedom*. New York, NY: Routledge.

hooks, B. (2003). *Teaching community. A pedagogy of hope*. New York, NY: Routledge.

hooks, B. (2010). *Teaching critical thinking. Practical wisdom*. New York, NY: Routledge.

Hostetter, C., & Busch, M. (2006). Measuring up online: The relationship between social presence and student learning satisfaction. *Journal of Scholarship of Teaching and Learning, 6*(2), 1–12. Retrieved from https://josotl.indiana.edu/article/view/1670

Jensen-Hart, S., & Williams, D. J. (2010). Blending voices: Autoethnography as a vehicle for critical reflection in social work. *Journal of Teaching in Social Work, 30*, 450–467. doi:10.1080/08841233.2010.515911

Kirby, E. G., & Hulan, N. (2016). Student perceptions of self and community within an online environment: The use of voicethread to foster community. *Journal of Teaching and Learning with Technology, 5*(1), 87–99. doi:10.14434/jotlt.v5n1.19411

Kurzman, P. A. (2013). The evolution of distance learning and online education. *Journal of Teaching in Social Work, 33*(4/5), 331–338. doi:10.1080/08841233.2013.843346

McGranahan, E. (2008). Shaking the "Magic 8 Ball": Reflections of a first-time teacher. *Journal of Teaching in Social Work, 28*, 19–34. doi:10.1080/08841230802178839

Nash, R. J., & Bradley, D. L. (2012). The writer is at the center of the scholarship: Partnering me-search and research. *About Campus, 17*(1), 2–11. doi:10.1002/abc.21067

National Association of Social Workers [NASW]. (2017). *Code of ethics.* Washington, DC: National Association of Social Workers. Retrieved from https://www.socialworkers.org/about/ethics

O'Neill, M., & Jensen, J. (2014). Comparison of student outcomes in a campus and a distributed learning class. *Journal of Technology in Human Services, 32,* 186–200. doi:10.1080/15228835.2014.908157

Palmer, P. J. (1997a). *The grace of great things: Reclaiming the sacred in knowing, teaching and learning.* Retrieved from http://www.CourageRenewal.org

Palmer, P. J. (1997b). *The heart of a teacher: Identity and integrity in teaching. Change, 29*(6), 14–21. Retrieved from http://www.jstor.org/stable/40165413

Paz-Armor, W. (2014). See me, see you. Finding and accepting your authentic self. In R. J. Nash & S. Viray (Eds.), *How stories heal. Writing our way to meaning and wholeness in the academy* (pp. 148–160). New York, NY: Peter Lang Publishing, Inc.

Saleebey, D., & Scanlon, E. (2005). Is a critical pedagogy for the profession of social work possible? *Journal of Teaching in Social Work, 25*(3–4), 1–18. doi:10.1300/J067v25n03_01

Sy, F. (2013). The artist, the activist, the academic: Building a critical pedagogy of embodied knowledge. *Reflections, 19*(3), 7–20. Retrieved from https://reflectionsnarrativesofprofessio nalhelping.org

Tinucci, M. E. (2017). *The place, function, and power of story in an evolving pedagogy* (DSW dissertation, St. Catherine University) Retrieved from http://sophia.stkate.edu/dsw/13).

Web-Based Social Work Courses: Guidelines for Developing and Implementing an Online Environment

BEVERLY ARAUJO DAWSON and JUDY FENSTER

Although web-based courses in schools of social work have prolifer-ated over the past decade, the literature contains few guidelines on steps that schools can take to develop such courses. Using Knowles's framework, which delineates tasks and themes involved in implementing e-learning in social work education, this article describes the cultivation of an online environment at one school of social work. We outline the steps and procedures used, as well as issues addressed in developing online and blended courses. Recommended strategies for creating a supportive environment for delivering social work content online are provided.

INTRODUCTION

During the past two decades, there has been a dramatic rise in offerings of online courses in schools of social work throughout the United States. Technological advances have made distance learning more feasible through the implementation of synchronous and asynchronous formats for online delivery (Reamer, 2013). Whereas the applicability of online education to social work initially was questioned (Collins, Gabor, Coleman, & Ing, 2002; Moore, 2005), it has received wider acceptance in the past decade and is now being used to deliver content across the social work curriculum (Flynn, Maiden, Smith, Wiley, & Wood, 2013; McFadden, Moore, Herie, & Schoech, 2005). A recent Council on Social Work Education survey of accredited social work programs found that, among 222 master's-level programs responding,

8% currently offered the entire MSW program online, 51% offered part of the program online, and another 16% were developing online offerings. Of the 471 BSW programs reporting, 2% offered full programs online, 38% had online courses, and 14% were developing online options (Council on Social Work Education, 2013).

Despite the proliferation of online offerings in social work, and evidence suggesting that web-based instruction is effective (Barnett-Queen, Blair, & Merrick, 2005; McAllister, 2013; Tallent-Runnels et al., 2006), there is little in the literature to describe the process by which schools of social work are creating their nascent online teaching and learning environments, along with issues that arise when doing so. Understanding the questions and challenges confronted, and the solutions explored by other schools transitioning to e-learning, can help social work programs currently developing (or contemplating the development of) online courses to create a supportive atmosphere in which to move forward.

This article provides an overview of the development of an online environment at one large school of social work located in the Northeast. We utilize A. J. Knowles's (2007) framework to describe the process through which our school developed and implemented an online learning environment, including challenges we confronted and strategies we used to address issues as they arose over a 2-year period. Suggestions for resolving dilemmas and working collaboratively to create a supportive environment in which to deliver social work content online are provided as well.

DEVELOPING AN ONLINE ENVIRONMENT

As noted, there is a dearth of literature suggesting how to develop an online environment. The exception is Knowles's (2007) research, which outlines environmental issues that schools of social work typically confront when shifting to online and blended course offerings. Surveying 30 faculty and administrators all closely involved in developing and implementing web-based courses at their schools, Knowles identified several themes: transformation, alignment, faculty engagement, coherence, resources, and leadership. His findings suggest that all of these areas require attention to ensure integration of online and blended courses into an existing social work program. Next we build on Knowles's findings to describe the various tasks and processes involved in our School of Social Work's quest to initiate and expand our online course offerings.

Transformation

Transformation refers to the modifications that instructors must make to teaching goals and techniques as they prepare to provide online instruction and changes that need to be made to a program's policies and structures. Teaching online demands a shift in one's view of knowledge transmission, from an emphasis on the instructor being the "sage on the stage" to "the guide on the side" (King, 1993). It also requires that faculty become proficient in using a number of rapidly changing information and communication technologies (Knowles, 2007). Significant changes at the organizational level may also be needed.

Social work programs have struggled with various aspects of transformation (Knowles, 2007), and our school was no exception. Our faculty, who varied in their comfort level with technology, recently had added a web-based component to the existing face-to-face classes so that instructors were now required to use Moodle[1] between class sessions to provide online activities ranging from discussions to quizzes to case assessments. However, few faculty had ever designed or taught an entire course in a blended or online format, and the majority either were not interested in or were opposed to the notion of teaching online.

It was within this context that two faculty members decided they wanted to develop and teach web-based courses. One had previous experience and training in online course development and teaching, and the other sought assistance from online resources for faculty, provided by the university. Both were financially compensated for developing the new online courses, one through the university's standard compensation and the other via a technology grant. These two faculty members served as "early champions" for the potential of online teaching, and as such they wanted to explore the feasibility of expanding online offerings more broadly.

To meet the challenge of making the organizational changes needed for such an expansion, an ad hoc Technology Committee was established within the school. The formation of a committee dedicated to technology and online teaching was an important tool in the transformation process. Comprised of social work faculty and administrators, the committee was headed by one of the authors, a tenured faculty member with experience in developing web-based courses. All faculty members were invited to participate, with attention paid to having diversity within the committee with respect to curriculum areas taught, experience designing and teaching online courses, and views regarding online education (ranging from one faculty member who favored the development of an entire MSW program online to another who strongly opposed further proliferation of online courses).

The Technology Committee was tasked with addressing everything from faculty's basic concerns about including web-based courses in the curriculum, to more specific questions regarding procedures for developing and offering certain online courses. Like other schools, we faced pressure from

---

[1]   Moodle is an open-source software learning management system used for blending learning and distance education.

university administrators to engage in online course development and teaching (Maidment, 2005), and this pressure may have contributed to faculty resistance to offering web-based instruction. Accordingly, one of the first topics addressed by the committee was faculty questions and concerns about the school's long-term goals regarding distance education. The majority of the faculty was opposed to the idea of a fully online program. The Technology Committee therefore convened discussion sessions with faculty regarding the issue and took the lead in communicating faculty concerns and preferences to the administration. When, after much discussion, a decision was made not to pursue a fully online program at this point in time, we were better able to focus on our goal of implementing the specific online courses we had agreed to develop.

The Technology Committee also helped devise a policy stipulating that, for a period of 1 year, only full-time faculty would be allowed to teach online and blended courses. This policy was designed to help us obtain feedback from our full-time faculty regarding student interest and feedback on the overall experiences of participating students and faculty so that we could move forward in a thoughtful way to plan courses and deliver them effectively.

Alignment

Alignment refers to the importance of ensuring that e-learning initiatives are connected to a school's mission, policies, and learning outcomes. As Knowles (2007) reported, programs developing online courses need to consider *philosophical* alignment (e.g., how the use of online pedagogy aligns with the school's mission to graduate competent and ethical social workers), *pedagogical* alignment (the need to examine curricula, integrate learning models, and develop assessment strategies to ensure that instruction methods are appropriate for both social work education and online learning), *policy* alignment (the need to develop policies addressing privacy and confidentiality, roles of faculty and administrators in creating and maintaining online materials, and other expectations and guidelines for students and faculty), and *organizational* alignment (e.g., how the financial costs of developing and delivering online courses will be recovered).

Our faculty had questions related to alignment: Can we deliver quality instruction online to help students attain the knowledge, skills, and values they will need to succeed as social work professionals? Which and how many courses should be offered online? How can we ensure equivalence between on-ground and online instruction? How should online learning be assessed? What incentives should be granted to faculty interested in developing online courses? Regarding intellectual property, who "owns" a course that was previously taught on-ground and now has been revised to be taught online? Because issues such as these need addressing at both program and university levels, Knowles (2007) recommended that schools formulate a strategic plan for technology integration; nevertheless, he also noted that, at the time of his study, only two out of the 12 participating social work programs had developed strategic plans for offering courses online.

To address concerns about equivalency of on-ground and online instruction, we decided that a course previously taught face-to-face should be reviewed and approved by our curriculum committee before it could be taught in a blended or online format. Regarding questions about intellectual property, we found that the university had previously stipulated that when faculty members are compensated to develop an online course, they can choose whether materials they develop will be their property or the university's. If the latter, administration would be free to share online materials with other faculty. Information such as this regarding policies and procedures implemented at the university level was disseminated to the entire social work faculty.

In line with *organizational* alignment, and issues related to financial costs, determining appropriate class sizes for online courses was a source of debate at our school. This experience echoes a larger debate in higher education about the appropriate class size for online courses, ranging from the conviction that smaller classes support instructor–student interaction, to the belief that larger class sizes facilitate group work within classes, to perceptions that the size of the class does not matter (Gilbert, 1995; Orellano, 2006; Simonson, 2004). Regarding class size, administrators often are concerned with cost–benefit factors and faculty workloads, as well as providing students with a high-quality online education (Simonson, 2004). Furthermore, administrators often view online education as having the potential to produce increased revenue, and therefore they may push for courseload or class size to be even higher than typically found in face-to-face courses (Tomei, 2006).

When determining the size of online and blended courses, it is important to consider the subject matter, the overarching mission of the school, and faculty members' online teaching aptitudes. Specifically, programs should consider whether large class sizes are conducive to training social workers to connect with others. In a community-based university such as ours, which aims to provide a sense of connection among students, between faculty and students, and between the academy and the larger community, it was apparent that larger classes would not likely support our mission and goals. Moreover, given that many of our faculty were still in the process of learning about available technological advances and other aspects of online learning, we agreed that large classes might interfere with their ability to teach to their strengths and therefore provide students with a quality learning experience. Keeping our mission in mind, and openly discussing our intention to stay aligned with it, helped us make decisions that we felt were in the best interest of our school and our students.

Faculty Engagement

Faculty engagement focuses on the processes required for faculty to decide how much they as individuals and the school should invest toward the goal of becoming instructors of online courses. In our view, this process should not be rushed, as it involves both a steep learning curve for instructors and what amounts to an identity change for the school. Participants in Knowles's (2007) study reported a sense of urgency at their schools to mount online offerings based on the fast-moving pace of technology and a need to maintain student enrollment in an increasingly competitive higher education environment. Such pressures may preclude in-depth dialogue regarding questions or concerns and may result in the work being shouldered by a few faculty and staff rather than shared by many. Rushing forward prematurely also may cause or exacerbate a rift between those supporting and those opposing the expansion of online offerings, which could lead to a stalemate.

One goal of the Technology Committee, therefore, was to ensure that the responsibility for planning and implementing online courses was "owned" by the faculty as a whole, which understood the need for an ample opportunity for dialogue and discussion. Thus, whereas the committee was tasked with articulating questions regarding policies and procedures, members used various venues to inform colleagues about emerging issues, solicit their ideas, and involve them in problem solving and decision making. Issues related to online teaching and learning were raised and discussed at curriculum area sessions, faculty meetings, in deliberations with the committee, and sessions of our monthly teaching discussion group. Informal conversations about online teaching and learning were encouraged as well. As a result, our faculty, while having diverse opinions about e-learning, was able to air their differences, reach some consensus, and share in the decision-making process.

Coherence

Another area that must be addressed when developing online courses is *coherence*, which is based on the question, "Does the use of e-learning alter values and standards?" (East, LaMendola, & Alter, 2014). At our school this question was examined simultaneously by the curriculum committee and the Technology Committee, which facilitated discussions with the faculty. The curriculum committee currently is pondering the appropriate procedures and criteria for evaluating online course proposals. For example, does *every* course, originally designed for on-ground instruction, now being revised for online instruction, need to be approved by the curriculum committee? Because teaching methods and assignments utilized by two different online instructors might vary considerably, does an online course that was previously developed, approved, and taught by one faculty member need to be re-reviewed if a different faculty member now wishes to teach it? In our discussions, we are attempting to balance our goal of ensuring quality instruction with our wish to avoid duplicative procedures that can cause unnecessary delays in development and implementation.

Throughout this process, some faculty have expressed concern about the possibility of a "watered-down" curriculum, echoing Reamer's discussion of a faculty member's report that, in the online social work practice methods courses he taught, "asynchronous assignments never seemed much more than 1/3 of the 75 minutes of 'class time' that they were supposed to occupy and the degree of challenge seemed extremely low" (Reamer, 2013, p. 374). Such concerns about the rigor of assignments, and the quantity and quality of student–faculty interaction in e-learning, need to be addressed head-on. Sharing successful models can be helpful, as can disseminating and openly discussing research demonstrating both the strengths and weaknesses of online learning. For example, a recent evaluation of four introductory BSW classes, taught by the same instructor, in which two sections were taught on-ground and the other two online, found that online students spent equal time reading and studying as those taking the class face-to-face and earned equivalent grades in the class. However, online students were less pleased with the quantity and quality of communication with faculty and classmates, and hence felt both less satisfied with the course and less well prepared to take additional social work courses (McAllister, 2013).

Yet another issue related to coherence is how to ensure that students have the technological and cognitive skills needed to succeed in an online course. Thus, schools should discuss and clarify requirements for enrolling in an online course. For example, should any prerequisites or other requirements be met before a student may register for an online course (e.g., second semester in the program, grade point average minimum, technology screening)? What are expectations for participation in an online class, and how should such participation be measured? Should there be standard policies about course activities; for example, should students be required to log in a certain number of times per week? Moreover, the larger question of who ultimately is responsible for quality control in online offerings needs to be discussed and answered, as well.

Resources

When implementing online courses, it is essential to have the requisite resources available. In our institution, several resources were present for faculty interested in developing online and blended courses. Our university's Faculty Center for Professional Excellence provided online trainings and one-on-one consulting on the development of online and blended courses, and on programs and tools—such as Turnitin, Google Chat, Prezi, Voicethread, and Moodle—to enhance teaching and augment learning. One such training,

"How to Create Narrated Power Point and YouTube Videos and Place Them on Moodle," was developed by a social work faculty member in collaboration with the Faculty Center for Professional Excellence and then offered to social work faculty and staff at all four sites. The training was very well attended, illustrating faculty interest in receiving information and training that they perceive to be relevant to their teaching goals.

Leadership

Finally, strong leadership will be needed in order to make the shift to offering online and blended courses. Many schools that have transitioned to offering online courses have created one or more leadership positions to spearhead online activities. At our university, an Assistant Provost of Online Learning was appointed and additional staff hired at the Faculty Center for Professional Excellence to assist those developing online courses. In addition, the university convened a Senate Task Force on Online Courses and Programs composed of faculty from each school and department, along with administrators who were charged with reviewing proposals for online courses and making suggestions for developing an online environment at the university. One of their major tasks this year was surveying faculty who had taught online and blended courses at the university and then disseminating the findings to faculty.

Within our school, the successful implementation of distance education courses has been supported by the Dean, Associate Dean for Academic Affairs, Admissions Coordinator, and the directors of our three satellite campuses. Because ours is a relatively large MSW program, with a main campus located in a suburban area, and three extension centers situated in urban, suburban, and rural areas, the cooperation of the site directors has been critical to our goal of ensuring equivalency for the students at all four sites.

The Associate Dean for Academic Affairs has played an instrumental role in getting our online courses up and running. As a member of our Technology Committee, he has distributed announcements of distance education offerings and worked with faculty teaching these courses in order to enroll students. This endeavor has required multiple e-mails and other outreach efforts to students, encouraging site directors to inform students at our branch campuses about online opportunities and preparing them to advise students regarding specific online offerings. In the 1st year that our online and blended courses were offered, enrollment was low, given that students often did not know about the availability of these courses or were wary of taking them. Last-minute cancellations of some online sections created a problem for faculty who needed to maintain their workload. In discussion, faculty requested that those volunteering to teach an online or blended course section be provided with a "backup" on-ground section in case the web-based version failed to get sufficient enrollment. This request was supported by the Associate Dean, which resulted in expanding the number of full-time faculty willing to try online teaching.

DISCUSSION

Developing an online environment has been a challenging but rewarding experience. In developing an online environment within our school, we learned three important lessons. First, in our context, process that is inclusive of faculty is crucial to achieving success. Unlike other schools that have taken a top-down approach to developing and implementing online environments (Maidment, 2005), for our school, having continuous discussions with faculty regarding the processes involved in offering online courses proved to be crucial to accomplishing our goal. Devising a process that is inclusive adheres to Knowles's framework, which stresses the importance of gaining faculty buy-in. Although including everyone in discussions and problem solving (and allowing for the expression of different points of view) may be time-consuming, the strategy is likely to pay off in wider ownership of the innovation. In addition, those leading discussions about online teaching must project an open attitude that is receptive to all points of view and should seek to understand rather than persuade others so that faculty can raise concerns, offer solutions, and feel that they have a say in how online and blended courses are developed and implemented.

Second, understanding and responding to students' needs, preferences, and technological skills is critical. Although some of our students were interested in online and blended courses, many were apprehensive at first about taking a course via this modality. Their initial hesitancy to enroll in our online course offerings taught us about the importance of providing greater information and guidance. To address concerns of students at the consideration stage, the school initiated workshops and in-class presentations to introduce them to online learning. These activities raised awareness about our online offerings and helped demystify distance education. To support those taking an online course for the first time, we are now collaborating with the university technology center to develop training specifically for students who enroll in online courses to address areas such as time management, technological skills, and how to best learn online.

Last, we learned about the importance of collaborating with the university at large in order to clarify policies, advocate for resources, and "have a voice at the table." In a recent speech, Senator Elizabeth Warren, rallying voters to support progressive women running for Congress, reminded them that "if you don't have a seat at the table, you're probably on the menu" (Oh, 2014). This advice is relevant for social work faculty wanting a voice in how their online courses are developed and implemented and how resources are allocated. We have found it beneficial to partner with colleagues from departments and professional schools, as well as with faculty and administrators at the university as a whole. These collaborations have included our faculty joining existing university committees focused on technology and teaching and forging relationships with senior university administrators and others interested in promulgating distance education. As a result, we have gained early access to various resources for developing online courses and have been able to influence university policy regarding distance education.

LIMITATIONS

Although the Knowles framework has been helpful in conceptualizing and analyzing our online learning environment, it may have limitations for some schools. For example, the framework fails to provide specific guidelines regarding best practices for the *selection* of courses to teach online. Understanding the process institutions engage in when selecting courses to be taught in this manner is important given the existing debate regarding the quality of online versus on-ground courses (Reamer, 2013). Over the past decade, this debate has moved from the question of "*Should* social work courses be taught online?" to "*Which* social work courses should be taught online?" with the most intense disagreements occurring around the question of whether clinical skills can be mastered in an e-learning format (Moore, 2005; Siegel, Jennings, Conklin, Napoletano, & Shelly, 1998). Although a few studies have appeared in the literature recently (Regan & Youn, 2008), more investigations of the effectiveness of teaching practice and other social work content online are needed to inform curriculum and pedagogical decisions.

Another limitation is the absence of information on how institutions can best select *online activities* for e-learning. This question needs addressing, as the quality of an online course often hinges on the quality of the learning resources, activities, and feedback provided by the online instructor. Finally, although Knowles's conceptual framework provides an important template for the steps that institutions have taken to develop an online environment, it does not distinguish between the needs and culture of smaller and larger institutions.

RECOMMENDATIONS

Building on Knowles's framework, and based further on our own experiences, we offer the following suggestions for schools of social work wishing to cultivate a supportive online learning environment:

1. Establish a technology committee within the school and invite faculty, administrators, and those with diverse views regarding online education to serve on this committee. Careful attention should be paid to engaging faculty, administrators, and students in all processes and phases related to making the transition to online teaching.
2. Start small and build from there, maintaining continual communication with all stakeholders. If the majority of the faculty is not interested in developing online or blended versions of their courses, begin with the few faculty who are. Share information, strategies, and perspectives. For example, the committee could conduct a literature review to obtain data on the effectiveness of online learning, helpful policies, and supportive processes and disseminate this information to colleagues. In addition, faculty members who have taught online can be invited to share with others their "lessons learned." Schools should consider and discuss formats that have worked well and that they believe will work best for their goals and be consonant with their culture. Initiating discussions about what social work content and courses would likely be most effective in an online format would be important and should happen early in the process
3. Become informed about your institution's vision and goals regarding distance education. Review existing distance education policies at your university and, when feasible, collaborate with staff from other schools and departments.
4. Continue to include students in feedback, planning, and information sharing. Consider collecting both formal and informal evaluation data on current online courses; surveying students about their interest in taking future online courses; preparing an advisement memo featuring forthcoming online and blended courses; and inviting students to sit on committees dealing with teaching, learning, curriculum, and technology.

CONCLUSION

Schools of social work interested in developing and implementing e-learning would do well to consider the organizational environment in which their new online offerings will take place. They also will need to attend to tasks and processes in order to ensure an effective transition in which the entire educational community is fully involved and engaged, working together cooperatively toward a significant pedagogical and environmental change We believe that Knowles (2007) framework for conceptualization and implementation will be helpful in this regard.

REFERENCES

Anderson, T. (Ed.). (2008). *The theory and practice of online learning*. Edmonton, Canada: Athabasca University Press.

Barnett-Queen, T., Blair, R., & Merrick, M. (2005). Student perspectives of online discussions: Strengths and weaknesses. *Journal of Technology in Human Services*, *23*, 229–244. doi:10.1300/J017v23n03_05

Collins, D., Gabor, P., Coleman, H., & Ing, C. (2002, July). *In love with technology: A critical review of the use of technology in social work education*. Paper presented at the Ninth International Literacy and Education Research Conference on Learning, Beijing, China.

Council of Social Work Education. (2013). *2013 statistics on social work education*. Retrieved from http://cswe.org/CentersInitiatives/DataStatistics/74475.aspx

East, J. F., LaMendola, W., & Alter, C. (2014). Distance education and organizational Environment. *Journal of Social Work Education*, *50*, 19–33. doi:10.1080/10437797.2014.856226

Flynn, M., Maiden, R. P., Smith, W., Wiley, J., & Wood, G. (2013). Launching the virtual academic center: Issues and challenges in innovation. *Journal of Teaching in Social Work*, *33*, 339–356. doi:10.1080/08841233.2013.843364

Gilbert, S. (1995). Quality education: Does class size matter? *CSSHE Professional File*, *14*.

King, A. (1993). From "sage on the stage" to "guide on the side". *College Teaching*, *41*, 30–35. doi:10.1080/87567555.1993.9926781

Knowles, A. J. (2007). Pedagogical and policy challenges in implementing e-learning in social work education. *Journal of Technology in Human Services*, *25*, 17–44. doi:10.1300/J017v25n01_02

Maidment, J. (2005). Teaching social work online: Dilemmas and debates. *Social Work Education*, *24*, 185–195. doi:10.1080/0261547052000333126

McAllister, C. (2013). A process evaluation of an online BSW program: Getting the student perspective. *Journal of Teaching in Social Work*, *33*, 514–530. doi:10.1080/08841233.2013.838200

McFadden, R. J., Moore, B., Herie, M., & Schoech, D. (2005). *Web-based education in the human services: Models, methods, and best practices*. New York, NY: Haworth.

Moore, B. (2005). Faculty perceptions of the effectiveness of web-based instruction in social work education: A national study. *Journal of Technology in Human Services*, *23*, 53–66. doi:10.1300/J017v23n01_04

Oh, I. (2014, September 25). Elizabeth Warren: Democratic women need a seat at the governing table. *The New York Times*. Retrieved from http://www.motherjones.com/mojo/2014/09/elizabeth-warren-donors-vote-democratic-women

Orellano, A. (2006). Class size and interaction in online courses. *The Quarterly Review of Distance Education*, *7*, 229–248.

Reamer, F. G. (2013). Distance and online social work education: Novel ethical challenges. *Journal of Teaching in Social Work*, *33*, 369–384. doi:10.1080/08841233.2013.828669

Regan, J., & Youn, E. (2008). Past, present, and future trends in teaching clinical skills through Web-based learning environments. *Journal of Social Work Education, 44,* 95–116. doi:10.5175/JSWE.2008.200600592

Siegel, E., Jennings, J. G., Conklin, J., Napoletano, F., & Shelly, A. (1998). Distance learning in social work education: Results and implications of a national survey. *Journal of Social Work Education, 34,* 71–81.

Simonson, M. (2004). Class size: Where is the research? *Distance Learning, 1*(4), 56.

Tallent-Runnels, M. K., Thomas, J. A., Lan, W. Y., Cooper, S., Ahern, T. C., Shaw, S. M., & Liu, X. (2006). Teaching courses on-line. *Review of Educational Research, 76,* 93–135. doi:10.3102/00346543076001093

Tomei, L. (2006). The impact of online teaching on faculty load: Computing the ideal class size for online courses. *Journal of Technology and Teacher Education, 14,* 531–541.

Part III

Ethical and Diversity Considerations

Digital Ethics in Social Work Education

Janet M. Joiner

ABSTRACT

Attention has been given to the revised National Association of Social Workers (NASW) Code of Ethics that guides social worker use of technology. The revision of the NASW Code of Ethics has signaled a transition in the profession toward ethical online practice using modern techniques and contemporary tools. Practicing social workers are applying these new ethical standards, and many social work educators are doing so when using information and communication technologies with students. However, little research focuses on teaching social work students about digital ethics and professional online conduct. This paper explores the importance of preparing social work students for ethical online behavior.

In the digital age, social work educators and their students have become adept at using information and communication technologies (ICT), including the Internet, social media, and smart devices (Chan & Holosko, 2016). ICT have proliferated in everyday life, with some social work faculty using these tools to engage students in teaching and learning. Groessl (2015) indicated that the Council on Social Work Education (CSWE), the national accrediting body for social work education, expects social work students to become ethically competent, but does not specify how ethics, including digital ethics, should be integrated across the curriculum.

Digital ethics

Digital ethics, a concept popularized by the Zur Institute (2018), is described as the use of sound moral and principled behaviors in online settings. Working collaboratively, the National Association of Social Workers (NASW), Association of Social Work Boards (ASWB), Council on Social Work Education (CSWE), and Clinical Social Work Association (CSWA) in 2017 promulgated the *Standards for Technology in Social Work Practice*. While social work practitioners are expected to follow these guidelines when using technology in their practice (Reamer, 2017), students are not required to use these standards to guide their online interactions.

Educating social work students about e-professionalism and digital ethics is essential, given the proliferation of technology in everyday life. In fact, McAuliffe and Nipperess (2017) argued that social workers who deploy technology with their clients must practice e-professionalism. E-professionalism involves using appropriate security safeguards to protect clients from potential harm, treating clients and others with respect and integrity, and being technologically proficient with the digital tools used with clients.

Students who are unfamiliar with the concept of e-professionalism may not be aware that their social media posts can be viewed by potential employers who may then make judgments about their level of competence. These seemingly private posts could be accessed by future clients and potential employers who may make judgments about their character based on content posted as a student (Boddy & Dominelli, 2017). Indeed, students may not fully appreciate that online posts, such as those made on social media, have the potential to live in cyberspace forever (Fang, Mishna, Zhang, Van Wert, & Bogo, 2014).

Faculty, therefore, must be willing to explore creative ways to integrate lessons about technology and ethics in the classroom to strengthen student moral and civic development while preparing them for professional practice (Reamer, 2019). Social work educators and experienced practitioners can help students understand that the imaginary line between the personal and professional self is no longer blurred, with professional and personal selves in effect becoming one online (Boddy & Dominelli, 2017). Karpman and Drisko (2016) maintained that social work students could benefit from classroom discussions and assignments related to digital engagement that involve comprehending the Code of Ethics; understanding responsible use of social media and technology with clients; recognizing the influence of social workers' online behavior with their clients, colleagues, and the organizations in which they work; and acknowledging their technological deficits while working to address them.

Technology in social work education

When social work programs of study were introduced in the early 1900s, American society was grappling with the consequences of technology and industrialization (Austin, 1997). Although social work education was in its infancy during this time, individuals and groups committed to advancing social change tended to use prevailing technology, including the offset printing press, to produce written content to educate and inform the community. Today, social work faculty and students are of course using technology in ways never imagined by previous generations of social workers (Regan, 2016; Selingo, 2016). Zilberstein (2015) noted that the relationship between people and technology is evolving quickly and technology is expected to continue influencing human behavior and social functioning.

While many social work students are proficient in using a variety of technologies, they may be unaware of the influence that using ICT could have on their evolving careers (Fang et al., 2014). Kreuger (1997) cautioned against the integration of technology in social work education, arguing, perhaps at the extreme, that the reliance on technology could result in "the end of social work" (p. 26). In contrast, Jarman-Rohde, McFall, Kolar, and Strom (1997) simply argued that for the profession to continue, it must evolve. This evolution must include social workers who are willing to address modern-day realities, such as using technology in practice, along with teaching students about current technology trends influencing human behavior and the broader society.

Literature review

A literature review identified an increasing number of faculty who used ICT to enhance teaching and learning, while building students' technological competence (Baker & Iverson Hitchcock, 2017; D'Cruz, Soothill, Francis, & Christie, 2002; Fang et al., 2014; Hitchcock & Young, 2016; Knowles & Cooner, 2016; Teixeira & Hash, 2017; Young, McLeod, & Brady, 2018). However, absent from the social work research is investigation focused on teaching students about digital ethics and the application of the *NASW Code of Ethics* (2017) in online settings. The research studies identified in this literature review simply supported the use of ICT in social work education, with an emphasis on technology literacy. Nevertheless, several of the researchers described ethical issues associated with using ICT, including privacy and confidentiality limitations, professional boundary concerns, and potential security breaches.

Social work students come from a variety of backgrounds that help shape their perspectives related to ethics and their engagement with others online. While student experiences influence their views and interactions with others, D'Cruz et al. (2002) reported that perceptions of ethics in social work did not differ significantly between male and female social work students, or older and younger ones. However, no research was found that compared differences in perceptions of ethical standards among students from diverse racial or ethnic groups.

Young et al. (2018) explored ethical challenges associated with educating social work students in the digital age and improving students' technological competency. These authors conducted a study with 76 undergraduate social work students enrolled in a nonprofit organizations and digital advocacy course. Young and colleagues argued that social work faculty have an ethical responsibility to promote student technology literacy, develop course assignments based on modern digital issues that students are likely to encounter as practitioners, and prepare students for ethical professional practice. Research findings indicated that students who completed the nonprofit organizations and digital advocacy course demonstrated higher levels of digital competence as determined by changes from pre to posttest.

Baker and Iverson Hitchcock (2017) conducted a study with 21 BSW students in a Human Behavior and the Social Environment (HBSE) course who used the social media platform, Pinterest, for professional development and engagement purposes. Baker and Iverson Hitchcock suggested that while social work students are using technology and social media in their everyday lives, they may not know how to use these tools appropriately in professional settings. Study results indicated that integrating social media assignments in certain social work courses could expand students' professional networks, raise awareness of digital resources, and strengthen their technological competency.

Teixeira and Hash (2017) conducted a study with 45 BSW students using the social media platform, Twitter, in a HBSE course. The students participated in an orientation that included content on ethical social media engagement; watched as faculty modeled appropriate online behavior for students; and completed an assessment of students' attitudes about the use of Twitter in the course. Study outcomes indicated that students enjoyed using Twitter, felt engaged with course content, and networked appropriately with classmates and faculty. Students also were encouraged to engage in online discussions with other classmates who could have opposing opinions (Teixeira & Hash, 2017). The authors did not indicate if participants were cautioned about posting criticisms about others on Twitter, or using other social media platforms to discuss their class experiences.

Hitchcock and Young (2016) conducted a study with 35 students, with 77% identifying as BSW and 23% as MSW. Students participated in a live Twitter chat to improve real-time engagement and professional networking. Study investigators explored perceptions of students regarding the use of Twitter chats for professional development, level of preparation for participating in a Twitter chat, and benefits resulting from Twitter chat participation. Study findings indicated that the Twitter chat experience helped participants develop professionally, connect with others, and build technology competence. Researchers (Baker & Iverson Hitchcock, 2017; Hitchcock & Young, 2016; Teixeira & Hash, 2017) however did not specify that participants received education related to ethical online engagement based on the *NASW Code of Ethics* (2017) and/or the NASW et al. (2017)*Standards for Technology and Social Work Practice.*

Knowles and Cooner (2016) conducted an inquiry with 80 undergraduate social work students from the United Kingdom (UK) and Canada. Study participants included 52 UK students and 28 Canadian students who participated in an asynchronous international learning collaborative with an emphasis on ethical online engagement based on the supplemental social media practice guidelines that are linked directly to the *Canadian Association of Social Workers Code of Ethics*

(CASW, 2005, 2013). Study findings revealed that students found participation in the collaborative worthwhile, learned to present themselves online professionally, and increased awareness of ethical challenges associated with using social media. Study authors recommended that faculty consider using social media to help students link classroom experiences with ethical social work practice and the *CASW Code of Ethics* (2005).

According to Fang et al. (2014), social work instructors are faced with a variety of challenges when teaching students about ICT. Faculty often struggle with integrating ICT into their courses, while ensuring that students learn to maintain client privacy and confidentiality. Fang and colleagues discussed ethical challenges associated with student levels of technology competency, as well as adequate preparation of students to practice in a world that is becoming increasingly virtual. Through their review of literature related to these concerns, no specific level of technology competency or literacy that students are expected to attain was established, although student use of ICT continues to increase.

Several studies advocated educating social work students about ICT (Baker & Iverson Hitchcock, 2017; Fang et al., 2014; Hitchcock & Young, 2016; Knowles & Cooner, 2016; Teixeira & Hash, 2017; Young et al., 2018). They presented a number of positive research findings, helped strengthen students' technology competence, and provided students with hands-on practice using social media. Knowles and Cooner (2016) indicated that their study participants received education related to understanding digital ethics based on the *CASW Code of Ethics*. However, little research has explored the extent to which social work faculty discussed expectations regarding student use of ICT, or whether social work students should be held to similar standards of ethical online behavior as professional practitioners.

This paper explores the importance of preparing social work students for ethical online conduct, specifically with regard to learning and following the *NASW Code of Ethics* (2017) and established standards for social workers use of technology in practice. The research questions addressed in this study were:

(1) What are students' perceptions regarding their preparation to follow the same ethical standards as professional social workers?
(2) What are students' perceptions regarding their level of preparedness to conduct themselves ethically when using social media, the Internet, and mobile technology?

Methods

A quantitative research design was used as the framework, and a researcher-developed survey was created specifically for this study. An online survey was made available to students enrolled in three online BSW classes at a single private university. (In addition, the survey also was completed by students in three traditional social work classes.) Prior to conducting the data collection, the Institutional Review Board of the university approved the study.

Participants

A total of 54 students completed the survey during the Winter 2019 semester. The participants ranged in age from 19 to 64 years of age, with a mean of 39.33 (*SD* = 15.21). The majority of students were female (*n* = 46, 85.2%). While students were at all levels of the BSW program, most were either seniors (*n* = 26, 49.0%) or juniors (*n* = 15, 28.3%). Most were enrolled full-time (*n* = 36, 66.7%) and 20 (37.0%) were working either full-or part-time. [Table 1 presents the student characteristics.]

Instrument

The students were asked to respond to 27 items that used multiple response formats, including forced choice responses and frequencies for demographics, and Likert-style items regarding their perceptions of digital ethics and perceived levels of preparation to engage others ethically online.

Table 1. Frequency distributions: student characteristics (N = 54).

Student Characteristics	N	%
Gender		
Female	46	85.2
Male	8	14.8
Academic Standing		
Freshman	3	5.7
Sophomore	9	17.0
Junior	15	28.3
Senior	26	49.0
Missing 1		
Enrollment Status		
Full-time	36	66.7
Part-time	18	33.3
Employment Status		
Full-time	20	37.0
Part-time	20	37.0
Not employed	14	26.0
Classes in Which Students Were Enrolled*		
Intro to Social Work	7	13.0
Social Welfare and Social Justice	12	22.2
Social Welfare Policy	16	29.6
Human Behavior II	23	42.6
Practice III	23	42.6
Seminar II	6	11.1
Social Work Ethics and Digital Advocacy	5	9.3

*Multiple responses, students could be enrolled in up to three courses, but only answered the survey once.

In addition to the quantitative items, students were asked to respond to one qualitative item regarding their perceptions of how prepared they were to use ICT ethically. The majority of items were taken from research on the topic, although some items were unique to the university where the study was conducted. The two scales (using a Likert response format) were tested for internal consistency. The obtained Cronbach alpha coefficient for digital ethics was .91, with an alpha coefficient of .93 for social work students' perceptions of faculty roles in learning ethical behavior. These alpha coefficients provide support for internal consistency as a measure of reliability.

Procedures

With the exception of those enrolled in the Social Work Ethics and Digital Advocacy course, the students did not have any specific intervention on digital ethics in their social work courses. Instead, faculty integrated general-ized ethics information across the curriculum. Following Winter term 2019, program faculty voted to integrate the digital ethics course in the curriculum as a required class for students admitted to the BSW program beginning in Fall 2019.

Students completed the survey in two ways. One group enrolled in online social work courses were given a link to SurveyMonkey. Nineteen students completed the survey online. The remaining 35 students were enrolled in traditional face-to-face courses and completed the survey in class. However, both surveys were identical. Students read the information sheet (online or on the paper survey) and asked any questions prior to participating. They were not required to sign or return the information sheet, assuring their anonymity. Regardless of method used to complete the survey, all were told that participation was voluntary and that their decision to participate or not participate would not influence their standing in their courses. (Students who were enrolled in multiple courses were asked to complete the survey in only one course to avoid duplicate reporting.)

Data analysis

Data collected from SurveyMonkey.com were downloaded into an Excel file and then transferred to an IBM-SPSS ver. 25 file for analysis. After the data from the paper surveys also were entered into the SPSS file, it was cleaned and checked for accuracy. Of the 62 surveys submitted, either electronically or on paper, eight surveys were eliminated due to incomplete data. Frequency distributions were used to summarize the responses to the demo-graphic questions, while inferential statistical analysis, including Pearson product moment correlations and logistic regression, were used to address the research questions. The responses to the open-ended item were analyzed using an instrument for content analysis to develop patterns and themes regarding perceptions of how prepared they were to use ICT ethically.

Findings

Pearson product moment correlations were used to determine the strength and direction of the relationships between student perceptions of instructors' roles in learning social work ethics, and perceptions of their preparation to use ethics with technology ($r = .89$, $p < .001$, 95% $ci = 82 - .93$), and perceptions of ethical standards for social work students ($r = .47$, $p < .001$, 95% $ci = .23 - .65$). The positive direction of the relationships indicated that students who had higher scores for their instructors' roles in learning social work ethics tended to have higher scores for their preparation to use ethics with technology and ethical standards for social work students. [Table 2 presents results of Pearson product moment correlations.]

A logistic regression was deployed to determine if preparation to use ethics with technology, ethical standards for social work students, and perceptions of instructors' roles in learning social work ethics could predict the educational level of students (freshman through junior and senior). The chi-square from the logistic regression was not statistically significant (χ^2 [3] $= 4.86$, $p = .182$), although students who were seniors were 8.17 times as likely to have positive perceptions regarding their instructors' roles in learning social work ethics than students in their freshman through junior years. [Table 3 presents results of logistic regression.]

The students answered an open-ended question that asked, "How prepared are you to conduct yourself ethically when using social media, Internet, and mobile technology (e.g., cell phones, tablets, etc.)." Student comments were transcribed and analyzed for patterns and themes that could be used to determine their self-reported level of preparedness to act ethically with technology. Three themes emerged from student comments, with most student responses directed at their perceived levels of preparation for engaging ethically with others using ICT. The themes were: (a) perceptions of preparedness to engage in ethical practice using ICT, (b) perceptions of ethical online behavior, and (c) perceptions of instructors' roles in learning social work ethics.

Table 2. Pearson product moment correlations: student perceptions of instructors role in learning SW ethics.

Variable	N	M	SD	r	p	95% *ci* Low	High
Preparation to use ethics with technology	54	4.56	.66	.89	<.001	.82	.93
Ethical standards for SW students	54	3.86	.91	.47	<.001	.23	.65

Table 3. Logistic regression: year in school and social work students' perceptions of digital ethics.

Variable	Odds Ratio	95% ci
Preparation to use ethics with technology	.15	.02–01.35
Ethical standards for SW students	1.13	.55–02.29
Perceptions of instructors' role in learning SW ethics	8.17	.96–69.63

Perceptions of preparedness to engage in ethical practice using ICT

Several students indicated they felt prepared to use technology ethically when interacting with other students or their professors. They also noted that they were aware of the *NASW Code of Ethics* (2017), including its standards associated with technology, and indicated they understood the importance of following ethical standards. One commented that the "ethics of using technology has been addressed in all my classes." Another student agreed, indicating "I feel we have really covered this [digital ethics] in every class. In contrast, a different student stated, "I am well prepared, but not from anything I have learned in class."

Perceptions of ethical online behavior

A second theme that emerged from student comments was related to their perceptions of ethical online behavior. For example, several students indicated the importance of being professional and respectful to others while engaged in using technology. One stated, "when it comes to using social media, I know what is right and what is wrong," and another remarked, "when I am on social media, I tend to use it for the right reasons and not wrong." A different student shared, "by simply knowing what is appropriate and what is not, I have prepared to conduct myself ethically." Other students indicated an awareness of the NASW Code of Ethics and the importance of following the profession's established ethics and standards.

Perceptions of their instructors' roles in learning social work ethics

A final theme that emerged was related to student perceptions of their instructors' roles in learning social work ethics. Several students remarked that faculty helped prepare them to use ICT ethically and that digital ethics had been discussed in each of their classes. One remarked, "I believe that my instructors have prepared me to conduct myself ethically using various outlets of technology." In contrast, some students suggested that, while prepared to engage others ethically online, they had not learned or practiced content related to digital ethics in their class, and another student stated, "I am well prepared, but not from anything I have learned in class." The overall pattern of student responses suggested that students were aware of the importance of engaging ethically while using ICT.

Discussion

This paper explored the importance of preparing social work students for ethical online conduct, specifically with regard to learning and following the NASW Code of Ethics (2017). Findings from the current study provided evidence that students held positive perceptions regarding their ability to engage ethically with others when using ICT, both personally and professionally. The majority of students indicated that they had been prepared to engage others ethically when using technology, although some equated ethical behavior simply with being nice, and knowing right from wrong. While the national accrediting body for social work education (CSWE) does not require social work instructors to include course content related to digital ethics and responsible online behavior, without the inclusion of this content in the curriculum, social work students may not be fully prepared for real world practice in the digital age. To help ensure that social work students attain competency in digital ethics, social work academics must look to CSWE to develop formal ethical expectations for the use of ICT in social work education.

Implications

Contemporary social workers are expected to use ICT ethically in direct practice, and many such practitioners develop their knowledge and skills by participating in continuing education workshops, engaging in personal study and research, as well as through direct practice with their clients. Nevertheless, early in their careers, practitioners generally lack work experience in the field and must rely on their classroom and fieldwork experiences to provide them with a foundation to engage clients ethically using online tools.

The lack of digital ethics education and instruction focusing on the use of ICT in direct practice could result in a future work force that is underprepared to address the ethical reality of the digital age. Hence, social work educators interested in integrating digital ethics and ICT content in their programs should consider the following: the existence of an institutional infrastructure to support increased student use of technology on campus; the knowledge levels of social work faculty regarding use of digital ethics and ICT in direct practice settings; and the capacity of campus instructional technology staff to support social work student ongoing ICT training needs.

Limitations

The current study presented several challenges, including small sample size, lack of participant demographic data (e.g., ethnicity, income level, religious preference), and social desirability influence. The first limitation was the small sample size that makes it not possible, of course, to generalize study results to students enrolled in social work courses at other colleges and universities. The current study simply was open to all students enrolled in BSW courses at one university. While 62 students submitted surveys for the study, 8 (13%) surveys had to be discarded as incomplete, and thus the study results were based on the 54 completed surveys. The second limitation is the lack of demographic data collected from participants beyond age, gender, academic standing, and employment status. The lack of available broad demographic data resulted in few substantive participant comparisons, since demographically, study participants were very similar. The final limitation of this study is related to student survey responses which could reflect socially desirable intent (Kelly, Harpel, Fontes, Walters, & Murphy, 2017). The authors note that social desirability response theory (Crowne & Marlowe, 1960) proposes that participants may respond in ways that they perceive will be viewed more positively by others, providing answers to survey questions that may be exaggerated or entirely untrue. However, study respondents here may have felt more relaxed when completing computer-based surveys, resulting in feedback that is truthful and authentic. Simply put, respondents may have felt comfortable in responding because of the perceived anonymity digital surveys could provide.

Conclusion

While the NASW *Code of Ethics* (2017) and the NASW et al. *Standards for Technology in Social Work Practice* (2017) provide social work practitioners with guidance related to responsible online engagement, integrating digital ethics content in the social work curriculum currently does not appear to be a priority. Social workers have long raised concerns about challenges associated with blurring personal identity with professional identity while online (Reamer, 2019), and social work students are not immune to this challenge. Indeed, with the absence of education related to digital ethics, they may lack the background to determine what constitutes ethical online behavior. Although CSWE currently does not require social work programs to include digital ethics content in the curriculum, some social work faculty have begun to develop course assignments to educate their students about ICT and responsible online behavior (Mishna, Tufford, Cook, & Bogo, 2013; Teixeira & Hash, 2017; Young et al., 2018). Providing education on the use of digital ethics in social work should help prepare students for principled online engagement with others, while offering innovative educational experiences based on today's practice realities.

Disclosure statement

No potential conflict of interest was reported by the author.

References

Austin, D. (1997). The institutional development of social work education. *Journal of Social Work Education*, *33*(3), 599–612. doi:10.1080/10437797.1997.10778897

Baker, L. R., & Iverson Hitchcock, L. (2017). Using Pinterest in undergraduate social work education: Assignment development and pilot survey results. *Journal of Social Work Education*, *53*(3), 535–545. doi:10.1080/10437797.2016.1272515

Boddy, J., & Dominelli, L. (2017). Social media and social work: The challenges of a new ethical space. *Australian Social Work*, *70*(2), 172–184. doi:10.1080/0312407X.2016.1224907

Canadian Association of Social Workers. (2005). *CASW code of ethics*. Ottawa, Canada: Author. Retrieved from https://www.casw-acts.ca/sites/default/files/attachements/casw_code_of_ethics_0.pdf

Canadian Association of Social Workers. (2013). *Social media use and social work practice*. Retrieved from http://www.caswacts.ca/sites/default/files/Social%20Media%20Use%20and%20Social%20Work%20Practice.pdf

Chan, C., & Holosko, M. J. (2016). A review of information and communication technology enhanced social work interventions. *Research on Social Work Practice*, *26*(1), 88–100. doi:10.1177/1049731515578884

Crowne, D. P., & Marlowe, D. (1960). A new scale of social desirability independent of psychopathology. *Journal of Consulting Psychology*, *24*(4), 349–354. doi:10.1037/h0047358

D'Cruz, H., Soothill, K., Francis, B., & Christie, A. (2002). Gender, ethics and social work: An international study of students' perceptions at entry into social work education. *International Social Work*, *45*(2), 149–166. doi:10.1177/00208728020450020501

Fang, L., Mishna, F., Zhang, V. F., Van Wert, M., & Bogo, M. (2014). Social media and social work education: Understanding and dealing with the new digital world. *Social Work in Health Care*, *53*, 800–814. doi:10.1080/00981389.2014.943455

Groessl, J. (2015). Teaching note—Conceptualization of a contemporary social work ethics course. *Journal of Social Work Education*, *51*(4), 691–698. doi:10.1080/10437797.2015.1076276

Hitchcock, L. I., & Young, J. A. (2016). Tweet tweet! Using live twitter chats in social work education. *Social Work Education: The International Journal*, *35*(4), 457–468. doi:10.1080/02615479.2015.1136273

Jarman-Rohde, L., McFall, J., Kolar, P., & Strom, G. (1997). The changing context of social work practice. *Journal of Social Work Education*, *33*(1), 29–46. doi:10.1080/10437797.1997.10778851

Karpman, H. E., & Drisko, J. (2016). Social media policy in social work education: A review and recommendations. *Journal of Social Work Education*, *52*(4), 398–408. doi:10.1080/10437797.2016.1202164

Kelly, N., Harpel, T., Fontes, A., Walters, C., & Murphy, J. (2017). An examination of social desirability bias in measures of college students' financial behavior. *College Student Journal*, *51*(1), 115–128. Retrieved from https://www.ingentaconnect.com/content/prin/csj/2017/00000051/00000001/art00013

Knowles, A., & Cooner, T. (2016). International collaborative learning using social media to learn about social work ethics and social media. *Social Work Education*, *35*(3), 260–270. doi:10.1080/02615479.2016.1154662

Kreuger, L. W. (1997). The end of social work. *Journal of Social Work Education, 33*(1), 19–27. doi:10.1080/10437797.1997.10778850

McAuliffe, D., & Nipperess, S. (2017). e-Professionalism and the ethical use of technology in social work. *Australian Social Work, 70*(2), 131–134. doi:10.1080/0312407X.2016.1221790

Mishna, F., Tufford, L., Cook, C., & Bogo, M. (2013). Research note–A pilot cyber counseling course in a graduate social work program. *Journal of Social Work Education, 49*(3), 515–524. doi:10.1080/10437797.2013.796855

NASW. (2017). *National association of social workers code of ethics.* Washington, DC: Author. Retrieved from https://www.socialworkers.org/About/Ethics/Code-of-Ethics.aspx

NASW, ASWB, CSWE, & CSWA. (2017). *Standards for technology in social work practice.* NASW Press. Retrieved from http://www.socialworkers.org/includes/newIncludes/home page/PRA-BRO33617.TechStandards_FINAL_POSTING.pdf

Reamer, F. G. (2017). Evolving ethical standards in the digital age. *Australian Social Work, 70* (2), 148–159. doi:10.1080/0312407X.2016.1146314

Reamer, F. G. (2019). Social work education in a digital world: Technology standards for education and practice. *Journal of Social Work Education,* 1–13. doi:10.1080/ 10437797.2019.1567412

Regan, J. A. C. (2016). Innovators and early adopters of distance education in social work. *Advances in Social Work, 17*(1), 113–115. doi:10.18060/21091

Selingo, J. J. (2016). *2026, the decade ahead: The seismic shifts transforming the future of higher education.* Washington, DC: Chronicle of Higher Education.

Teixeira, S., & Hash, K. M. (2017). Teaching note–tweeting macro practice: Social media in the social work classroom. *Journal of Social Work Education, 53*(4), 751–758. doi:10.1080/ 10437797.2017.1287025

Young, J. A., McLeod, D. A., & Brady, S. R. (2018). The ethics challenge: 21st century social work education, social media, and digital literacies. *The Journal of Social Work Values and Ethics, 15*(1), 13–22. Retrieved from http://jswve.org/download/15-1/15-1-Articles/13-The-Ethics-Challenge-15-1.pdf

Zilberstein, K. (2015). Technology, relationships and culture: Clinical and theoretical implications. *Clinical Social Work Journal, 43*(2), 151–158. doi:10.1007/s10615-013-0461-2

Zur Institute. (2018). *What is digital ethics?: Clinical & ethical considerations.* Retrieved from https://www.zurinstitute.com/clinical-updates/digital-ethics-101/

Globalization or Colonization in Online Education: Opportunity or Oppression?

Melanie Reyes ⓘ and Elizabeth A. Segal

ABSTRACT
A proliferation of student enrollment in online higher education, particularly in social work, may reflect a neoliberal shift from public good to private commodity. Critical theory is an excellent lens to assess whether there has been such a shift. While online higher education represents opportunities for information globalization, consciousness-raising, and social justice, it may also be an instrument of colonization related to profit generation, reliance on market transactions, and power related to discourse. Recommendations made here include targeted student recruitment and accessibility, geographically and culturally grounded knowledge integration, cultivation of market skills and student voice, and intentional outcome measures.

Introduction

More than six million students participate in online courses, educational degrees, and other learning opportunities offered by a variety of educational institutions (Allen & Seaman, 2017). The recent rise of online education creates the possibility of expansion of American higher education structure, knowledge, and influence around the world. With this opportunity comes the responsibility of examining the purpose, accessibility, and delivery of online higher education. Is this proliferation of educational opportunities an asset for those who may in the past not have had access to expanding education globally, or is it a pathway for American hegemony, creating a dominant pedagogy? To better understand this dichotomy, it is helpful to use a theoretical lens that considers such factors as power and influence over national and international debates. Analysis of power imbalances and whether online education is a global breakthrough, or a way of further colonizing and oppressing other cultures, can best be assessed through the lens of critical theory.

History of online education

Throughout the history of the United States and across the globe, access to higher education has been available predominantly to those with the social and economic means to attend courses on a college or university campus. In the United States, there have been efforts over time to expand this limited access to a wider population, starting with the establishment of correspondence programs in the 1870s. Early distance education programs were implemented with the intent of broadening accessibility for those who would not otherwise enroll in higher education. Programs, such as Illinois Wesleyan University, the Society to Encourage Studies at Home, the Correspondence University, and the Chautauqua Literary and Scientific Circle provided a variety of courses and degree opportunities to a student population that included women and other non-traditional college students, namely blue-collar and agricultural workers (Lee, 2017; Portman, 1978).

With criticism emerging from the academic community questioning the standards of correspondence education, some of these programs were closed in the early 1900s while others continued to thrive, including the International Correspondence Schools of Scranton, a for-profit enterprise that by 1920 served a cumulative student population of more than two million individuals. These types of profit-generating educational institutions were viewed by some critics as exploitative with high-pressure recruitment, expensive tuition, inadequate instruction, and often confusing degree completion expectations (Knowles, 1962). Interestingly, in the same time period, there was an emerging trend among universities to develop extension programs as a way to teach classes in communities outside the universities and campuses (Portman, 1978).

As technology advanced in the twentieth century, radio and television joined textbooks as popular delivery platforms for distance education programs (Lee, 2017). In the 1930s and 1940s, support for distance higher education strengthened with federal funding of university correspondence courses for members of the Civilian Conservation Corps and the United States Armed Forces Institute (Portman, 1978). Amidst the public outcry for a well-trained workforce in the 1960s, universities promoted new educational opportunities via independent correspondence courses, with the primary beneficiaries of this accessibility expansion remaining the dominant university student population, as opposed to prospective non-traditional students historically excluded from higher education (Lee, 2017).

Technology advances in the decades leading up to the twenty-first century opened the door to creative pedagogical approaches, including incorporation of the Internet and electronic learning management systems as a means for delivering programs. These advances corresponded with a decline in government financial support for higher education and the concurrent emergence of private business interests in the delivery of online learning (Lee, 2017). With momentum from software development and Internet infrastructure expansion, distance education shifted toward becoming largely digital immersion.

In the early twenty-first century, Massive Open Online Courses (MOOCs) constituted an emerging experimental pedagogical structure intended to weave together open access principles with digitally immersed instruction. These MOOCs were designed to achieve accessibility that had until that time not been possible until digital infrastructure connected global networks; however, student retention became a challenge (Leire, McCormick, Richter, Arnfalk, & Rodhe, 2016). While these MOOCs advanced student learning around the world, operational costs to support these courses decreased significantly (after the initial investment in course design, development, and delivery) due to the practice of repeatedly offering courses without needing to recreate content after the initial investment (Leire et al., 2016). While initially viewed as a revolutionary threat to 85 traditional delivery of higher education due to anticipated challenges related to low course completion rates and the lack of critical thinking, many MOOCs were offered by elite higher education institutions that were otherwise inaccessible to many, and other universities which discounted insurmountable costs of completion certifi-cates (Bennett & Kent, 2017). However, if MOOC students were unable to transition to a degree-granting program, they were not likely to access the social and economic capital that accompanies a college degree. Successful MOOC students reflected the traditional dominant student population able to navigate access, hidden participation costs, and integration into a degree program (Bennett & Kent, 2017).

By 2016, there were 5.8 million students engaged in some form of distance learning, including online education. This represented a 263 percent increase in the number of online students from 2002. Seventy-seven percent of higher learning institutions providing online courses and programs report incorporating online learning into their institutional long-term strategies (Online Learning Consortium, 2017).

The movement of online higher education in social work

The Council on Social Work Education, the accrediting body for social work programs, reports that there are 27 undergraduate and 78 graduate accredited social work programs that are currently offered in some version of online, distance, or hybrid format in the United States (CSWE, 2019). Of these accredited programs, approximately 19 percent offer a Master of Social Work and 24 percent offer a Bachelor of Social Work as an entirely online degree option. Meanwhile, partial and hybrid options are available in nearly 35 percent of graduate and 32 percent of undergraduate accredited programs (CSWE, 2018). Research shows that students who enroll in online programs are disproportionally nontraditional, socially disempowered, and isolated, as opposed to traditional students who tend to be younger, recent high school graduates who can afford attending college full time and in person. To these students, higher education represents a valuable cultural currency that paves the way to employment opportunities that may previously have been unobtainable (Chick & Hassel, 2009). The growth in online alternatives in social work, therefore, can be seen in part as an attempt to create pathways to the profession for nontraditional students.

Critical theory as a framework for analysis

Rooted in the interpretive work of Marxism conducted by Horkheimer and the Frankfurt School, critical social science emerged from the influence of ideologies studied by Max Weber, Sigmund Freud and Friedrich Nietzsche combined with tenets from feminism, postmodernism, and social constructionism (Bentz & Shapiro, 1998; Payne, 2014). Through the analysis of complex structures of power, critical theory provides a philosophical, political, and social lens to examine and critique social institutions, societal disparities, and oppressive systems to identify internal contradictions between policy and practice and to better impact change (Bentz & Shapiro, 1998; Cimino, 2015; Rexhepi & Torres, 2011). Because dominant institutions and structures maintain power through the persistent acceptance of cultural and societal norms supported by the ruling hegemony, investigation of these norms is essential within the complex context of class, race, ethnicity, gender, and other differences of the human experience (Payne, 2014; Rexhepi & Torres, 2011). Critical theory is an excellent lens through which the impact of interventions, in this case, higher education disseminated widely through online learning, may be assessed in light of who holds power and who does not.

In addition, critical theory provides the foundation for raising consciousness through praxis and conscientization to support people in determining and taking reflective action to change systems of oppression and inequality, resulting in the expansion of freedom and justice vital for cultural emancipation (Bentz & Shapiro, 1998; Freire, 1973; Payne, 2014). This perspective is attuned to social work values and professional commitment, which further reinforces the value of using a critical theory lens to consider the potential strengths and weaknesses of providing social work education through the medium of online learning (Moya-Salas, Sen, & Segal, 2010). The power of reflection moves forward the integration process for individuals and communities, and combats the emergence of dissonance, while building social responsibility and community engagement. In higher education, key components include active participant observation, as well as educator–learner interactions that encompass dialogue, choice, and reciprocity (Freire, 1973).

The shift in higher education from public good to commodity

A key shift in the power balance in society (and thus in higher education) over the past several decades has been the strengthening of neoliberal trends in the economy, including the free market, globalization, deregulation, and restructuring of institutional systems to meet the perceived needs of student consumers (Nerad, June, & Miller, 1997; Payne, 2014). Neoliberalism relies on a cost-benefit analysis that evaluates the benefits of investment returns to society and considers higher education to be a personal choice to develop skills and knowledge to meet the demands of employers (Hensley, Galilee-Belfer, & Lee, 2013).

Prior to the influence of neoliberalism, higher education was viewed as a public good which benefited society overall. Public funding and support were perceived as investments in future financial and mobility currency stemming from higher salaries and revenues consistent with an educated workforce (Hensley et al., 2013). As neoliberalism has extended into education, public opinion increasingly has viewed higher education institutions as incapable of incorporating cost-savings measures without resulting in a substantial impact on the quality of education (Baum, Kurose, & McPherson, 2013; Rexhepi & Torres, 2011). Within this context, online education may be a revenue-generating opportunity when viewed from a business model perspective that defines higher education transactions as profit-based, and therefore may be quantified as dollars, as opposed to the softer measure of public good.

Accompanying the shift toward neoliberalism has been the growing perception that higher education primarily benefits the private individual; therefore, public funding cuts over recent decades have purposefully shifted the cost of higher education to the individual student while state appropriations for higher education have evolved as uncertain and unstable (Hensley et al., 2013). At the same time, higher education tuition has exceed inflation increases over the past several decades, leaving students more reliant on tuition discounts and financial aid (Baum et al., 2013; Kvaal & Bridgeland, 2018). These new realities are complicated by federal funding formulas for higher education institutions being based on student enrollment, as opposed to course completion or rates of graduation (Bridgeland & Kvaal, 2018). This rise in tuition, motivation of higher education institutions to enroll greater numbers of students, and decrease in support for higher education as a public good increasingly put much pressure and responsibility on the individual student.

Higher education costs are impacted by expenses incurred with the delivery of online education, including the implementation of technology, provision of remedial courses for students who are under prepared but have access to higher education, enactment of new governmental regulations, and presence of increased marketing and recruitment efforts to compete for students beyond the traditional borders of the university. Higher education institutions today increasingly tend to employ contractual part-time adjunct faculty, thereby avoiding hiring and employment costs present with tenure-track faculty. Notably, from 1970 to 2007, during the time frame associated with the shift to neoliberalism, the average percentage of full-time faculty decreased from 80 to 51.3 percent in institutions of higher education (Baum et al., 2013).

With the transition to neoliberal efficiency, online courses are viewed as advantageous because they tend to be developed in a universal structure conducive to the attainment of employment skills while being delivered in a consistent manner by different, often part-time, instructors. While this is a highly cost effective strategy, the technology underlying online courses does not automatically accommodate the needs of students with diverse learning styles without significant changes that would require the new allocation of resources. The highly structured learning present in digitally immersed courses also may not be conducive to supporting critical thinking, free inquiry, or an integrated emphasis on cognitive development and a learning process.

Opportunity or oppression?

When examining online education and associated power dynamics through the lens of critical theory, it is possible to analyze whether such education presents as an opportunity for globalization or reenacts oppressive colonization. This debate calls for a critique of the impact and dominance of technology, the development of critical thinking and cognitive skills, the cultivation of social justice, the goals of higher education as a profit-generating commodity, the transactional nature of online education, and power dynamics related to discourse.

Online education as an opportunity

Online higher education presents several opportunities related to globalization. The geographic reach of distance education allows for knowledge to be disseminated around the world, thereby facilitating networking and resource sharing on a previously unparalleled level. As global discourse occurs in an online education environment, consciousness-raising may emerge to lay the groundwork for the promotion of social justice.

Opportunities for globalization of information

With institutions of higher education investing in global partnerships with other educational and business enterprises, the possibilities for the growth of scientific and professional knowledge, as well as the sharing of resources, are unparalleled. Over the past several decades, technological innovations (such as the Internet) have facilitated communication and networking, with a direct impact on professional connections being initiated and strengthened on both community and global levels. Around the world, students and instructors engage in educational transactions that bring together ideas, knowledge, and experiences of unique cultures and many nations.

Such globalization of information sharing has a direct impact on online education delivery. Opportunities include increased networking and professionalism, broad discourse and the development of critical consciousness, and the advancement of social justice through access to local and global opportunities. However, technological advancements have been rapid and complex; students must have access to the relevant technologies and infrastructure, as well as the skills required to take advantage of them.

Opportunities for consciousness-raising

Research shows that higher education degree completion not only benefits the economy as a public good in the form of enhanced income from taxes, improved health, happiness, and civic engagement but also through the emergence of innovative ideas and the building of tolerance for diversity (Hensley et al., 2013). Opening an educational dialogue on national and international levels is a powerful move toward consciousness-raising, and higher education institutions are positioned to promote a call to action through support of praxis, discourse, and conscientization. As diverse cultures and communities engage in the educational opportunities presented through the globalization of online learning, systems of oppression may be identified as targets for change in order to achieve greater equality. As noted by Freire (1973), this may create an opportunity for disadvantaged populations to build community responsibility and engagement.

Opportunities for increasing social justice

In higher education, promoting social justice is at the heart of expanding access to advanced educational programs for nontraditional college student populations, including women and students from marginalized communities. In fact, Kurzman (2013) advances that online higher education has a "quintessentially democratic spirit" (p. 335), which allows more students to pursue higher education. It creates opportunities for those who would not otherwise have the chance to pursue higher education to expand their understanding of social conditions and thereby raise their levels of awareness. Such consciousness is an essential means of acquiring the tools to succeed in local and global economies and social structures. In this educational environment, technology may be harnessed to incubate ideas to alleviate poverty, separation, and oppression.

Online education as an instrument of colonization

While online higher education offers opportunities for globalization, it also opens the door to be an instrument of colonization through the promotion of profit-making enterprises, an emphasis on transactions instead of transformative development, and increasing the present power imbalance between institutions and students.

The oppressive nature of the profit-making elements

The prioritization of higher education delivery in a format that maximizes the generation of operations revenue is in fundamental conflict with the categorization of higher education as a public good, capable of opening opportunities for oppressed populations, and the social justice notion of universal accessibility. Reamer (2013) specifically calls for social work to attend to the ethics of online education, and for program decisions to be "a matter of conscience not revenue," (p. 381). Lee (2017) asserts that the development of online education does not directly equate open access to higher education because accessibility is much more complex than simply offering digitally immersed courses. Students must have the relevant technological tools, knowledge, and skills to succeed in an online environment, and their communities need to provide and support the global networking infrastructure that serves as a foundation for the technology. In order to determine if accessibility is globally broadening, it is crucial to examine whether higher education is being expanded to new student populations or simply giving greater choice and opportunities to those who already have access.

Concerns regarding higher education trends include the technocracy that represents the movement toward business models of education through the hiring of part-time consultants to teach and the propagation of positivist thinking that centers on value-free research separate from politics (Rexhepi & Torres, 2011). This distinction is important when evaluating whether digitally immersed programs are delivering the same content and quality education as campus-based programs. An additional consideration is if quality instruction is consistent in both campus and online programs when online instructors are primarily part-time adjunct faculty, as opposed to tenure-track faculty immersed in academic service and research. The extension of a perceived lower quality education through digital immersion may create a second-class category of students.

Higher education as a transaction, not as intellectual growth

Digital immersion requires a different level of metacognition, and students who do well in the online learning environment typically possess a high level of academic skill and cultural capital and have access to many resources, including technology, cultural support, self-regulation, motivation, time, and financial resources (Bennett & Kent, 2017; Lee, 2017). The data show that there are higher dropout rates associated with online learning than campus-based educational program (Lee, 2017). Moreover, in the current higher education culture that is influenced by neoliberalism, the opportunity for critical inquiry is in danger of not being realized, resulting in education being viewed solely as the ticket to job entry and advancement, as opposed to the opportunity for conscientization. Hence, students enrolled in these online programs may be more motivated by the perceived transactional value of the degree in the marketplace, as opposed to the educational value of the degree. Through higher education, however, students should be advancing in their cognitive development to become deeper, more critical thinkers and not simply conforming to the ideas presented to them in their coursework. This process of cognitive development relies on dialogue that supports the exposure to rich language, introducing new concepts, and promoting critical inquiry that may be absent in the digitally immersed classroom environment.

Replicating colonization: providers dictate the discourse

There is a distinct power imbalance in higher education on several levels. From a macro perspective, this power dynamic reflects neoliberalism in the current culture, with economic forces increasingly at the heart of higher education decisions. The cost-benefit prioritization of institutional leadership may result in the prioritization of financial goals toward propelling the delivery of academic programs in the digitally immersed environment. Nonetheless, faculty may resist the trend to move higher education programs to online formats as negatively impacting the quality and rigor of instruction. A reality, of course, is that providers of higher education possess the bulk of the power in the transactional relationships with the student learners. The institutions oversee the development of the courses and curriculum, while students are limited to controlled participation in the prepared classroom environment.

With the expansion of online higher education beyond the borders of the United States into the global student market, there has been an accompanying proliferation of American-centric ideas distributed through the common distance education models. This fact becomes important given that the 50 higher education institutions which have the largest student fully online enrollments host 38.4 percent of the total student population that enrolls solely in online courses. Of these 50 institutions, 14 are private nonprofit, and 17 are public (Seaman, Allen, & Seaman, 2018). The remaining 19 are private for-profit institutions and they currently educate 48.8 percent of the solely online students. Furthermore, in the global online education market, only seven institutions in the United States have distance enrollment of more than a thousand international students, with only one university serving more than five thousand students online globally (Seaman et al., 2018). With such a small number of higher educational organizations providing the online pedagogy to a large percentage of students, these institutions wield a virtual monopoly on curriculum delivered, both domestically and internationally, to nontraditional students who are likely less advantaged and more marginalized.

At risk are diverse approaches to learning, indigenous ways of teaching, and unique perspectives on how knowledge is transmitted and received within different cultures. Because technology design and development accelerate exponentially, countries which have fewer resources, infrastructure, and knowledge base become set in the role of education consumers, and those countries which have greater technology resources continue to benefit as the producers and deliverers of higher education on a global level. This producer–consumer relationship increases dependency upon Western approaches to higher education and further promotes a growing power differential among nations and cultures.

Recommendations

Critical theory can assist in the assessment of higher education, to challenge the existing structure through examination of the purpose and values of online higher education and promoting the commitment to a supportive relationship between educators and learners in the development of a critically transitive global consciousness. This pursuit is particularly important for social work education. The profession's educational competency commitment "to ensure that social goods, rights, and responsibilities are distributed equitably and that civil, political, environmental, economic, social and cultural human rights are protected" (CSWE, 2015, p. 7) applies to all our educational efforts, including online learning. Our delivery of higher education is a social good, and therefore we must ensure that it is done in a manner consistent with our professional commitment to social justice, one of the core values that comprise the foundation of our profession (National Association of Social Workers [NASW], 2017). Equally as important is the expansion of student capacity for choice and the creation of accurate and meaningful options for learning in order to avoid a degree of colonization (Freire, 1973). We believe all of these outcomes may be supported and achieved through the integral components of online education.

Student recruitment and accessibility

There are multiple challenges when addressing the structure of online higher education. Recruitment efforts must target diverse, nontraditional populations as opposed to focusing primarily on the dominant mainstream student community. This prospective cohort may be first-generation students in higher education, those from a working or lower socio-economic class, and students living in developing countries (Bennett & Kent, 2017). In the opening of accessibility to higher education, colleges cannot solely rely on standard online course structure and delivery to meet the needs of students who may not have had prior access. Nontraditional students may need support in navigating the American system of higher education (Bennett & Kent, 2017). Unique partnerships with communities, such as Native American tribes and refugee enclaves, could promote accessibility by removing barriers to higher education that will enable cohorts of students to study together in digitally immersed environments in a way that is culturally syntonic and without a presence of colonization.

Geographically and culturally grounded knowledge integration

The needs of the students should drive the design and delivery of online programs via a bottom-up approach that incorporates personalized educational delivery (Lee, 2017). Rexhepi and Torres (2011) argue that academic rigor in knowledge acquisition and expansion is connected with the ability to engage and affect change on a local and global stage. The instructor–student relationship must incorporate the delivery of strong research-based knowledge, grounded in both experience and rich interaction to promote integration into the students' understanding. This means that knowledge relevant to students (based on their geographic and cultural place) may be more important than the top-down approach of classic higher education models that tell students what they need to know.

Market skills and student voice

In this neoliberal era, students should maintain an awareness of the need to incorporate skills for the marketplace while also achieving critical thinking development and the discovery of voice that are so vital to active civic engagement. In this context, it is time to carefully analyze whose voice is being cultivated through the delivery of online education to ensure the reflection and representation of the student's culturally and historically specific human experience. Such personalization will allow for active participation in coursework and the integration of concepts into the student learner's expertise. Without the student voice being secured as central, online higher education could be on the brink of appearing to cultivate Western thought and institutions as dominant in online delivery in a manner more reflective of colonization.

Outcome measures

As opposed to focusing on the collection of outcome statistics related to the number of students enrolled and graduating, a more accurate measure of student learning achievement and civic engagement is needed as outcome documentation that includes but goes well beyond measuring preparation to enter the marketplace (Bridgeland & Kvaal, 2018). These outcome measures would assure cognitive development and personal growth in students. Giving students a seat at the table in planning these higher education outcomes will allow for the interweaving of student cultural and academic needs with institutional requirements for accountability and efficiency.

Conclusion

By and large, online higher education programs present an opportunity for quality academic transactions to occur both in the global setting and our domestic educational system. Nevertheless, attention must be paid to resolving challenges stemming from present neoliberal trends in higher education to avoid historic tendencies toward colonization. Only via analysis through a critical inquiry lens, and the incorporation of a conceptual framework that ensures operation of social goods and social justice competencies, may online social work education be poised to achieve globalization, as opposed to the promotion of colonization through neoliberal approaches to higher education.

Disclosure statement

No potential conflict of interest was reported by the authors.

ORCID

Melanie Reyes ⓘ http://orcid.org/0000-0003-3282-6117

References

Allen, I. E., & Seaman, J. (2017). *Digital learning compass: Distance education enrollment report 2017*. Retrieved from the Babson Survey Research Group website: https://www.onlinelearningsurvey.com/reports/digtiallearningcompassenrollment2017.pdf

Baum, S., Kurose, C., & McPherson, M. (2013). An overview of American higher education. *The Future of Children, 23*(1), 17–39.

Bennett, R., & Kent, M. (2017). Any colour as long as it's black! MOOCs, (post)-Fordism and inequality. In R. Bennett & M. Kent (Eds.), *Massive open online courses and higher education: What went right, what went wrong and what next?* Chapter 2 (pp. 11–25). New York, NY: Routledge.

Bentz, V. M., & Shapiro, J. J. (1998). *Mindful inquiry in social research*. Thousand Oaks, CA: Sage.

Bridgeland, J., & Kvaal, J. (2018). We can help more college students graduate – At lower cost. *The Hill*. Retrieved from http://thehill.com/opinion/education/368500-we-can-help-more-college-students-graduate-at-lower-cost

Chick, N., & Hassel, H. (2009). Don't hate me because i'm virtual: Feminist pedagogy in the online classroom. *Feminist Teacher, 19*(3), 195–215. doi:10.1353/ftr.0.0049

Cimino, A. (2015). Feminist and critical theories. In C. L. Langer & C. A. Lietz (Eds.), *Applying theory to generalist social work practice: A case study approach* Chapter 13 (pp. 245–271). Hoboken, NJ: Wiley.

CSWE. (2018). *2017 statistics on social work education in the United States: Appendix*. Retrieved from https://www.cswe.org/CMSPages/GetFile.aspx?guid=190ec3c2-1163-46bb-b0c3-717bd8434572

CSWE. (2019, January 25). *Online and distance education: Online and distance education offerings by accredited programs [Website]*. Retrieved from https://www.cswe.org/Accreditation/Directory-of-Accredited-Programs/Online-and-Distance-Education

CSWE Commission on Educational Policy and the CSWE Commission on Accreditation. (2015). *2015 education policy and accreditation standards for baccalaureate and master's social work programs [CSWE]*. Council on Social Work Education.

Freire, P. (1973). *Education for critical consciousness*. New York, NY: Continuum Publishing Company.

Hensley, B., Galilee-Belfer, M., & Lee, J. J. (2013). What is the greater good? The discourse on public and private roles of higher education in the new economy. *Journal of Higher Education Policy and Management, 35*(5), 553–567. doi:10.1080/1360080X.2013.825416

Knowles, M. S. (1962). *The adult education movement in the United States*. New York, NY: Rinehart and Winston.

Kurzman, P. A. (2013). The evolution of distance learning and online education. *Journal of Teaching in Social Work, 33*(4/5), 331–338. doi:10.1080/08841233.2013.843346

Kvaal, J., & Bridgeland, J. (2018). Moneyball for higher education: How federal leaders can use data and evidence to improve student outcomes. *Results for America.* Retrieved from https://results4america.org/tools/moneyball-higher-education-federal-leaders-can-use-data-evidence-improve-student-outcomes/

Lee, K. (2017). Rethinking the accessibility of online higher education: A historical review. *Internet and Higher Education, 33*, 15–23. Retrieved from https://www-sciencedirect-com.ezproxy1.lib.asu.edu/journal/the-internet-and-higher-education/vol/33/suppl/C

Leire, C., McCormick, K., Richter, J. L., Arnfalk, P., & Rodhe, H. (2016). Online teaching going massive: Input and outcomes. *Journal of Cleaner Production, 123*, 230–233. doi:10.1016/j.jclepro.2015.12.014

Moya-Salas, L., Sen, S., & Segal, E. A. (2010). Critical theory: Pathway from dichotomous to integrated social work practice. *Families in Society: the Journal of Contemporary Social Sciences, 91*(1), 91–96. doi:10.1606/1044-3894.3961

National Association of Social Workers (NASW). (2017). *Preamble to the code of ethics.* Retrieved from https://www.socialworkers.org/About/Ethics/Code-of-Ethics

Nerad, M., June, R., & Miller, D. S. (1997). Volume introduction. In M. Nerad, R. June, & D. S. Miller (Eds.), *Graduate education in the United States volume introduction* (pp. vii–xiv). New York, NY: Garland Publishing.

Online Learning Consortium. (2017). *2016 higher education online learning landscape* [Infographic]. Retrieved from https://onlinelearningconsortium.org/read/olc-infographic-higher-education-online-learning-landscape/

Payne, M. (2014). *Modern social work theory* (4th ed.). Chicago, IL: Lyceum Books.

Portman, D. N. (1978). *The universities and the public: A history of higher adult education in the United States.* Chicago, IL: Nelson-Hall.

Reamer, F. G. (2013). Distance and online social work education: Novel ethical challenges. *Journal of Teaching in Social Work, 33*(4/5), 369–384. doi:10.1080/08841233.2013.828669

Rexhepi, J., & Torres, C. A. (2011). Reimagining critical theory. *British Journal of Sociology Education, 32*(5), 679–698. doi:10.1080/01425692.2011.596363

Seaman, J. E., Allen, I. E., & Seaman, J. (2018). *Grade increase: Tracking distance education in the United States.* Retrieved from the Babson Survey Research Group website: https://www.onlinelearningsurvey.com/highered.html

Diversity and Difference in the Online Environment

Jeanna Jacobsen

ABSTRACT

The online environment challenges social work educators in their approach to developing students' cultural awareness and culturally competent skills. To develop student competencies, it is important for accredited social work programs to consider both their explicit and implicit curricula. Although research has focused on the influence of multicultural classrooms and engaging diverse students, scant literature has been focused on teaching about diversity and difference in the online environment. This article hopes to fill this gap in knowledge by providing recommendations for social work programs to consider as they look to teach diversity and difference in the online environment.

Online social work programs face challenges in teaching diversity and ensuring students develop cultural awareness and culturally competent skills. To address these challenges, accredited social work programs need to assess their ability to develop student competency to *engage diversity and difference in practice* and *advance human rights and social, economic, and environmental justice* by evaluating their curricula (Council on Social Work Education [CSWE], 2015). This article discusses considerations related to diversity in the virtual world and how the online environment affects the experience of difference. Recommendations in this article are based on literature and practice experiences in an online social work program.

Background

Online education continues to grow throughout higher education, minimizing some barriers but introducing new challenges. It can provide accessibility to students with disabilities, working adults, and individuals in faraway geographic locations who would otherwise not be able to pursue a social work education. Distance education also has the benefit of bringing diverse students together such as students in remote or rural areas, minorities, and nontraditional students who might not otherwise have an opportunity to pursue graduate education (Quinn & Barth, 2014; Schwartz, Wiley, & Kaplan, 2016). However, online education also introduces challenges expressed through workload demands on both students and instructors, access to bandwidth to connect to online courses and tech support resources, and opportunities to engage in events and to build relationships essential to challenging personal bias (Smith, Jeffery, & Collins, 2018). Further, though diversity affects the learning environment – and is inherent to the online classroom because it attracts learners from various geographic settings and different social/cultural groups (Schwartz et al., 2016) – such diversity is not necessarily a central topic of the learning environment.

Although literature shows the influence of leading multicultural classrooms, designing inclusive classrooms, and engaging diverse students (McLoughlin, 2001), there is little written on teaching about diversity and difference in the online environment. However, one of the few studies on this topic showed no significant difference in pre- and post-test measures of competency to engage in diversity between students who took a diversity course online versus face-to-face (Stauss, Koh, & Collie, 2018), suggesting that concepts and skills related to diversity can be taught in an online environment. But engaging in discussion about diversity is already difficult, and the online environment may lead to additional barriers to engagement because some students experience defensiveness as they challenge their own privilege (Gayles, Kelly, Grays, Zhang, & Porter, 2015). To successfully engage students, faculty need to create an environment for difficult dialogs, perceive students as coproducers of knowledge, recognize student dissonance, and address instructor positionality (Gayles et al., 2015). Doing so in an online setting requires programs to consider curriculum design related to resources, discussions, assignments, faculty facilitation, and online presence. Before building such a curriculum, programs need to consider how to approach design through cultural awareness and sensitivity.

Cultural humility in curriculum design

Approaching social work curriculum design with cultural humility involves developing student skills related to cultural awareness and sensitivity while having them retain a humble attitude about their self-assessment of cultural understanding. Cultural humility places the social worker as learner and clients as experts in their own experience, rather than expecting practitioner mastery of cultural knowledge (Sue, Sue, Neville, & Smith, 2019). In addition, cultural humility addresses oppressive social structures within social systems and how these structures influence experience (Fisher-Borne, Cain, & Martin, 2015). Teaching social work students to utilize cultural humility further includes social work instructors demonstrating and modeling cultural humility. Designing learning opportunities for diversity and difference requires social work faculty to reflect on their own positionality and consciously step into teachable moments. It is important as well to consider the intersectionality of the student population whose diverse social identities both bring them to online learning and may equip them with expertize beyond textbook descriptions.

Social work instructors can build on the multiculturally diverse classroom to create an effective learning community in which to teach about diversity and social justice. Yet building community in the online environment requires more effort than required in a face-to-face classroom in order to engage students and make connections among individuals behind a computer (Farrel et al., 2018; Schwartz et al., 2016). Social work faculty therefore must create an online learning community both at the individual class and programmatic level. Within an accredited educational program, this goal requires consideration of both the explicit and implicit curriculum.

Explicit curriculum

The explicit curriculum includes the courses offered, resources provided, and requirements of the coursework (CSWE, 2015). Some programs have a course focused on aspects of diversity, but programs should also consider how diversity is interwoven through the entire curriculum which may require larger program oversight to monitor and maintain aspects of diversity, ensuring representation, for example, of sexually and gender diverse populations (Craig, Iacono, Paceley, Dentato, & Boyle, 2017; Mclnroy, Craig, & Austin, 2014), religious and spiritual diversity (Oxhandler & Giardina, 2017), and respect for indigenous peoples (Nedegaard, Barkdull, Weber, & Jayasundara, 2018), to name a few underrepresented populations. A well-designed explicit curriculum will consider representation (i.e., who is present and how are they depicted) of diverse social identities, for instance, in case studies assigned to students. Online programs may have a better capacity to ensure representativeness because the courses are often predesigned, which ensures a consistent delivery of content, rather than variations dependent on the idiosyncrasies of an instructor. In addition to representation, the explicit curriculum includes forms of learning activities and classroom interaction. Activities, such as experiential learning, provide rich engagement with diversity and difference that may lead to deep learning. Similarly, enhancing classroom interaction through video and active discussion can make visible the diversity that already exists within the classroom. The next sections of this paper will expand on representation, experiential activities, and classroom interaction as essential components of explicit curriculum.

Representations of diversity

Social work programs work to ensure that their curricula represent a diversity of voices, images, and perspectives. Accurate representation signals to students of diverse identities acceptance of their characteristics within the social work profession and confidence that students enrolled in the program can be trained to work competently with diverse groups. But, if a program only relies on text-based resources, important aspects of diversity may be diminished because students often do not "see" difference in written formats.

Social work programs may consider using video, podcasts, and other media to present both visual and auditory diversity in the classroom, in addition to difference of experience. However, the ability to integrate media may depend in part on copyright issues and a program's financial ability to pay for content. Although some colleges and universities have legal or media personnel to review content recommendations, not all social work programs have access to these resources. Instead, utilizing media through the program's institutional library, and free online resources such as TedTalks (https://www.ted.com/talks) or StoryCorps (https://storycorps.org/), can be used to find appropriate resources, although this takes time.

Resource accessibility also needs to be considered to ensure that the program not only is representing diversity, but also ensuring that those resources can be accessed by students with diverse abilities. Many videos available on social media sites use automated closed-captioning, which is never 100% accurate. Addressing accessibility does more than fulfill the Americans with Disability Act requirements in an education setting; it also models expectations for accessibility in social work practice.

It is important as well for social work programs to consider how to ensure that their diversity content remains up-to-date. Conscious instructional design can create coursework that promotes learning while being flexible within a predesigned curriculum. For example, aspects of diversity become more or less salient due to their sociohistorical context. Current events focus on different groups or social problems disproportionately affecting a specific minority population. An online course may be designed during the height of a social event and may emphasize experiences that resonate with current national dialog (e.g., Katrina, #Metoo movement). However, as social movements shift or different communities are impacted by new disasters, prominence of diverse identities shift as well, and curriculum therefore needs to be designed with this in mind.

Experiential activities

Engaging students in the classroom is an additional challenge to teaching diversity online. It is important for courses to create opportunities for experiential learning rather than merely relying on read-and-write responses. Experiential exercises frequently offer enhanced learning about diversity and difference (Ando, 2017; Deepak & Rountree, 2015; Nilson, 2016). Research on teaching methods suggests that having contact with diverse individuals, in addition to teaching anti-racist practices, may be important in developing a variety of culturally competent skills (Stough-Hunter, Guinan, & Hart, 2016).

Designing experiential activities often means entering a virtual world, or asking students to engage in their local community for an experience and return to report. Virtual experiential activities may include the use of avatars (Lee, 2014), virtual worlds such as Second Life (Reinsmith-Jones, Kibbe, Crayton, & Campbell, 2015), and deployment of virtual reality (Blakeman, 2018). Virtual worlds provide simulated experiences that allow social work practice in a physically safe and accessible online environment prior to working in the field. At the same time, online virtual worlds may reinforce stereotyping in the characterization of avatars. Nonetheless, virtual worlds may provide students with culturally appropriate knowledge and skills, but it may be costly, or require a level of technical skill that challenges faculty or students with less technical ability. However, by mastering these challenges in advance, technology can be used to expand student access to diverse experiences that they otherwise would not have.

Naturally, the benefit of asking students to experience events in their community is that they will learn more about the community within which they will most likely continue to work upon graduation. Yet, students may have limited opportunities in rural areas, or time constraints, as a working adult learner, or a family care provider, which is the reason many students choose online education in the first place. Instructors also may have difficulty motivating students to plan ahead, since these types of assignments require time for finding an appropriate event and producing a high-quality report. It may also be more challenging for an instructor to help a student find an activity that meets expected guidelines of an assignment because students are in different geographical areas. To address these barriers, instructors can attempt to engage students early and often in thinking about and looking toward an experiential assignment.

Classroom interaction

Classroom interaction, of course, is an important part of the explicit curriculum as it relates to how students demonstrate the knowledge, values, skills, and cognitive/affective processes they are gaining. Many programs rely on written responses, such as essays, reflection papers, or discussion posts, but these avenues do not allow demonstration of learning through other student strengths such as oral presentation or skill demonstration. One option in the online environment is the use of videos which can be deployed to record presentations, role-plays, or student collaborations. Video can be used both for assignments and asynchronous discussions (see, Clark, Strudler, & Grove, 2015). Video recording offers opportunities for diverse learners to demonstrate their strengths and provides access to simulated practice evaluation that cannot be replicated in a written response. It also permits instructors to assess behavioral or nonverbal skills that are difficult to convey through writing. In addition, video may allow increased interaction, as students present more of themselves in the classroom. However, video recording may also bring up issues related to personal trauma or religious objections. For this reason, online programs should consider how to address student concerns; the purpose of video recording; and if some form of alternative assignment could meet the learning objective.

Another part of classroom interaction for online programs is virtual discussion, whether asynchronous on a discussion board, or synchronous in tele- or video-conference. There are pros and cons to each approach (Watts, 2016). Synchronous video conferences allow for exchanges most similar to those in face-to-face settings, whereas asynchronous discussions permit them to communicate in their own time, and with opportunities to reflect and formulate responses. Regardless of the discussion design, it is important for social work educators to facilitate the online discussion. Given the greater body of knowledge of facilitating synchronous discussions, this article focuses primarily on asynchronous discussion posted on the classroom discussion forum.

Facilitating asynchronous online discussions

Facilitating online discussions may enhance the explicit curriculum through implementation of active teaching strategies. On the other hand, passive facilitation can lead to an implicit curriculum where students do not feel supported in their diverse identities or feel safe disclosing these identities in the virtual classroom. This observation is important because the social work profession is committed to serving vulnerable populations and seeking social justice for those who may be oppressed, including clients with diverse identities (National Association of Social Workers [NASW], 2017). As students develop their understanding of the social forces of oppression, they may experience (a) cognitive dissonance as they challenge previously unexamined personal bias; (b) defensiveness at feelings of personal accusation (whether directed toward themselves as students or at the concept of privilege); (c) guilt or shame related to place within institutional systems of oppression, and possible unearned privilege; and (d) anger at others (including classmates or facilitators) about being formerly "unaware." In addition to the individual process, differential awareness and understanding among classmates in the same course may lead to miscommunication or activation of potential triggers. In fact, as students process material, they may share biased or stereotypical beliefs. This is more likely to occur if the classroom is treated as an online public forum in which students respond to discussions with opinions or personal beliefs, rather than with an appropriate academic debate. For example, students may share that they don't believe in "the gay lifestyle," refer to undocumented immigrants as "aliens" or "illegals," or support their comments with references to their religious leader. These types of comments or attitudes, of course, may similarly be displayed in the face-to-face classroom; however, the dynamics shift online when the interaction is not occurring in real time. When these issues occur in a learning environment, it is the role of the facilitator to ensure that all students have a safe space to engage in reflection and dialogue.

Online instructors can build a climate of mutual respect here by establishing guidelines and group norms at the start of the course, just as they would in a face-to-face classroom. The expectations of interaction can be normed through the social work Code of Ethics that provides guidelines to ensure professionalism and respect toward colleagues (NASW, 2017). Additionally, students appreciate quality instruction (Secret, Bentley, & Kadolph, 2016), which supports instructors providing response posts that indorse critical reflection. Hence, faculty who make minimal or unsubstantial posts do not facilitate the discussion or model the behavior that they are expecting from students.

Classroom presence

Faculty need to maintain a presence in the class (Bentley, Secret, & Cummings, 2015). An asynchronous class means that students can participate at any time on any day. Although it naturally is not expected for the instructor to be in the classroom 24/7, it is important for them to check in on class discussions often. Allowing several days between check-ins could create a situation where a student comment has created toxic interactions between students. At the same time, an instructor must find a balance between responding to every student immediately and allowing them the freedom to respond. This may mean flagging a comment and returning in a day or two to see if another student has responded. If not, the instructor should provide an appropriate response. Alternatively, an instructor may want to make a preliminary reply asking others to comment before returning later with a more thorough response. This allows students to know their instructor is present in the conversation.

Talking about diversity is difficult and can be both uncomfortable and challenging (Constantine & Sue, 2005). Students may respond based on their emotions, which remain present in the discussion even if a post goes unacknowledged in further replies. Acknowledging emotions opens the door to further discuss diverse perspectives. For instance, the instructor may wish to be the first to challenge bias and misconception before allowing students to challenge one another. Allowing a biased statement to go unaddressed may create an implicit approval of what was said. Further, not all students will feel comfortable challenging their peers or telling the instructor that they have been hurt by a comment. Moreover, a student who holds an underrepresented group identity should not be the only one to challenge bias or present diverse perspectives (Constantine & Sue, 2005;

Craig et al., 2017; Hubain, Allen, Harris, & Linder, 2016). Faculty have power to set the standard in the classroom in respecting diverse groups, which is how they demonstrate being advocates and allies to others.

Part of an instructor's presence in addressing bias involves considering how they might respond to inappropriate comments made in an online discussion. Taking a culturally humble approach, instructors may assume that students are working from their current place of knowledge and awareness. When appropriate, faculty can provide guidance via a direct reply to a specific post, a general comment, end of week summary post in the discussion board, or through a class announcement. These methods will allow the entire class to benefit and learn. Depending on how offensive a comment is, it is important that a direct statement is made on the discussion board, reminding students of the ground rules for safe space and expectations for respectful interaction. In rare situations, an instructor may consider editing or deleting a post. Deleting a student's post is better done after deliberation with regard to potential harms – both in censoring a comment and harm to others in being exposed to the offending post. If the decision is to alter the post in any way, the instructor can contact the student as appropriate to explain why the post was edited or removed. In addition, the instructor should consider providing further feedback to the offending student privately when grading the discussion.

Grading

Grading discussions or assignments related to diversity content can be challenging, as students may feel penalized because the instructor simply disagreed with their opinions. Feedback should address the challenge through acknowledgment of student strengths and specific feedback about how students can develop knowledge, values, skills, and cognitive processes related to appropriately engaging in diversity and difference.

Implicit curriculum

Designing an implicit curriculum requires creating culture and community in an online environment. A diverse student and faculty body bring multicultural expectations to an online environment, which adds an additional layer of culture. Cultural rules governing online behavior (e.g., not using all CAPS to indicate yelling or emojis that may be construed as culturally insensitive) can mitigate misunderstandings about tone and intent when students or faculty have not learned online culture through other Internet interactions. The implicit curriculum is developed within this larger virtual milieu.

Implicit curriculum is defined as "the learning environment in which the explicit curriculum is presented" and includes "the program's commitment to diversity" (CSWE, 2015, p. 12). Creating an implicit curriculum for diversity and difference involves social work educators making multiformity visible in the classroom. The instructor's role includes modeling of social positionality, vulnerability, and accessibility. In addition, the implicit curriculum includes admission standards and resources for retention, which should demonstrate the value the program places on the diversity of the student body. Finally, the implicit curriculum includes extracurricular offerings to enhance learning outside of the classroom.

Making diversity visible in the classroom

Online education introduces challenges for the implicit curriculum because it can obscure diversity in ways not possible in a traditional classroom setting. For example, most of the visible identities can now remain hidden. Every time I step into a face-to-face classroom, my identities as a white, middle-aged, able-bodied, woman are immediately disclosed, but my identities as a queer person in a same-sex marriage with a genderqueer partner remains hidden until I choose to self-disclose. For some students, masking visible identities is a reason for choosing to pursue an online education. Removing physical signals that can trigger implicit bias in others may allow students more confidence in pursuing their educational goals. Students from historically underrepresented groups have expressed discomfort posting photographs due to concern that their picture would disclose their racial identity, or ability status, and result in a negative response by peers or instructors. Given research suggesting that implicit bias occurs toward gender and racially diverse faculty and students (Boring, 2017; Jacoby-Senghor, Sinclair, & Shelton, 2016), taking away identity cues can mean that online participants would only be judged on the quality of the ideas shared in a text-based forum. However, further research needs to be conducted to determine whether removing visible identity cues increases unbiased assessments.

Despite not having visible difference, without images of students or instructors, there are still stereotypical beliefs and biased interactions that occur online due to implicit diversity. Other cues, such as names (Conaway & Bethune, 2015), writing style, or descriptions of past experience still may trigger stereotypical and biased beliefs. On the other hand, students may egocentrically assume that everyone in class thinks and looks like them. If such beliefs or biases about other identities in the classroom are not addressed, microaggressions may occur. Therefore, it is important to not diminish social identity or visibility since students may not have an opportunity to address their personal bias if they "ignore" that difference exists. Further, social work students may not be prepared to address how clients or coworkers perceive and respond to their social identity. Though visibility has different risks, depending on privilege, it is important to encourage more visibility, rather than marginalization, and to create a safe space through identifying minority presence.

Instructor role in the implicit curriculum

Unfortunately, not every social work instructor is equally prepared to address issues related to diversity and difference. Reamer (2013) noted inconsistency of instructor competence and training in this arena within social work education. This reality is significant because teaching diversity can create tension in the classroom (Garran, Kang, & Fraser, 2014), which requires faculty to assess their own values and beliefs (Gay, 2013). Although social work faculty may be committed to issues of diversity, faculty are often left unprepared with limited faculty development (Garran et al., 2014). Faculty need pedagogical support and development opportunities which may include regular meetings throughout the term to discuss challenges and share best practice (Baran & Correia, 2014).

To create a safe space for students, faculty can acknowledge the impact of their identity, and how it is important for a learning community to have difficult conversations of diversity and difference. Believing that it is helpful for instructors to name their positionality and subjectivity, I use my experience as a model to demonstrate the critical reflection in which I encourage social work educators to engage. Pedagogically, I make a conscious effort to come out in face-to-face and online classrooms. I come out as a minority, even though it exposes me to potential bias, because I know that others in the LGBTQ+ community do not have the luxury of hiding their identity. For faculty or students who hold other minority identities, an online environment may be their first experience with the "coming out" process. From microaggressions they experience every day, they may feel safer choosing to not be open; however, being visible can create a safe space for other students to share their identities and start conversations about diversity and difference.

One of the ways to "come out" is by choosing whether to share a picture. Not sharing images is analogous to color blind ideology, which does not change the racialized experiences of minority groups and can cause more harm than good (Edwards, 2017). Educators should not ignore the diversity of experiences in students and themselves, and is relevant for the online classroom. Students from underrepresented backgrounds may see these examples and feel capable of reaching academic goals.

Instructors both can model and show vulnerability in sharing identity and impact of identity. Beyond posting a photo, this includes posting videos that allow students access to the instructor's social identity. Faculty may feel reluctant to share information about themselves in this way, but it will likely allow for better identification and connection. Social work educators can also model accessibility by ensuring closed captioning or providing a transcript in addition to a recording. Ensuring accessibility adds time and effort; however, modeling the commitment to accessibility, even if no students in class will benefit, draws attention to social work values and supports principles of universal design that allow nonassumption of student ability, and values diverse identities related to ability.

Admission standards and resources for retention

In addition to faculty representation, the implicit curriculum includes the diversity of the student body. The diversity of online social work programs is based on who gets admitted and who gets denied admission. Given the lack of substantial evidence suggesting effective predictors of graduate success (Hughes, McNabb, Ashley, McKechnie, & Gremillion, 2016), allowing broad access to social work programs addresses social injustices caused by institutional discrimination. Reaching groups underrepresented in the social work profession ensures that all individuals have an equal opportunity to receive high quality social work services and all communities to have skilled social workers able to advocate for social justice. In short, broad access missions can enhance the social justice efforts of the social work profession by increasing representativeness of diverse groups in the social work profession. However, students also need resources to be successful at the graduate level and should be held accountable to graduate standards and achieving outcome competencies.

Extracurricular events

Having a diverse student body becomes an even greater strength when that student body has opportunities to interact together, which may be more difficult when there is no campus, per se. Online programs nevertheless may consider offering extracurriculars that traditional programs use to bring interactive and diverse voices to their campus, such as guest presenters from diverse cultural communities (Morgan Consoli & Marin, 2016; Quinn & Barth, 2014). Creating additional learning opportunities outside of the classroom also allows students the opportunity to "connect in-school learning to out-of-school living" (Gay, 2013, p. 49) and may become part of the implicit curriculum.

Synchronous video conferencing

One of the ways to facilitate synchronous events as part of the implicit curriculum involves use of video conferencing tools that allow discussion despite different geographic locations. Emerging evidence shows the effectiveness of using live-streaming to increase cultural competency scores for students (Lau, Woodward-Kron, Livesay, Elliott, & Nicholson, 2016). But facilitating these types of events requires different skills than in a face-to-face setting, as well as flexibility in discussion facilitation. For example, students may be more comfortable using chat than using a microphone and voicing their experiences. This means faculty moderators of such events may need to adapt their facilitation style to manage and integrate verbal and text-based conversation, rather than having two distinct parallel conversations.

Though synchronous events can add variety to essentially asynchronous programs, considerations need to be made about the type of student who chooses an online program which tends to attract working adult students because of the flexibility they need to continue to meet family and employment responsibilities while pursuing their higher education goals. These realities also mean that students may not be able to meet synchronously for optional events, even if they would like to do so. Programs can address this variable by recording events. Students will not have the full benefit of interaction but at least can participate in some way. As with other educational approaches, the format must alter to meet the difference of the virtual world and the diversity of the students.

Creating inclusive online environments

Engaging in diversity, difference and social justice is an important part of social work education whether the program is delivered through a traditional brick-and-mortar format or in an online environment. Creating an inclusive learning environment requires attention to the class climate surrounding diversity, including instructor ability to create a safe space and facilitate students' comfort with disclosing personal experiences to one another (Morgan Consoli & Marin, 2016).

The explicit curriculum must design diversity into resources and activities so students can engage in reflection and in diverse activities. This requires creativity and effort at planning and execution. The explicit curriculum, in turn, is enhanced by the administrative support and resources that allow construction of the implicit curriculum, including learning opportunities outside of the classroom and shaping the culture within the classroom.

Acknowledgments

Special acknowledgment goes to Dr. Kathy Goodridge-Purnell who co-created a best practices guide for facilitating difficult discussions for our MSW program, from which sections of this article developed. While not a coauthor on this project, she deserves to be recognized for the significant contribution of her ideas and work.

Disclosure statement

No potential conflict of interest was reported by the author.

References

Ando, S. (2017). Teaching note—Inclusion of diversity content in MSW curriculum using a diversity event. *Journal of Social Work Education, 53*(1), 72–78. doi:10.1080/10437797.2016.1237911

Baran, E., & Correia, A. P. (2014). A professional development framework for online teaching. *TechTrends, 58*(5), 95–101. doi:10.1007/s11528-014-0791-0

Bentley, K. J., Secret, M. C., & Cummings, C. R. (2015). The centrality of social presence in online teaching and learning in social work. *Journal of Social Work Education, 51*(3), 494–504. doi:10.1080/10437797.2015.1043199

Blakeman, P. (2018). Virtual reality: What it offers, and how it can be used easily (and inexpensively) by health & social care tutors. *Journal of Practice Teaching & Learning, 16*(1), 81–93.

Boring, A. (2017). Gender biases in student evaluations of teaching. *Journal of Public Economics, 145*, 27–41. doi:10.1016/j.jpubeco.2016.11.006

Clark, C., Strudler, N., & Grove, K. (2015). Comparing asynchronous and synchronous video vs. text based discussions in an online teacher education course. *Online Learning, 19*(3), 48–69. doi:10.24059/olj.v19i3.510

Conaway, W., & Bethune, S. (2015). Implicit bias and first name stereotypes: What are the implications for online instruction? *Online Learning, 19*(3), 162–178. doi:10.24059/olj.v19i3.452

Constantine, M. G., & Sue, D. W. (2005). *Strategies for building multicultural competence in mental health and educational settings*. Hoboken, NJ: John Wiley.

Council on Social Work Education. (2015). *2015 educational policy and accreditation standards educational policy and accreditation standards for baccalaureate and master's social work programs*. CSWE. Retrieved from https://www.cswe.org/getattachment/Accreditation/Standards-and-Policies/2015-EPAS/2015EPASandGlossary.pdf.aspx

Craig, S. L., Iacono, G., Paceley, M. S., Dentato, M. P., & Boyle, K. E. (2017). Intersecting sexual, gender, and professional identities among social work students: The importance of identity integration. *Journal of Social Work Education, 53*(3), 466–479. doi:10.1080/10437797.2016.1272516

Deepak, A. C., & Rountree, M. A. (2015). Delivering diversity and social justice in social work education: The power of context. *Journal of Progressive Human Services, 26*(2), 107–125. doi:10.1080/10428232.2015.1017909

Edwards, J. F. (2017). Color-blind racial attitudes: Microaggressions in the context of racism and White privilege. *Administrative Issues Journal, 7*(1), 5–18.

Farrel, D., Ray, K., Rich, T., Suarez, Z., Christenson, B., & Jennigs, L. (2018). A meta-analysis of approaches to engage social work students online. *Journal of Teaching in Social Work, 38* (2), 183–197. doi:10.1080/08841233.2018.1431351

Fisher-Borne, M., Cain, J. M., & Martin, S. L. (2015). From mastery to accountability: Cultural humility as an alternative to cultural competence. *Social Work Education, 34*(2), 165–181. doi:10.1080/02615479.2014.977244

Garran, A. M., Kang, H. K., & Fraser, E. (2014). Pedagogy and diversity: Enrichment and support for social work instructors engaged in social justice education. *Journal of Teaching in Social Work, 34*(5), 564–574. doi:10.1080/08841233.2014.952868

Gay, G. (2013). Teaching to and through cultural diversity. *Curriculum Inquiry, 43*(1), 48–70. doi:10.1111/curi.12002

Gayles, J. G., Kelly, B. T., Grays, S., Zhang, J. J., & Porter, K. P. (2015). Faculty teaching diversity through difficult dialogues: Stories of challenges and success. *Journal of Student Affairs Research and Practice, 52*(3), 300–312. doi:10.1080/19496591.2015.1067223

Hubain, B. S., Allen, E. L., Harris, J. C., & Linder, C. (2016). Counter-stories as representations of the racialized experiences of students of color in higher education and student affairs graduate preparation programs. *International Journal of Qualitative Studies in Education, 29*(7), 946–963. doi:10.1080/09518398.2016.1174894

Hughes, C., McNabb, D., Ashley, P., McKechnie, R., & Gremillion, H. (2016). Selection of social work students: A literature review of selection criteria and process effectiveness. *Advances in Social Work and Welfare Education, 18*(2), 94–106.

Jacoby-Senghor, D. S., Sinclair, S., & Shelton, J. N. (2016). A lesson in bias: The relationship between implicit racial bias and performance in pedagogical contexts. *Journal of Experimental Social Psychology, 63*, 50–55. doi:10.1016/j.jesp.2015.10.010

Lau, P. M. Y., Woodward-Kron, R., Livesay, K., Elliott, K., & Nicholson, P. (2016). Cultural respect encompassing simulation training: Being heard about health through broadband. *Journal of Public Health Research, 5*(657), 36–42. doi:10.4081/jphr.2016.657

Lee, E.-K. O. (2014). Use of avatars and a virtual community to increase cultural competence. *Journal of Technology in Human Services, 32*(1/2), 93–107. doi:10.1080/15228835.2013.860364

McInroy, L., Craig, S., & Austin, A. (2014). The perceived scarcity of gender identity specific content in Canadian social work programs. *Canadian Social Work Review, 31*(1), 5–21.

McLoughlin, C. (2001). Inclusivity and alignment: Principles of pedagogy, task and assessment design for effective cross-cultural online learning. *Distance Education, 22*(1), 7–29. doi:10.1080/0158791010220102

Morgan Consoli, M. L., & Marin, P. (2016). Teaching diversity in the graduate classroom: The instructor, the students, the classroom, or all of the above? *Journal of Diversity in Higher Education, 9*(2), 143–157. doi:10.1037/a0039716

National Association of Social Workers. (2017). *Code of ethics of the National Association of Social Workers*. Retrieved from https://www.socialworkers.org/About/Ethics/Code-of-Ethics/Code-of-Ethics-English

Nedegaard, R. C., Barkdull, C., Weber, B. A., & Jayasundara, D. S. (2018). Lessons our BSW students taught us about teaching social work in a reservation community. *Journal of Teaching in Social Work, 38*(1), 73–87. doi:10.1080/08841233.2017.1414097

Nilson, L. B. (2016). *Teaching at its best: A research-based resource for college instructors*. Hoboken, NJ: John Wiley & Sons.

Oxhandler, H. K., & Giardina, T. D. (2017). Social workers' perceived barriers to and sources of support for integrating clients' religion and spirituality in practice. *Social Work, 62*(4), 323–332. doi:10.1093/sw/swx036

Quinn, A., & Barth, A. M. (2014). Operationalizing the implicit curriculum in MSW distance education programs. *Journal of Social Work Education, 50*(1), 34–47. doi:10.1080/10437797.2014.856229

Reamer, F. G. (2013). Distance and online social work education: Novel ethical challenges. *Journal of Teaching in Social Work, 33*(4–5), 369–384. doi:10.1080/08841233.2013.828669

Reinsmith-Jones, K., Kibbe, S., Crayton, T., & Campbell, E. (2015). Use of second life in social work education: Virtual world experiences and their effect on students. *Journal of Social Work Education, 51*(1), 90–108. doi:10.1080/10437797.2015.977167

Schwartz, S. L., Wiley, J. L., & Kaplan, C. D. (2016). Community-building in a virtual teaching environment. *Advances in Social Work, 17*(1), 15–30. doi:10.18060/20875

Secret, M., Bentley, K. J., & Kadolph, J. C. (2016). Student voices speak quality assurance: Continual improvement in online social work education. *Journal of Social Work Education, 52*(1), 30–42. doi:10.1080/10437797.2016.1112630

Smith, K., Jeffery, D., & Collins, K. (2018). Slowing things down: Taming time in the neoliberal university using social work distance education. *Social Work Education, 37*(6), 691. doi:10.1080/02615479.2018.1445216

Stauss, K., Koh, E., & Collie, M. (2018). Comparing the effectiveness of an online human diversity course to face-to-face instruction. *Journal of Social Work Education*, *54*(3), 492–505. doi:10.1080/10437797.2018.1434432

Stough-Hunter, A., Guinan, J., & Hart, J. P. (2016). A comparison of teaching methods building cultural competency informed by contact theory. *Journal of Cultural Diversity*, *23*(3), 91–98.

Sue, D. W., Sue, D., Neville, H. A., & Smith, L. (2019). *Counseling the culturally diverse: Theory and practice* (2nd ed.). Hoboken, NJ: John Wiley and Sons.

Watts, L. (2016). Synchronous and asynchronous communication in distance learning: A review of the literature. *Quarterly Review of Distance Education*, *17*(1), 23–32.

The Teacher–Learner Relationship: Considerations for Social Work in the Digital Age

Jennifer Spitz

ABSTRACT

In light of a rapidly changing educational landscape, this paper will discuss the implications of online education for the teacher–learner relationship, which is a critical aspect of academic and professional development for the social work student. As technology revolutionizes relationships, how will we ensure the intra- and interpersonal nature of social work education? The pursuit of accessible and flexible educational opportunities presently driving social work education threatens to undermine this important alliance. The centrality of relationship is discussed here in the context of current trends in distance learning. Relational-Cultural Theory and Transactional Distance Theory are posited to provide evidence for the significance of relationship in learning.

Distinguishing marks of [social caseworkers] were, first, skill in discovering the social relationships by which a given personality had been shaped; second, ability to get at the center core of difficulty in these relationships; and third, power to utilize the direct action of mind upon mind in their adjustment. (Richmond, 1917, p. 399)

Introduction

Mary Richmond was the first to identify the centrality of relationship in social work practice (Richmond, 1917). Through her work with Charity Organization Societies, she focused on ensuring that families received essential services. Her method centered upon relationship building, she with her clients, and her clients, in turn, with their resources. The seeds planted by Richmond have taken deep root and should continue to ground social work and social work education.

Despite changing social and political climates and technological innovation, human connection remains at the foundation of social work. While *how* we connect has changed, the *need* for human connection is innate and timeless (Perlman, 1979). The importance of relationship is most often spoken about with respect to practice, but the teacher–learner relationship is important in social work education as well.

In traditional brick and mortar social work education settings, the teacher–learner relationship is seen as essential for fostering a safe and dynamic environment in which students can explore their own self-awareness (Smith & Wingerson, 2006) and experience in vivo interactions which model the client–worker relationship. These interactions highlight concepts such as transference and countertransference, boundaries, and the building of trust that are critical themes in the helping relationship. With the growth of distance learning, how will we retain the intra-and interpersonal nature of social work education and the centrality of relationship in our work? Students require a different skill set to thrive in an autonomous and dispersed online learning environment, changing the nature of traditional teacher–learner relationships. Through the perspectives of Relational-Cultural Theory (Miller, 1986) and Transactional Distance Theory (Moore, 1997), this paper will discuss relational themes in distance learning. We begin with a brief discussion of the emergence of distance learning and the impact of technology on social work education as a context for the exploration of relational implications in the teacher–learner relationship.

Trends in distance education

Distance education is defined in many ways. In traditional face-to-face courses, technologies such as videos, PowerPoint presentations, and the limited use of course management systems such as Blackboard or Moodle are seen as adjunctive teaching tools (Blackmon, 2013). Alternatively, some courses are taught entirely through web-assisted technology, with or without the presence of an instructor (i.e., synchronous or asynchronous). Hybrid courses offer a blend of online and face-to-face components, a model that is increasingly attractive (Zidan, 2015). For this discussion, online education will refer to instruction in which teachers and learners are at a distance, but connected through the internet (Conceicāo, 2006). The terms online and distance learning will be used interchangeably.

The literature on online learning strongly supports its cost-efficiency, access, and educational effectiveness (Kurzman, 2013; Selingo, 2016). Financial benefit (Blackmon, 2013), wider reach to non-traditional students (Zidan, 2015) and those who reside in remote areas (Moore et al., 2015) make online education appealing to colleges and universities. The need for digital literacy in the current workplace is often cited as another motivation (Conceicāo, 2006). For those students looking to upgrade skills or to change careers, online learning can be more economically and logistically feasible.

Other studies highlight notable limitations (Conceicāo, 2006; Jones, 2015; Knowles, 2007; Phirangee, 2016). The temporal dimension and design elements of an online course can raise both complex and nuanced issues that require careful consideration. As an example, although asynchronous engagement is thought to enhance opportunities for thoughtful and reflective participation

(Harasim, 1996), much of the learning activity is solitary and not in real time (Trammell & LaForge, 2017), limiting spontaneous feedback. Synchronous online learning generally provides a more dynamic and interactive environment; however, it is resource-intensive and less cost-effective (Sawikar, Lenette, McDonald, & Fowler, 2015). Serdyukov (2015) further suggests that the online student often has little time or desire for deep learning, but rather is on a fast track to a degree. While the successful online student is likely to be highly skilled and motivated, this is not true of a significant portion of enrollees (The Trouble with Online College, 2013). Many students are seen to prefer online learning for its convenience. This perception could be detrimental to rigor and may affect students' attitudes toward learning (Serdyukov, 2015).

Trends in social work education

In 2017, approximately 22% of BSW programs accredited by the Council on Social Work Education (CSWE) were fully online, while roughly an additional one-third was partially online (CSWE, 2018). Approximately 20% of MSW programs were fully online and 35% offered part of their program at a distance. Along with the rapid evolution of technology, accessibility and flexibility are frequently cited benefits of online programs (Kurzman, 2013; Selingo, 2016; Zidan, 2015), and distance learning affords access to students in remote and rural areas (Moore et al., 2015), as well as those encumbered by the demands of work, family, and other responsibilities (Selingo, 2016). The literature provides evidence of these advantages and documents the comparability of educational outcomes for social work students in face-to-face and online settings (Kurzman, 2013).

Accordingly, the National Association of Social Workers (NASW), in collaboration with the Council on Social Work Education (CSWE), Association of Social Work Boards (ASWB) and Clinical Social Work Association (CSWA) recently disseminated standards for technology in social work practice and education. Section 4 of these standards provides guidance on the use of technology in education and supervision. The standards suggest that technology can enhance skill development, engagement, and learning outcomes, and can be used to the extent that it enables students to "master core and essential professional skills." (National Association of Social Workers [NASW], 2018, p. 45). Substantial growth in online social work education affirms its permanence and warrants the dissemination of these standards.

The role of relationship and learning in social work

Teaching and learning in social work occur within the context of relationships. As in the client-worker dyad, starting where the learner is can facilitate this transformative experience (Anastas, 2010). Teacher–learner relationships connect coursework to students' emotional lives and classroom learning. The educator's attunement further helps to facilitate an affective learning environment in which students can examine themselves, their values, and emotional responses (Ikebuchi & Rasmussen, 2014).

Whether in the classroom or online, a student's sense of the teacher is critical to their success (Woods & Baker, 2004). While the teacher's online presence is cited as a critical factor in student engagement and satisfaction (Bentley, Secret, & Cummings, 2015; Higgs, 2012), how presence is developed and perceived by students varies. For each student, the teacher will, of course, be different, with perceptions based upon that student's past experiences and current interactions. Thus, it is the patterns of teacher-student and student–student interaction that create a student's sense of the teacher. However, Dockter (2016) cautions that there is danger in expecting that the teacher is solely responsible for creating a presence. "Within any class, in any domain, information is shared, and meaning is created between students and a teacher through the give and take of information – a transaction." It is these transactions which are the underpinning of the teacher–learner relationship, and, ultimately, the client-worker alliance. Navigation of this transactional space largely will be influenced by the learning modality (classroom or online), thereby shaping the relationship (Woods & Baker, 2004). Regardless of the learning environment, interpersonal contact that imbues a sense of community must be a central focus of course design and implementation (Arasaratnam-Smith & Northcote, 2017). Failure to prioritize relational needs may increase isolation and diminish satisfaction and performance (Woods & Baker, 2004).

The need for connection: relational-cultural theory

Aligning with John Bowlby's theory of attachment (1951), Relational-Cultural Theory (RCT) suggests that we are "hardwired" for connection (Trepal & Duffey, 2016). Whether online or in the classroom, this is a "pre-existing condition," which is inherent in human nature. According to attachment theory, students think, interpret, and behave in accordance with their attachment styles and internal working models (Fleming, 2008). The student's perceptions of the educator's availability and responsiveness can be determined by these templates. Similarly, Relational-Cultural Theory (RCT) suggests that it is these "relational templates," developed through life experiences, that shape one's ideas about relationships. Templates are still further influenced by the intersection of social identities which engender themes of privilege and oppression (Comstock et al., 2008). Accordingly, RCT identifies the sociocultural and contextual challenges that impede one's ability to create and sustain growth-fostering relationships (Comstock et al., 2008), which are validated by neuroscience (Frey, 2013) and affirmed by the innate need for connection.

Relational-Cultural Theory provides a framework for understanding the significance of teacher-learner connections in online learning. It offers a lens for viewing the development of social work knowledge and skills within the context of relationship. With similarities to the client–worker relationship (Jensen, 2017), teacher–learner interaction engenders attachment, trust, and interpersonal themes. Students' attachment styles will contribute to their comfort and success in embracing new ideas and achieving learning goals (Carr, Colthurst, Coyle, & Elliot, 2013). Attachment style and relational templates, as explicated by RCT, will underpin students' trust in new learning situations and relationships. Secure and positive relational experiences will enhance the capacity for student engagement and success. On the contrary, insecurity or ambivalence will amplify mistrust, a fear of failure, and have implications for motivation and participation (Carr et al., 2013).

Emphasizing the innate need for connection, RCT asserts that individual development occurs within the context of relationships, in other words, the development of self-with-others (Edwards & Richards, 2002). This concept of development aligns with social work values which uphold the importance and centrality of human relationships (NASW, 2018). Thus, the affordances of autonomy and flexibility in online learning should be balanced with the development of self-with-others, prioritizing opportunities for connection separate and apart from learning activities.

Edwards and Richards (2002) suggest that this process requires mutual engagement and mutual empathy, key ingredients for connection. Smith (2015) notes that this occurs through a "reciprocal, mutually influencing process of attunement" (p. 238). Establishment of connections between teachers and learners should be addressed before the start of a course as a critical element of student engagement and learning. This will involve specific actions pertaining to teacher-learner communication and interaction *prior* to a student's initiation to online learning. Suggestions for these activities will be made later in this discussion.

RCT supports thinking about the social work classroom (whether online or on the ground) as providing a secure base for learners (Fleming, 2008), a "holding space" (Jensen, 2017) for the emotional dimensions of social work education. This point is particularly important in bridging field learning to the classroom where students examine, question, and challenge existing assumptions and world views. Consequently, dynamics related to social identity, privilege, oppression, and other systemic inequities should be surfaced. RCT asserts that the teacher–learner relationship provides the context and support for students to critically engage in these emotionally demanding aspects of learning (Edwards & Richards, 2002).

The importance of a connection between teacher and learner in online learning has been cited often in the social work education literature. Social presence (Bentley et al., 2015) and teaching presence (Dockter, 2016) are indicated to be key factors in student engagement, satisfaction, and success. Woods and Baker (2004) note, however, that the presence of dyadic communication does not guarantee genuine interpersonal and contextual interaction. RCT supports this thinking, suggesting that connection requires more than presence. It encourages us to give greater attention to reducing psychological and social distance between and among teachers and learners (Arbaugh, 2000; Stein, Wanstreet, Calvin, Overtoom, & Wheaton, 2005), an especially important consideration for online course design.

Transactional distance theory

Influenced by philosopher and psychologist John Dewey's thinking about social dynamics and learning frameworks, Moore (1997) theorized that distance was a "pedagogical phenomenon" (p. 2) rather than a function of geographical separation, and may exist in face-to-face as well as distance classes (Woods & Baker, 2004). He referred to this phenomenon as "transactional distance" (Moore, 1997), or a "psychological and communication space" (Giossos, Koutsouba, Lionarakis, & Skavantzos, 2009). Within this space, the teacher and learner develop patterns of behavior and interaction, which are influenced by their *dialogue* with each other, the *structure* of the distance program, and the extent to which the learner exhibits *autonomy* in the learning process (Giossos et al., 2009). Transactional Distance Theory (TDT) posits that these three elements are in shifting proportional relationships within the transactional space.

Dialogue is the communication between the instructor and learner. Structure refers to course design, such as learning activities, prescribed interaction, and evaluation. Autonomy refers to the ability of a learner to manage learning in a self-directed way. The theory posits that high structure and low dialogue increase transactional distance, requiring greater learner autonomy (Stein et al., 2005). Low structure and high dialogue decrease transactional distance, as well as learner autonomy. More autonomous learners may require additional structure and less dialogue, which will increase transactional distance. In turn, learners with low autonomy may need increased dialogue, lessening transactional distance, but at the cost of structure.

A great deal of attention is given to structure of online courses which is cited as an important feature for student engagement and success (Goldkind & Wolf, 2015). However, according to TDT, this could have unintended consequences for relationships, learning, and satisfaction (Dockter, 2016). Hence, a relational approach in social work education online requires a thoughtful balance of these elements.

TDT provides a useful framework for online learning. On a broad level, reducing transactional distance is particularly important in the beginning stages of a student's experience. Developing a connection to the course, classmates, the instructor, and college or university culture is important in facilitating engagement and ensuring retention. Continuous monitoring of transactional distance vis-à-vis student participation enables the instructor to be proactive in identifying how the elements defined above may need realignment from time to time for a particular student due to a change in life circumstances, or a greater awareness of specific learning needs (Major & Sumner, 2018). In such cases, the student and instructor may co-create a success plan in which increased structure *and* dialogue serve to decrease transactional distance (Stein et al., 2005). Within this framework, course structure can be fluid, especially at the beginning, allowing students to identify their learning needs and work with the instructor to lessen the transactional distance. At the same time, the teacher–learner relationship remains central in the learning process.

The concept of immediacy (Mehrabian, 1967) also deserves mention since it suggests that selective communication behaviors can enhance physical or psychological closeness in relationships, thereby reducing perceived distance between people. Structure, dialogue, and immediacy can positively impact student satisfaction and sense of community in online courses (Arbaugh, 2000), while also enhancing learner autonomy.

Considerations for online social work education

The current online educational environment has radically altered the relationship of the learner to the teacher and the content to be learned (Harasim, 1996). Interactional limitations on the ability to see or hear emotions and tone (along with the absence of body language and eye contact) represent considerable challenges. Students tend to feel supported by an instructor's eye contact and body language, which can be constrained by distance and technology (Markova, Glazkova, & Zaborova, 2017). Thus, pedagogical approaches that facilitate teacher–learner interaction are important in the design and implementation of distance courses.

Given their relevance to the dynamic nature of teacher–learner relationships, RCT and TDT both offer valuable frameworks for developing online social work courses. As they begin, and throughout their coursework, students can benefit from opportunities for teacher–learner interactions that should help to navigate the new learning environment. The following are recommendations for such activities.

The importance of orientation

The literature reflects the value of online orientation programs in helping students to feel welcomed, to best understand expectations for a course, and to increase comfort with technology (Cascio & Gasker, 2001; Jensen, 2017). Most online orientation programs focus on technological issues, such as hardware, learning management systems, and technical proficiency. However, there is a need, as well, to focus on issues beyond just the technical ones (Jensen, 2017).Such orientation for online students can be a critical first step toward establishing effective teacher–learner relationships. First and foremost, orientations should assess student readiness for online learning (Murphy, Mahoney, Chen, Mendoza-Diaz, & Yang, 2005). It is risky to presume that all students who seek an online education format are prepared to effectively navigate the nuanced relationships and inherent time management demands. In addition, well-designed orientation programs can help students articulate their goals for online learning; why did they choose it and what are their expectations? These are important questions, the responses to which may help surface potential misconceptions and clarify relational and academic expectations.

A role for mentoring

A mentor is defined as a trusted counselor or guide (Merriam-Webster's online dictionary, 2018). In the education literature, mentoring refers to a "one-to-one relationship in which a more experienced faculty member guides and supports the career development of a new or early-career faculty member" (Sorcinelli & Yun, 2007, p. 58). The social work literature also suggests that mentoring of students by faculty can be influential in their professional development and cites the benefits of peer mentoring as well (Jensen, 2017; Murphy et al., 2005). Effective mentors greatly influence their mentees, inculcating professional values and modeling professional identity and effective use of self (Cascio & Gasker, 2001). Mentoring can help students see themselves and the world in a new way. Mentors also can support students through unsettling experiences and promote new ways of knowing, assisting students with this transformative process by creating a "holding space" for self-reflection. Mentors can also be the link to campus support services (academic, disability, psychological, social) which may sustain student enrollment in online programs. This reality is particularly salient for first generation, non-traditional, and young undergraduate students for whom simultaneous orientation to the profession and an online learning environment can be overwhelming (Jensen, 2017).

Mentoring for online students aligns with the tenets of RCT and TDT in fostering growth-promoting relationships and managing transactional distance. Distance learning social work programs will need to determine who is best suited for this role, and whether additional human, financial, and institutional resources are necessary. Instructors may simultaneously be mentors, which can provide a more seamless transition for students. Students report preferring face-to-face meetings with mentors, when feasible, although email and/or telephone calls often are more realistic (Bozarth,

Chapman, & LaMonica, 2004). One might, therefore, infer that advanced technological systems may not provide the same feeling of connection to teachers that students seem to feel with more traditional means of communication (Jensen, 2017).

RCT and TDT also suggest the value of increasing synchronous and blended learning opportunities where students have more opportunities for interaction and creating interpersonal relationships. Indeed, several studies have demonstrated the effectiveness of these approaches in increasing connection and student satisfaction while reducing the transactional distance (Czerkawski, 2014; Major & Sumner, 2018).

Ethical considerations

While the National Association of Social Workers and Association of Social Work Boards standards (2018) frame the ethical issues embedded in the use of technology in social work practice and education, interpretation of these standards can be subjective and influenced by modes of practice, populations served, treatment settings, and other aspects of delivery. Consequently, diverse methods of utilization of technology by practitioners and educators make it difficult to ascertain relevant, consistent, and credible "protections" for clients, students, and practitioners. Assessment of the scope of utilization can inform a strategic plan to more directly address the ethical risks. Such could be an undertaking of the profession, coordinated by various constituencies (geographical locations, practice modalities, fields of practice, schools of social work) in order to develop cohesive and coherent approaches for operationalizing the NASW and ASWB standards.

Ethical considerations are salient for students, many of whom are heavily engaged with social media (Major & Sumner, 2018). Technology has been their norm for communication and interpersonal connection. This may, of course, raise complicated boundary issues in working with clients and colleagues. Reamer (2013) raises many other critical issues, such as dual relationships, informed consent, documentation, and risk management, that warrant attention for practitioners, and for students whose "technological life course" may dilute their ability to discern the nuances and complexities inherent in these risks. Distance learning programs are positioned to take up these topics, utilizing the online environment as a platform for teaching about them.

Conclusion

Future social workers increasingly are being educated in online, consumer-driven environments, which has shifted the dynamics and expectations of the teacher–student relationship. Curtailment of a traditional bricks-and-mortar format of education, coupled with a sense of urgency among students to complete a degree, have made online learning a convenient and desirable alternative (Serdyukov, 2015). Relational-Cultural Theory and Transactional Distance Theory reinforce the importance of relationship and connection in learning and provide frameworks for developing online educational programs that promote effective teacher–learner relationships as well as foster student engagement and persistence.

"As a discipline based on advocacy for the successful titration between people and the systems and environment that surround them, social work is uniquely situated to offer a human compass in the conversation about technology, and to represent the essential ethical values of social justice and connection in a reality whose constant engine is change" (Goldkind & Wolf, 2015, p. 87). We suggest that RCT and TDT can guide a digital strategic plan for social work education to promote pedagogical, professional, and institutional frameworks for change that will help us to maintain the relational foundations of our profession that Mary Richmond laid before us more than a century ago.

Disclosure statement

No potential conflict of interest was reported by the author.

References

Anastas, J. (2010). *Teaching in social work: An educator's' guide to theory and practice.* New York, NY: Columbia University Press.

Arasaratnam-Smith, L. A., & Northcote, M. (2017). Community in online higher education: Challenges and opportunities. *Electronic Journal Of E-Learning, 15*(2), 188–198.

Arbaugh, J. B. (2000). Virtual classroom characteristics and student satisfaction with Internet-based MBA courses. *Journal of Management Education, 24*, 32–54. doi:10.1177/105256290002400104

Association of Social Work Boards [ASWB]. (2018). *Technology standards in social work practice.* Retrieved from https://www.aswb.org/news/technology-standards-in-social-work-practice/

Bentley, K., Secret, M., & Cummings, C. (2015). The centrality of social presence in online teaching and learning in social work. *Journal of Social Work Education, 51*(3), 494–504. doi:10.1080/10437797.2015.1043199

Blackmon, B. (2013). Social work and online education all with deliberate speed. *Journal of Evidence-based Social Work, 10*(5), 509–521. doi:10.1080/15433714.2012.663672

Bowlby, J. (1951). *Maternal care and mental health.* Geneva, Switzerland: World Health Organization Monograph.

Bozarth, J., Chapman, D. D., & LaMonica, L. (2004). Preparing for distance learning: Designing an online student orientation course. *Educational Technology & Society, 7*(1), 87–106.

Carr, S., Colthurst, K., Coyle, M., & Elliott, D. (2013). Attachment dimensions as predictors of mental health and psychosocial well-being in the transition to university. *European Journal of Psychology of Education, 28*(2), 157–172. doi:10.1007/s10212-012-0106-9

Cascio, T., & Gasker, J. (2001). Everyone has a shining side: Computer mediated mentoring in social work education. *Journal of Social Work Education*, *37*(2), 283–293. doi:10.1080/10437797.2001.10779054

Comstock, D., Hammer, T., Strentzsch, J., Cannon, K., Parsons, J., & Salazar, G. (2008). Relational-cultural theory: A framework for bridging relational, multicultural and social justice competencies. *Journal of Counseling and Development*, *86*(3), 279–287. doi:10.1002/j.1556-6678.2008.tb00510.x

Conceição, S. (2006). Faculty lived experiences in the online environment. *Adult Education Quarterly*, *57*(1), 26–45. doi:10.1177/1059601106292247

Council on Social Work Education [CSWE]. (2018). *Annual statistics on social work education in the United States*. Retrieved from https://www.cswe.org/getattachment/992f629c-57cf-4a74-8201-1db7a6fa4667/2015-Statistics-on-Social-Work-Education.aspx

Czerkawski, B. (2014). Designing deeper learning experiences for online instruction. *Journal of Interactive Online Learning*, *13*(2), 29–40.

Dockter, J. (2016). The problem of teaching presence in transactional theories of distance education. *Computers and Composition*, *40*, 73–86. doi:10.1016/j.compcom.2016.03.009

Edwards, J. B., & Richards, A. (2002). Relational teaching: A view of relational teaching in social work education. *Journal of Teaching in Social Work*, *22*(1/2), 33–48. doi:10.1300/J067v22n01_04

Fleming, T. (2008). A secure base for adult learning: Attachment theory and adult education. *Adult Learner: the Irish Journal of Adult and Community Education*, *25*, 33–53.

Frey, L. (2013). Relational-Cultural Therapy: Theory, research, and application to counseling competencies. *Professional Psychology: Research and Practice*, *44*(3), 171–185.

Giossos, Y., Koutsouba, M., Lionarakis, A., & Skavantzos, K. (2009). Reconsidering Moore's transactional distance theory. *European Journal of Open, Distance and E-Learning*, *2*, 1–6.

Goldkind, L., & Wolf, L. (2015). A digital environment approach: Four technologies that will disrupt social work practice. *Social Work*, *60*(1), 85–87.

Harasim, L. (1996). Online education: The future. In T. Harrison & T. Stephen (Eds.), *Computer networking and scholarly communication in the twenty-first-century university* (pp. 203–214). New York: SUNY Press.

Higgs, A. (2012). e-Learning, ethics and 'non-traditional' students: Space to think aloud. *Ethics & Social Welfare*, *6*(4), 386–402. doi:10.1080/17496535.2012.654496

Ikebuchi, J., & Rasmussen, B. M. (2014). The use of emotions in social work education. *Journal of Teaching in Social Work*, *34*(3), 285–301. doi:10.1080/08841233.2014.909378

Jensen, D. (2017). Mentoring in a distributed learning social work program. *Journal of Social Work Education*, *53*(4), 637–650. doi:10.1080/10437797.2017.1287026

Jones, S. H. (2015). Benefits and challenges of online education for clinical social work: Three examples. *Clinical Social Work Journal*, *43*(2), 225. doi:10.1007/s10615-014-0508-z

Knowles, A. (2007). Pedagogical and policy challenges in implementing e-learning in social work education. *Journal of Technology in Human Services*, *25*(1/2), 17–44. doi:10.1300/J017v25n01_02

Kurzman, P. (2013). The evolution of distance learning and online education. *Journal of Teaching in Social Work*, *33*, 331–338. doi:10.1080/08841233.2013.843346

Major, A., & Sumner, J. (2018, March 1). *Reducing transactional distance: Engaging online students in higher education*. The evoLLLution. Retrieved from https://evolllution.com/

Markova, T., Glazkova, I., & Zaborova, E. (2017). Quality issues of online distance learning. *Procedia - Social and Behavioral Sciences*, *237*, 685–691. (Education,Health and ICT for a Transcultural World). doi:10.1016/j.sbspro.2017.02.043

Mehrabian, A. (1967). Orientation behaviors and nonverbal attitude communication. *Journal of Communication*, *17*, 324–332. doi:10.1111/j.1460-2466.1967.tb01190.x

Mentor [Def. 1]. (n.d.). *In Merriam webster online*, Retrieved from https://www.merriamwebster.com/dictionary/mentor?utm_campaign=sd&utm_medium=serp&utm_source=jsonld.

Miller, J. B. (1986). *Toward a new psychology of women* (2nd ed.). Boston, MA: Beacon.

Moore, M. (1997). Theory of transactional distance. In D. Keegan (Ed.), *Theoretical principles of distance education* (pp. 22–38). New York, NY: Routledge.

Moore, S., Golder, S., Sterrett, E., Faul, A., Yankeelov, P., Weathers, M., & Barbee, A. (2015). Social work online education: A model for getting started and staying connected. *Journal of Social Work Education, 51*, 505–518. doi:10.1080/10437797.2015.1043200

Murphy, K., Mahoney, S., Chen, C., Mendoza-Diaz, V., & Yang, X. (2005). A constructivist model of mentoring, coaching, and facilitating online discussions. *Distance Education, 26* (3), 341–366. doi:10.1080/01587910500291454

National Association of Social Workers [NASW]. (2018). *Standards for technology in social work practice.* Retrieved from https://docs.google.com/document/d/1tgd-oq 7rvDIPQMueXWuIoQtq83zDmPbTww7GIc7CWW4/edit

Perlman, H. H. (1979). *Relationship: The heart of helping people.* Chicago, IL: The University of Chicago Press.

Phirangee, K. (2016). Students' perceptions of learner-learner interactions that weaken a sense of community in an online learning environment. *Online Learning, 20*(4), 13–33. doi:10.24059/olj.v20i4.1053

Reamer, F. (2013). Social work in a digital age: Ethical and risk management challenges. *Social Work, 58*(2), 163–172.

Richmond, M. (1917). *The social caseworker's tasks.* New York, NY: Russell Sage Foundation. Russell Sage Foundation Reprints.

Sawikar, P., Lenette, C., McDonald, D., & Fowler, J. (2015). Don't silence "the dinosaurs": Keeping caution alive with regard to social work distance education. *Journal of Teaching in Social Work, 35*, 343–364.

Selingo, J. J. (2016). *2026, The decade ahead: The seismic shifts transforming higher education.* Washington, DC: Chronicle of Higher Education. Retrieved from https://www.uky.edu/ universitysenate/sites/www.uky.edu.universitysenate/files/The-Decade-Ahead-Chronicle-of -Higher-Education1.pdf

Serdyukov, P. (2015). Does online education need a special pedagogy? *Journal of Computing and Information Technology, 23*, 61–74. doi:10.2498/cit.1002511

Smith, P. R., & Wingerson, N. W. (2006). Is the centrality of relationship in social work at risk with IVT? *Journal of Technology in Human Services, 24*(2/3), 23–37. doi:10.1300/J017v24n02_02

Smith, W. (2015). Relational dimensions of virtual social work education: Mentoring faculty in a web-based learning environment. *Clinical Social Work Journal, 43*(2), 236–245. doi:10.1007/s10615-014-0510-5

Sorcinelli, M., & Yun, J. (2007). From mentor to mentoring networks: Mentoring in the new academy. *The Magazine of Higher Learning, 39*(6), 59–61. doi:10.3200/CHNG.39.6.58-C4

Stein, D., Wanstreet, C., Calvin, J., Overtoom, C., & Wheaton, J. (2005). Bridging the transactional distance gap in online learning environments. *The American Journal of Distance Education, 19*(2), 105–118. doi:10.1207/s15389286ajde1902_4

Trammell, B. A., & LaForge, C. (2017). Common challenges for instructors in large online courses: Strategies to mitigate student and instructor frustration. *Journal of Educators Online, 14*(1), 1–10.

Trepal, H., & Duffey, T. (2016). Everything has changed: An interview with Judy Jordan. *Journal of Counseling & Development, 94*(4), 437–441. doi:10.1002/jcad.12102

Trouble with Online College [Editorial]. (2013, February 19). The New York Times.

Woods, R., Jr., & Baker, J. (2004). Interaction and immediacy in online learning. *The International Review of Research in Open and Distributed Learning, 5*(2). doi:10.19173/ irrodl.v5i2.186

Zidan, T. (2015). Teaching social work in an online environment. *Journal Of Human Behavior In The Social Environment, 25*(3), 228–235. doi:10.1080/10911359.2014.1003733

Part IV

Strategies for Engagement

Introducing Social Work to HyFlex Blended Learning: A Student-centered Approach

Benjamin R. Malczyk

ABSTRACT

The HyFlex blended learning model is a student-driven approach that allows students to determine what blended learning they prefer to meet their unique needs. In a HyFlex course, students are presented with a choice with each class session – whether to attend face-to-face or participate online. This article introduces social work educators to the HyFlex blended learning model and presents the results from a five-week experiment utilizing the HyFlex blended approach in an undergraduate social welfare policy course. Benefits and challenges of the model are presented and discussed.

Introduction

The body of literature on online social work education continues to expand (Kurzman & Maiden, 2014; Racovita-Szilagyi, Carbonero Muñoz, & Diaconu, 2018). Recent articles and research on blended learning, which includes instruction that incorporates elements of both face-to-face and online instruction (Garrison & Kanuka, 2004) also have grown over the past several years (Carter et al., 2018). Indeed, blended learning is often portrayed as an ideal modality of instruction that can outperform fully online classes or even traditional face-to-face classes (Bernard, Borokhovski, Schmid, Tamim, & Abrami, 2014), and presents students with the opportunity to have face-to-face interactions with faculty and colleagues that can lead to meaningful relationships and sense of community (Rovai & Jordan, 2004) while still offering the time and space benefits of having some class sessions online. Blended learning also promises to better align with the challenges working adults and part-time students may face when time and space constraints make weekly brick-and-mortar classes a challenge to attend (Campbell, Davis, Phelan, & Hanley, 2018; Rodriguez-Keyes & Schneider, 2013).

Blended learning is a broad term that incorporates numerous variations and modalities of instruction (Bersin, 2004). Institutions and researchers have varying definitions that can be properly classified as blended learning (Graham, 2013). For instance, one may call a course blended if it includes any online learning. Students in such classes may meet face-to-face for every meeting, except for one, and the course could be considered blended since all content was not delivered face-to-face, nor was it all delivered online. Other institutions have specific ratios to more clearly codify what is meant by blended learning. For instance, at the author's university, a blended course is one that includes both online and face-to-face delivery but where students meet no more than one-third of class sessions in a face-to-face modality. In the social work literature, blended learning has also been defined in different ways, but at the core is its purposeful combination of synchronous and asynchronous learning (Bonk & Graham, 2005; Levin, Whitsett, & Wood, 2013) and generally a combination of face-to-face and computer-aided learning. The current study specifically seeks to introduce social work educators to HyFlex blended learning, a unique form and approach.

The vast array of blended learning research and offerings is primarily faculty or institution driven, and it generally is the institution or faculty member that determines how the blend of face-to-face versus online instruction will be implemented. Blending may occur according to faculty members' preferences or schedule, or institutional policies may dictate the form that blending takes. While students who have time and distance constraints may be advantaged by online learning, compared to traditional face-to-face courses, they may not fully benefit from a blended schedule when face-to-face attendance requirements do not match their schedules. When faculty or institutions decide how and when to blend, it usually is up to students to adapt their schedules.

Rationale

The HyFlex blended learning model is this student-centered approach (Beatty, 2007). Hyflex blended learning has received some attention in other areas and disciplines such as adult education (Abdelmalak, 2014), but little in the existing social work education literature. The intent of this article therefore is to introduce the social work education community to the Hyflex blended model of learning. The current article will define HyFlex blended learning and then present results from its utilization in an undergraduate social welfare policy course at a mid-size midwestern public university. Through the use of a pre-test post-test design, and a 5-week intervention, this research seeks to answer the following question: When given an opportunity to enroll in a HyFlex blended learning course, will students utilize varying modalities in order to meet their unique needs?

Defining HyFlex blended learning

As defined and implemented by Beatty (2006), hyflex blended learning is a combination of *hybrid* learning and *flexible* learning. *Hybrid* learning is incorporated as class content is offered in both face-to-face and online modalities. *Flexibility* is introduced since the power to choose what blended learning means is placed in the hands of each student who can choose on a continuous basis whether to attend online or in the traditional face-to-face classroom (Beatty, 2014).

Students not only can choose to come in a traditional face-to-face modality but may alternatively choose to join synchronously, but remotely, via a video-conference platform. In addition, they may choose to complete asynchronous online learning exercises throughout the week. (Furthermore, after making this choice for a given class session, students are given the same option for each future class session.) This format offers participants the power to choose what blended learning looks like for them, and provides flexibility for students facing changing constraints such as a new work schedule, challenging family situation, illnesses, or a myriad of other challenges. Providing students with such choices and autonomy aligns well with demands adult students frequently face (Kyei-Blankson, Godwyll, Nur-Awaleh, & Keengwe, 2011), as well as with the technologies which students routinely encounter in their daily lives (Miller, Risser, & Griffiths, 2013).

Beatty (2010) outlines several core principles of effective HyFlex blended learning, which bear mentioning, to include 1) learner choice, 2) equivalency, 3) reusability, and 4) accessibility. Learner choice places the power to decide what blended learning will look like in the hands of each student. Providing students with this power is crucial, and comprises the "flex" portion of the model. Equivalency guides instruction as faculty must design alternative approaches to learning that challenge students in order for them to remain engaged, regardless of the modality choose. Reusability is the principle that as students develop and utilize artifacts such as videos, podcasts, discussion board posts, etc., they are consuming and producing valuable learning resources regardless of the chosen modality to produce or consume it. Finally, accessibility underscores serving students in the way that they need it. If they cannot attend face-to-face then they need a viable alternative. If they do not have reliable internet connectivity then a different alternative is required. Each of these principles goes back to the core tenets of the HyFlex blended learning model – capitalizing on technologies through hybrid learning, and providing students with greater flexibility by giving them ongoing opportunities to choose the learning modality that will work best for them at any given time.

While discussion of this learning model can be found in publications as early as 2006 (Beatty, 2006), the overall body of literature is not extensive, and in social work education, virtually non-existent. It should be noted that the current deployment was purposely delimited to providing a basic definition of HyFlex blended learning and to implementing a pilot use of the approach in a social work education setting.

Current study

With no readily apparent utilization of the model in social work education and a minimal amount of research on HyFlex blended learning in general (Miller et al., 2013), the current research sought to examine the following questions: 1) Given the opportunity to participate in various modalities, will students preferences for different instructional modalities change? 2) When given an opportunity to participate in a HyFlex blended learning course, will students blend varying modalities to meet their unique and changing needs? 3) When given a choice of modality, which format will students actually select? 4) What benefits and challenges did students experience with each modality? 5) What are students' overall attitudes toward HyFlex blended learning? And 6) Do students feel that the rigor and quality of the different modalities are comparable?

The author implemented the HyFlex model for a five-week segment of a traditional face-to-face course. (Given the lack of evidence to support this model in social work, a 5-week trial was seen as a more appropriate experiment rather than an entire course.) Students were briefed on the research project and signed the requisite IRB human subjects forms. Students were offered a choice on a week to week basis to attend class in one of three ways: 1) they could attend face-to-face as they originally registered to do; 2) attend synchronously via video-conference using Zoom software; or 3) complete asynchronous online exercises that were the equivalent of the tasks students in the face-to-face section completed through the learning management system. Students completed a preference survey prior to the five-week experiment. Students then had the freedom to choose on a weekly basis which modality to participate in that particular week. Following completion of the five-week experiment, the class resumed meeting face-to-face and students completed a follow-up survey. It should also be noted that, given the basic level of research of this project, student learning outcomes in terms of grades on examinations or other assignments were not assessed in this experiment.

Methods

Sample

All 18 students participating in a required undergraduate social policy course were invited to participate and all chose to do so. Students in the course were enrolled in a face-to-face program, and only one reported commuting more than 10 miles to class. All of the 18 students either were social work majors, minors, or enrolled in a similar major.

Course structure

As previously noted, this 5-week experiment served as a preliminary foray into the HyFlex Blended learning approach in one social work course taught by one faculty member. It is acknowledged that such learning may look different for each course and each instructor (Miller et al., 2013), and thus it is necessary to outline how the 5-week section of this course was taught from a pedagogical standpoint.

Prior to beginning the 5-week portion of the course, the faculty member prepared lesson plans for each of the five modules (weeks). The class was taught in a block format for 3 hours for those who choose to come face-to-face. Students choosing to attend face-to-face would download a worksheet at the beginning of the class from the Learning Management System [LMS] that had question and exercise prompts to be utilized during the class session. During the three-hour block, the instructor would proceed from one exercise to the next while students took notes and completed tasks as outlined on the worksheet. For example, after a brief lecture on a new concept about policy analysis, participants would complete an exercise such as a matching or sorting activity or response to a brief writing prompt. Some exercises were to be completed individually while others were done in three seven-member teams. At the end of the face-to-face class, students would upload their completed worksheets that would serve as their notes from the class as well as evidence of their engagement during the class session. Those who chose to attend remotely via Zoom would participate in the same way. These students would watch brief lectures synchronously on their computers and complete worksheets on their own, or in small groups, when appropriate.

Students who chose to participate asynchronously would complete the same exercises as those attending face-to-face but would do so on their own time and at their own pace so long as they abided by established due dates. Generally, two due dates were provided, with several exercises being due on Tuesday and the remaining exercises, including follow-up discussions, being due on Thursday. The Thursday to Thursday due dates for each module ensured that students could stay caught up and still choose each week to attend classes via their preferred modality.

Measures

Utilizing an online survey platform, students completed a brief survey the week prior to the experiment and again the week after the end of the experiment.

Student modality preference

Both in the pre and post-test, students were asked the following questions:

- If you could only choose one modality for a course which modality would you choose?
- Of these three approaches, rank them from most to least preferred (1 = favorite, 3 = least favorite)

() Face-to-face
() Video Conference
() Asynchronously

Student-driven blending expectations and actual attendance

In order to assess if students would take advantage of the flexible course options, they were asked to predict their choice for modalities for the varying class periods. Students were presented with a list of dates that class would be offered and asked to predict whether they would attend each session face-to-face, online via video-conference, or online at their own pace and time. (They also were presented with an "Other" option if they wanted to combine two modalities for a specific week.) The original intent was to offer the students a choice over six consecutive weeks. However, due to attendance at a conference, one of the 6 weeks was offered in the online asynchronous modality for all students. Student choices for actually participating each week were monitored by either taking attendance in class or completion of exercises in the LMS which would constitute a post-test measure of student-driven blending. Student attendance also was categorized based on the ratio of online versus face-to-face classes that they attended.

Benefits and challenges of each modality

Students were asked to identify both the benefits and challenges they experienced from those in which they actually participated.

Student attitudes toward HyFlex blended learning

Students were presented with the following question:

- Assess your views on the following statements:

If a full course were to be offered where you could choose on a weekly basis to participate online or face-to-face, (choose all that apply)

- I would choose this type of format over a face-to-face course
- I would choose this format over a fully online course
- I would pay an additional fee (<$100) to have the option to choose each week if I could attend online or face-to-face
- I would choose this format but I would not pay extra to have this option

Students also responded to the following question as a means of assessing their perceptions of the rigor associated with each modality:

- True or False: I felt like the rigor and quality of the online coursework was equal to rigor and quality of the work in the face-to-face section.

Results

Student modality preference

Overall, students reported that their preferred modality was the face-to-face format. However, when comparing these rankings between the pre and post-test, there was movement toward more students preferring an asynchronous modality. Some clearly had a positive experience in the asynchronous modules as evidence by an increased preference for such instruction, when comparing the pretest and posttest preferences. [See Table 1]

Student-driven blending expectations versus actual attendance

A comparison of students' <u>predicted</u> choice of modality each week and their <u>actual</u> selections are presented in Table 2. The table shows the number of students that predicted and utilized each modality of instruction during the five-week experiment. [See Table 2]

Generally, student predictions did not match their actual choices. Overall, students predicted that they would attend more face-to-face than online sessions. However, more of them decided to participate via online asynchronous modules. In fact, when comparing student predictions of their choice of attendance, only 3 of the 18 students actually followed their prediction for all 5 weeks. Two students predicted completing all sessions online and followed through; one student predicted attending all classes face-to-face and chose to participate in this manner.

Table 3 further outlines the ratio of online to face-to-face classes that each student chose to participate in. While several completed the bulk of the modules in face-to-face sessions, the majority of students ultimately chose to participate more often online. Specifically, 72% completed the majority of class sessions online while 28% selected to attend the majority of sessions in a face-to-face format. Some students chose to complete everything online (44%), while others chose to complete everything face-to-face (17%). The remaining 39% of students chose to blend their learning according to their personal needs.

Table 1. Student rankings of preferred modalities.

Modality	If students could only choose 1 modality	Pretest average rank	Posttest average rank
Face-to-face	10	1.3	1.5
Video conference	1	2.6	2.9
Asynchronous	7	2.1	1.6

Table 2. Student predicted attendance compared to actual attendance.

| | Week 1 | | Week 2 | | Week 3 | | Week 4 | | Week 5 | |
	Predicted	Actual	Predicted	Actual	Predicted	Actual	Predicted	Actual	Predicted	Actual
Face-to-face	11	8	12	6	10	7	8	6	12	6
Online	5	10	4	12	6	11	9	12	5	12
Video Conference	2	0	2	0	2	0	1	0	1	0

Table 3. Student blending choices.

Ratio of Online to Face-to-face	Number of Students	Percent of Students
100% Online 0% Face-to-face	8	44%
80% Online 20% Face-to-face	1	6%
60% Online 40% Face-to-face	4	22%
40% Online 60% Face-to-face	0	0%
20% Online 80% Face-to-face	2	11%
0% Online 100% Face-to-face	3	17%

Benefits and challenges

Table 4 outlines student responses when asked about perceived benefits and challenges they experienced from the varying modalities.

Attitudes toward HyFlex blended learning

Finally, Table 5 presents participants' responses as they relate to future HyFlex blended course offerings.

Table 4. Student reported benefits and challenges of the different learning modalities.

Benefits of the asynchronous online modality
- Opportunity to pick up more work hours or spend time on school work that was more urgent
- Ability to move at own pace – complete work faster or slower if needed, take breaks when needed
- Able to still participate when faced with illness or having feelings of anxiety
- Opportunity to remain at home
- Chance to replay videos if content was not understood the first time

Benefits of the face-to-face modality
- Complete tasks in class at a consistent time
- Easier to stay caught up on coursework
- Matches the learner's preference of interacting face-to-face
- Chance to share and learn in groups and from fellow classmates and enjoy regular interactions with classmates
- Chance to ask questions and get immediate feedback rather than waiting for email replies
- Easier to focus

Challenges of face-to-face instruction
- Took more time and offered less flexibility for breaks
- Left less time to work (for pay) or for other activities with family
- The 2–5 pm timing was not ideal as it was hard to maintain focus
- Language challenges for non-native English speakers

Challenges of asynchronous online learning
- Learning exercises were time-consuming and there were many tasks to complete
- Procrastinating online tasks or forgetting them altogether
- Feeling like students have to learn more on their own

Challenges with technology
- Not as many interactions with classmates or chances to learn from them
- Delayed response to questions – no immediate feedback

Table 5. Student views on HyFlex blended learning.

Statement	% of student agreement
I would choose this type of format over a face-to-face course	28%
I would choose this format over a fully online course	39%
I would pay an additional fee (<$100) to have the option to choose each week if I could attend online or face-to-face	22%
I would choose this format but I would not pay extra to have this option	39%

Rigor

Eleven of the eighteen (61%) students said that they felt the rigor and quality of the online coursework was equal to that of the face-to-face section. In informal discussions with the seven students who felt that the rigor did not match, some stated the online work was easier, while others described the online work as being challenging.

Discussion

The current study is small in scale but may serve as a useful starting point for examining the utilization of the HyFlex model in social work education. While additional research (across a full course and additional sections) would make a stronger case for generalizability to other courses and programs, we feel that important conclusions perhaps may be drawn from this pilot research. Four will be discussed.

Complexity of life

Results highlight that students' intentions to attend or complete coursework using a specific modality clearly did not match their actual decisions. Students' lives often change from week to week due to challenges arising from home life, work expectations or illness. The sheer complexity of life, as well as the reality that many students now are working more hours outside of school than ever before (Carnevale, Smith, Melton, & Price, 2015) suggest a need to offer greater flexibility of instruction. It is unrealistic to make an early one-time decision regarding attending in-person versus online when unanticipated events occur in adult lives.

Known preferences

Nevertheless, there were some students who clearly knew their preferred learning modality and were able to align their choices with such stated preferences. For example, 11 students identified face-to-face instruction as their preferred modality. Most of these students then made plans and followed through with their intention to attend face-to-face for four or five of the sessions. Additionally, some students described a preference for the asynchronous option and proceeded to complete assignments this way for each of the 5 weeks.

General optimism

Overall, students expressed a positive view toward the HyFlex model and felt that it yielded favorable results. While some recognized that they were not always able to participate in their preferred modality of instruction, they felt that they were still able to learn the course content in a way that fit well with their current life circumstances.

Synchronous instruction not utilized

Despite the fact that several students intended to participate via videoconference, not one single student participated via this modality. This outcome suggests that while a synchronous paradigm may sound good in theory, at least in this sample, students more often chose to participate online because of time, rather than distance constraints. Perhaps these numbers would be different if the class were to consist of more students commuting a greater distance.

Benefits

HyFlex blended learning is student-driven (Kyei-Blankson & Godwyll, 2010). Students can decide on a week to week basis which modality best fits their circumstances at a given time. The HyFlex approach offers even greater flexibility, especially as unanticipated challenges arise such as illness, issues with transportation, unexpected child or elder-care needs, or whatever unique and unanticipated situation comes up. Students who participate in a HyFlex blended course may experience enhanced levels of satisfaction (Miller et al., 2013) and increased participation (Kyei-Blankson, Godwyll, & Nur-Awaleh, 2014), while still performing at the same academic level (Lakhal, Khechine, & Pascot, 2014).

Challenges

Although the HyFlex blended approach may be ideal for student autonomy, such offerings demand additional planning and preparation by faculty. While traditional approaches to blended learning mandate a unique faculty skill set, training (Ma'arop & Embi, 2016), and additional work to be effective (McGee & Reis, 2012; Pelech et al., 2013), HyFlex blending requires additional technical ability, and commitment to a flexible approach to learning. Faculty cannot easily plan in advance how many students will actually come to face-to-face sessions on a given day which can complicate specific instructional plans such as group activities or simulation. Instructors may have to alter the class exercises they deploy as different numbers of students may impact the types of learning exercises that students can best participate in (Pelech et al., 2013). Faculty who seek to implement a HyFlex approach also may be required to redesign course content in order to have online equivalents for all learning exercises (Wright, 2016). Consistent with previous research regarding online learning, the social work program may also require additional financial resources (Stotzer, Fujikawa, Sur, & Arnsberger, 2013). In this light, the HyFlex blended learning model may not be ideal for all classes, instructors, or institutions. Given general concerns around online education in social work education as a whole among many faculty (Levin, Fulginiti, & Moore, 2018), a new and even more complex approach may not likely have widespread support.

Implications and limitations

However, Hyflex blended learning is an approach to instruction that is slowly beginning to gather an evidence base (Lakhal et al., 2014). Despite the challenges and additional work that may be imposed on faculty to adopt such a model, we feel it is still an approach worth considering. The HyFlex blended model may, in fact, garner more attention as faculty roles change and online education continues to impact pedagogy in various ways, reshaping traditional in-class versus online boundaries (Dziuban & Moskal, 2011). Institutions that choose to adopt it may also be able to offer courses to online and traditional students at the same time without having to offer multiple sections of the same course (Beatty, 2014).

It should be noted that the HyFlex approach is not ideal for all classes, institutions or contexts. The current study was conducted at the BSW level with a sample of traditional college-aged students. While further research would be necessary to validate the model at the MSW level as a whole, or in a graduate policy course, it is anticipated that MSW students also would benefit from the flexibility offered through a HyFlex blended format. Research indeed suggests that MSW students may display greater preparedness for online learning (Buchanan & Mathews, 2013) and thus be more likely to succeed with a HyFlex blended learning format.

The HyFlex blended paradigm may not be universally applicable, but it does challenge current approaches that are still unable to respond adequately to the multi-faceted needs of today's students. HyFlex blended learning can be viewed simply as another tool social work programs can implement to better recruit and serve their students. The approach can enable social work faculty to offer blended learning in a way that enables more students to complete their social work degrees. Bonk and Graham (2005) suggest that one of the main drivers and benefits of offering blended instruction is to facilitate access. The HyFlex blended model may well expand access to an even broader array of students than more traditional approaches to blended learning.

Hence, this article serves as an introduction of the Hyflex model for social work education. Findings from one class with one instructor and only 18 students are not generalizable across institutions, courses, programs or instructors. Additionally, the 18 students in this study fit the traditional college mold, being between the ages of 18–22. Additional research with non-traditional students of varying ages and circumstances might offer more generalizable data for the universe of BSW programs. While such limitations, of course, must be kept in mind, the current research seeks to introduce the model and offer a starting point for further research and discussion.

Disclosure statement

No potential conflict of interest was reported by the author.

References

Abdelmalak, M. (2014, March). Towards flexible learning for adult students: HyFlex design. In M. Searson & M. Ochoa (Eds.), *Proceedings of SITE2014–Society for Information Technology & Teacher Education International Conference* (pp. 706–712). Jacksonville, Florida: Association for the Advancement of Computing in Education (AACE).

Beatty, B. (2006, October). *Designing the hyFlex world - hybrid, flexible courses for all students.* Paper presented at Association for Educational Communication and Technology International Conference, Dallas, TX.

Beatty, B. (2007, June). Transitioning to an online world: Using HyFlex courses to bridge the gap. In C. Montgomerie & J. Seale (Eds.), *EdMedia: World conference on educational media and technology* (pp. 2701–2706). Chesapeake, VA: Association for the Advancement of Computing in Education (AACE).

Beatty, B. (2010). *Hybrid courses with flexible participation – the HyFlex design. Draft v2.2.* Retrieved from http://itec.sfsu.edu/hyflex/hyflex_course_design_theory_2.2.pdf

Beatty, B. (2014). Hybrid courses with flexible participation: The HyFlex course design. In L. Kyei-Blankson & E. Ntuli (Eds.), *Practical applications and experiences in K-20 blended learning environments* (pp. 153–177). Hershey, PA: IGI Global.

Bernard, R. M., Borokhovski, E., Schmid, R. F., Tamim, R. M., & Abrami, P. C. (2014). A meta-analysis of blended learning and technology use in higher education: From the general to the applied. *Journal of Computing in Higher Education, 26*(1), 87–122. doi:10.1007/s12528-013-9077-3

Bersin, J. (2004). *The blended learning book: Best practices, proven methodologies, and lessons learned.* San Francisco, CA: Pfeiffer.

Bonk, C. J., & Graham, C. R. (2005). *The handbook of blended learning: Global perspectives, local designs.* San Francisco, CA: Pfeiffer.

Buchanan, R. L., & Mathews, D. A. (2013). A comparison of student knowledge and attitude toward research: Are main campus students different from those in a hybrid environment? *Journal of Teaching in Social Work, 33*(4–5), 467–480. doi:10.1080/08841233.2013.828668

Campbell, J., Davis, M., Phelan, A., & Hanley, D. (2018). Dealing with the learning needs of child welfare social and health care workers: an interdisciplinary approach to blended learning with part time students. *Social Work Education, 37*(6), 746–760. doi:10.1080/02615479.2018.1479384

Carnevale, A. P., Smith, N., Melton, M., & Price, E. (2015). *Learning while earning: The new normal.* Washington, DC: Georgetown University Center on Education and the Workforce. Retrieved from https://cew.georgetown.edu/wp-content/uploads/Working-Learners-Report.pdf

Carter, I., Damianakis, T., Munro, S., Skinner, H., Matin, S., & Nash Andrews, T. (2018). Exploring online and blended course delivery in social group work. *Journal of Teaching in Social Work, 38*(5), 486–503. doi:10.1080/08841233.2018.1523824

Dziuban, C., & Moskal, P. (2011). A course is a course is a course: Factor invariance in student evaluation of online, blended and face-to-face learning environments. *The Internet and Higher Education, 14*(4), 236–241. doi:10.1016/j.iheduc.2011.05.003

Garrison, D. R., & Kanuka, H. (2004). Blended learning: Uncovering its transformative potential in higher education. *The Internet and Higher Education, 7*(2), 95–105. doi:10.1016/j.iheduc.2004.02.001

Graham, C. R. (2013). Emerging practice and research in blended learning. In M. J. Moore (Ed.), *Handbook of distance education* (3rd ed., pp. 333–350). New York, NY: Routledge.

Kurzman, P. A., & Maiden, R. P. (Eds.). (2014). *Distance learning and online education in social work.* New York, NY: Routledge.

Kyei-Blankson, L., & Godwyll, F. (2010, October). An examination of learning outcomes in HyFlex learning environments. In J. Sanchez & K. Zhang (Eds.), *E-Learn: World conference on E-Learning in corporate, government, healthcare, and higher education* (pp. 532–535). Chesapeake, VA: Association for the Advancement of Computing in Education (AACE).

Kyei-Blankson, L., Godwyll, F., Nur-Awaleh, M., & Keengwe, J. (2011, March). The New Blend: When students are given the option to choose. In M. Koehler & P. Mishra (Eds.), *Society for information technology & teacher education international conference* (pp. 433–436). Chesapeake, VA: Association for the Advancement of Computing in Education (AACE).

Kyei-Blankson, L., Godwyll, F., & Nur-Awaleh, M. A. (2014). Innovative blended delivery and learning: exploring student choice, experience, and level of satisfaction in a hyflex course. *International Journal of Innovation and Learning, 16*(3), 243–252. doi:10.1504/IJIL.2014.064728

Lakhal, S., Khechine, H., & Pascot, D. (2014). Academic students' satisfaction and learning outcomes in a HyFlex course: Do delivery modes matter?. In T. Bastiaens (Ed.), *E-Learn: World conference on E-Learning in corporate, government, healthcare, and higher education* (pp. 1075–1083). New Orleans, LA: Association for the Advancement of Computing in Education (AACE).

Levin, S., Fulginiti, A., & Moore, B. (2018). The perceived effectiveness of online social work education: insights from a national survey of social work educators. *Social Work Education, 37*(6), 775–789. doi:10.1080/02615479.2018.1482864

Levin, S., Whitsett, D., & Wood, G. (2013). Teaching MSW social work practice in a blended online learning environment. *Journal of Teaching in Social Work, 33*(4–5), 408–420. doi:10.1080/08841233.2013.829168

Ma'arop, A. H., & Embi, M. A. (2016). Implementation of blended learning in higher learning institutions: A review of literature. *International Education Studies, 9*(3), 41. doi:10.5539/ies.v9n3p41

McGee, P., & Reis, A. (2012). Blended course design: A synthesis of best practices. *Journal of Asynchronous Learning Networks, 16*(4), 7–22.

Miller, J., Risser, M., & Griffiths, R. (2013). Student choice, instructor flexibility: Moving beyond the blended instructional model. *Issues and Trends in Educational Technology, 1*(1), 8–24.

Pelech, W., Wulff, D., Perrault, E., Ayala, J., Baynton, M., Williams, M., … Shankar, J. (2013). Current challenges in social work distance education: Responses from the Elluminati. *Journal of Teaching in Social Work, 33*(4–5), 393–407. doi:10.1080/08841233.2013.834863

Racovita-Szilagyi, L., Carbonero Muñoz, D., & Diaconu, M. (2018). Challenges and opportunities to eLearning in social work education: perspectives from Spain and the United States. *European Journal of Social Work, 21*(6), 1–14. doi:10.1080/13691457.2018.1461066

Rodriguez-Keyes, E., & Schneider, D. (2013). Cultivating curiosity: Integrating hybrid teaching in courses in human behavior in the social environment. *Journal of Teaching in Social Work, 33*(3), 227–238. doi:10.1080/08841233.2013.796304

Rovai, A. P., & Jordan, H. M. (2004). Blended learning and sense of community: A comparative analysis with traditional and fully online courses. *International Review of Research in Open and Distance Learning, 5*(2). Retrieved from http://www.irrodl.org/index.php/irrodl/article/view/192/274.

Stotzer, R. L., Fujikawa, K., Sur, J., & Arnsberger, P. (2013). Cost analysis of a distance education MSW program. *Journal of Teaching in Social Work, 33*(4–5), 357–368. doi:10.1080/08841233.2013.826318

Wright, D. (2016). The HyFlex course design: A case study on adult and career education courses. *National Social Science Journal, 48*(2), 88–93.

Teacher as Client Therapy (TACT): A Model for Simulated Learning for Traditional and Online Delivery Models

Jason S. McKinney

ABSTRACT

The movement towards competency-based education in social work has required a shift in delivery to more experiential learning opportunities for students. Looking forward, the Council on Social Work Education [CSWE] has instituted a Futures Task Force, exploring roles social workers may play in the future, with particular attention to the evolution and revolution in technology. It is clear that social work programs will need to consider opportunities for ensuring the development of competency in an ever changing digital landscape. This article presents the evolution of a simulation model for use in various delivery models, including traditional face-to-face campus-based offerings, off-campus satellite classes, and hybrid or fully online courses. It documents the origin of the model in an off-campus format, highlighting the attributes afforded with its application on a traditional campus, and proposes an online solution to the resource dilemma endemic to many off-campus satellite models.

Introduction

The movement to competency-based social work education, with emphasis on measurable practice skills and behaviors, can be complemented via simulation experiences in social work classes, which has been touted as a promising practice both for preparing *and* assessing readiness for practice (Linsk & Tunney, 1997; Mooradian, 2007, 2008). Through the work of its Futures Task Force, the Council on Social Work Education (CSWE) has directed special attention to the evolution and revolution of technology, recognizing that the requisite roles of social workers will and must change to meet the needs of individuals, families, and communities in the future. The Task Force Report is a call to action to social work programs to join in the endeavor to respond to the contexts that shape practice (CSWE, 2018, April). This consideration of technology is not a new phenomenon, but rather one that dates to the origins of the profession. Consider the seminal work of Mary Richmond, who, more than one hundred years ago, urged fearful social workers to consider the telephone as a useful tool for social work practice (Richmond, 1917). Still today, the apprehension of educators toward instructional technology is reminiscent of the fear of the telephone in the past; yet, many faculty are already embracing the affordances of technology as a useful tool for learning. Clearly, preparing students for the future of social work requires both building upon the past *and* anticipating the future.

One such approach is the use of simulation experiences in the online arena which mimics the growing use of tele-therapy by clinical social work practitioners. This article will detail the use of the Teacher as Client Therapy (TACT) simulation model, developed for use in multiple delivery models (i.e., traditional campus-based, distance campuses, and online instruction), as an innovative approach with potential to augment a student's sense of competence as well as increase the opportunity to supervise, evaluate, and provide individual feedback on the development of practice skills.

The TACT simulation model: continuous improvement leading to online delivery

As is the case with many discoveries, the TACT model was not intentionally crafted, but rather was an incremental realization that began during an attempted class role play activity, at an off-campus satellite location, within a required course, Advanced Clinical Practice with Individuals, in the second year of an MSW program. During a face-to-face evening class, students were asked to practice a prescribed clinical technique in dyads, a common pedagogical practice of this author, which materialized differently this particular evening. The all-to-common issue during partner work in the classroom is the odd number of students in a class, requiring a student to join another dyad, or dividing the class into triads. Although viable options, I instead volunteered to be one student's partner, allowing the student to practice the technique as if I were the client; and when the others in the class were instructed to switch roles, I provided feedback to the student in a supervisory manner. Although this student reported initial anxiety at the notion, it was considered an extremely valuable learning experience – so much so, that I began purposefully working with a different student during each subsequent class session. This section will present the general evolution of the simulation experience, as it developed from its conception at the off-campus location to the traditional campus, and finally back to the off-campus site with the addition of online simulation as a proposed solution to a resource problem.

Version 2.0: traditional campus

Based on student reports of an increased sense of competence after having regular opportunities for experiential learning and immediate feedback, the approach was incorporated into the syllabus as a clinical demonstration assignment and an in-class activity. In a quest to provide a more realistic simulation experience of clinical practice, and considering that traditional campuses often offer more resources (such as office space) than leased classrooms off campus, the utilization of private office space provided the necessary environment for the new-and-improved simulation. Students found the experience of having a private office to be far more comfortable due to the decreased distraction and the increased privacy.

Version 3.0: online simulation for off-campus

After teaching at the traditional on-campus site, I returned to an off-campus location to teach another section of the course with the new-and-improved version 2.0 in the syllabus. Although the experience was more organized now that it was clearly conceptualized in the syllabus, providing focused super-vision, with the teacher as client for every student, the encounter was substandard in contrast to version 2.0. Without private office space, the process was not a simulation at all, but was classroom role play. Some students were noticeably distracted by the voices of other students practicing, looking over their shoulders in response to what sometimes sounded like a classroom of parrots as the students echoed one another, practicing the technique at differential rates. The addition of a portable white-noise machine in the center of the classroom reduced some of the noise, but naturally could not remove the visual distractions or replicate the quiet environment of private office space. Once again, the quest for continuous improvement commenced, and it was eventually realized that synchronistic online platforms could not only address the issue of distraction, but could also offer a private space while mimicking the practice of tele-therapy.

Online education programs, such as Zoom, offer the ability for real-time, face-to-face video interaction with students via the online platform. A key educational feature of Zoom is that it allows the instructor to assign students to dyads (or groups), and with a mere click students can privately practice the clinical technique with the assigned partner. Once the allotted time for the session has ended, the instructor can reconvene the entire class for a plenary discussion. While the physical office space will continue to be utilized on the traditional campus, where the resource is available, using Zoom (or similar online educational software) became a highly effective alternative for hybrid courses at off-campus sites.

Method

As a graded assignment, students are required to participate in six simulated sessions, dispersed over six classes, which are labeled "Clinical Exercises and

Table 1. Class Time Utilization.

Class Time Utilization	
30 Minutes	Theory Review
30 Minutes	Demonstration of Technique
1 Hour	Simulated Practice and Supervision
1 Hour	Critical Reflection

Demonstrations" in the syllabus. In the three hours of class time, the first thirty minutes are spent reviewing a theory and another thirty minutes demonstrating practice technique(s). An hour is dedicated to the simulation and practice sessions during which time each student spends twenty-five minutes practicing before switching partners. The last hour of class includes a period of critical reflection, using the DEAL model (Ash & Clayton, 2009), *describing* the experience of the simulation, *examining* how it went (e.g., What went well? What didn't? How did the client experience the session?), and *articulating learning*. See Table 1 for specific details on the proposed use of class time.

Theory review

The first thirty minutes of each class, during which the simulated exercises occur, is dedicated to reviewing theory, namely the theory and/or practice model from which the particular technique to be simulated is derived, such as psychoanalytic, person-centered, cognitive-behavioral, solution-focused, narrative, or trauma-informed. Although this constitutes a review for students, having already taken a course on theory, the connection between theory and practice is emphasized with the expectation that students will move beyond preferring *how-to* knowledge, or a "cook book approach," – favoring intervention strategies over theory – and develop an appreciation for the reasons *why* we intervene in particular ways – that is, the theory behind the interventions, which offers more generalizable knowledge toward developing new interventions based on theoretical understanding.

During this time, questions are explored such as, "What does this theory suggest is the origin of presenting problems? What is the connection between the view of presenting problems and the assumptions about potential solutions? How are solutions to presenting problems approached from this perspective?" As answers to these questions unfold, the discussion naturally turns to techniques for assessment and intervention based on the theory in consideration.

Demonstrating technique

A student volunteer is solicited to partner with the instructor to facilitate the demonstration of the technique(s) for the class. Refer to Table 2 for select

Table 2. Select Techniques.

Theory/ Model	Technique(s)
Psychoanalytic	Float Back
Person-Centered	Non-directive Questions, Reflections, Summaries
Cognitive-Behavioral	CBT Triangle: Thinking, Feeling, Doing
Solution-Focused	Miracle Question, Exceptions
Narrative	Reauthoring and Remembering
Trauma-informed	Trauma History, Containment

techniques. In the front of the class, the professor demonstrates the technique(s) to be simulated for the class period, which are as follows:

Psychoanalytic

The float back technique is the first simulated session and is an intentionally simple approach to help students make the connection between a client's past experiences and present functioning. Students are instructed to explore the client's feelings related to the presenting problem and to ask the client to consider his or her earliest memory of feeling this way with the goal of helping the client develop insight regarding the connection between early life experiences and the present situation.

Person-centered

The person-centered approach is often difficult for students who desire a more scripted method, while others prefer the flexibility within the style. Students are asked to explore the presenting problem while simply attempting to gain an in-depth understanding of the client's experience and perspective of the problem, without offering advice or proposing solutions, and practicing the art of being non-directive. They practice open-ended questions and attentive listening, using reflections of feelings and summaries of what the client has discussed.

Cognitive-behavioral

The cognitive-behavioral triangle is presented as both an assessment tool as well as intervention technique. Considering the presenting problem, students are asked to explore the three domains while assessing, in no particular order, while taking notes in the categories of thinking, feeling, and doing as they emerge in the discussion. Examples of the types of questions include, "So while this is happening, what thoughts are running through your mind? How do you feel when this is happening? How do you typically respond when this occurs?" Once students have explored each of these areas with furthering questions, attention is shifted to help clients see the interplay between their thoughts, feelings, and actions.

Solution-focused

Using a variation of Insoo Kim-Berg and Steve De Shazer's (cf de Shazer & Dolan, 2012) approach, students are asked to use the "miracle question," asking the client to imagine waking up in the morning, when the problem no longer exists, and to note what would be the first few clues that things were different. Students also are asked to search for exceptions to the problem by strategically asking about times when the problem did not exist, preferably without asking directly in order to avoid defense mechanisms, or the subjective experience of the enduring nature of the problem. For example, if asked directly, "Can you think of a time when this wasn't happening?" A client may assert, "It seems like this has been going on forever!" In order to avoid this outcome, students are directed to use more creative questioning, such as "How long has this been going on? And before that? What was life like then?"

Narrative

The demonstration of *reauthoring* and *remembering* is adapted from a Narrative Therapy training that the author attended during which Micheal White demonstrated these techniques (White, 2007). Reauthoring included the deconstruction of the client's presenting problem by considering the dominant storyline, which includes the negative and traumatic aspects often remembered, and the subordinate storyline, which adds the client's values and commensurate actions within the story. *Remembering*, or "re-membershipping," as White called it, entails exploring the sources of the values and the reconnection to those aspects of the client's identity that often are overshadowed by the problem the client is experiencing (M. White, personal communication, October, 2007). For example, White shared how one person with whom he consulted noted how a particular children's book was an inspiration, and so he encouraged the client to write a letter to the author and note the impact of the story. The author replied to the letter, which further reinforced the client's identity.

Trauma-informed

In this practice session, Greenwald's (2013) Progressive Counting scripts are used to take a brief trauma history, using a "Best Things/ Worst Things" scenario, and deep breathing containment exercises, to help the client practice mindfulness at the end of the session. The session is not intended to explore the client's trauma history in detail, as in other approaches, but rather to create a brief bulleted version, preventing the client from prematurely exploring unresolved traumas.

Often the most anticipated portion of the simulation experience is the demonstration of the technique during which students hope to learn *precisely* how to perform the intervention themselves which, depending on the topic, may or may not be feasible. For example, if discussing a person-centered approach the *sorts* of non-directive questions would be demonstrated, rather than the *exact* questions students should quote. In such cases, students are directed to focus on the concepts, such as non-directive, open-ended questions, rather than on replicating practice techniques verbatim.

Simulated practice and supervision

With assigned partners, students are provided a private office to replicate the environment of clinical practice. They practice up to three techniques from the particular model or theory with their client, who is assigned a presenting problem from the instructor, which is often something benign such as the stresses of graduate school. The topic is safe enough for practicing students, yet real enough for the clients to understand their role in the simulation and comfortably embody the character. After twenty-five minutes the students switch roles *and* partners. (Students who were social workers become clients, and students who were clients become social workers.) It is most effective to have students switch partners, rather than simply switching roles with the same partner, so that students aren't the client of a social worker who just was in the role of the client and vice versa. The most efficient way of organizing this transition is to have students who were the clients remain in their offices to become the social worker in the next simulation, and the students who were the social workers rotate to the next office. The benefit of this approach is twofold: 1) the experience is more highly organized causing less wasted time with confusion regarding the dyads, and 2) having the client remain in the same office allows for a nice transition as they become the new social worker. As those who were previously the social worker migrate to the next office to become the client, they can enter the office and be welcomed by their social worker as if it is the beginning of a session.

The symbolic beginning and ending of the sessions (i.e., entering and exiting offices) are helpful for embracing the character of social worker and client. In addition to the office changes, a script is used for beginning and ending the session. Students are directed to begin by welcoming the client to the office, inviting them to sit down, and then asking, "So tell me what brings you in today?" In the same way, students are directed to end each session with a summary of what has been discussed, and then to state, "Thank you for coming in today. I will see you next week." Such a "book ends" approach to beginning and ending sessions curtails the awkwardness of getting started with role play (e.g., "umm okay? What were we supposed to do again?") or ending (e.g., "Yeah ummm … I don't know what else to say, so I think we're done?").

While students are practicing, the instructor also serves as the client for one or two students, depending on the size of the class, so that students will have worked with their teacher as the client during the course. The author offered the same presenting problem to each student: reporting feeling over-whelmed with work, graduate school, and recent conflict in their marriage relationship. Using a common presenting problem not only ensures a similar experience for all students, but more importantly, that the instructor will have a consistent means of evaluating student performance. On occasion, a student may commit whole-heartedly to "fixing" the marriage, while for-getting that the presenting problem actually is the stress of balancing work, school, and family, which causes the client to feel frustrated and misunder-stood. Such a scenario offers a valuable opportunity for learning through immediate supervisory feedback.

Supervision and consultation are provided both during and after the session. If a student needs direction, the instructor can say "cut" and step out of the role to offer suggestions to keep the student on track; or, after the session, at which point the instructor can evaluate how it felt to be the client, as well as identify strengths and areas for growth.

Critical reflection

The last hour of class is used to critically reflect on the experience, to highlight learning, surprises, and challenges, and to explore solutions. Using the DEAL model (Ash & Clayton, 2009) the instructor structures the discussion to tease out and solidify the learning. The first task of the DEAL model is to ask students to *describe* the experience of the simulation, simply to portray what happened, without evaluation of the experience as negative or positive. This request is often difficult for students, as feelings and judge-ments, likes and dislikes, are typically at the forefront of discussion; there-fore, it is important to help students delay their evaluations, at least for a moment, until the next portion of discussion, which involves *examining* how it actually went (e.g, What went well? What didn't? How did it feel to be the social worker versus how did it feel to be the client?).

Although the *examine* portion of the discussion represents an evaluation, it constitutes a *critical* evaluation, It is therefore important to scaffold the discussion with the "examining" questions, in order to move beyond whether or not a student enjoyed the approach or not, toward a more sophisticated assessment and analysis of the session. The goal is to uncover the cognitive dissonance, which may have allowed for some of the most meaningful discussion and realizations for students. They are encouraged to resist con-clusions based purely on comfort or discomfort related to the particular techniques. Students are reminded that they are not simply "trying on for size" the various techniques to determine fit, but are practicing a new language for the first time, which is almost guaranteed to feel awkward and uncomfortable. When asked "how it went," students tend to fall into two camps, the "I liked it" and the "I didn't like it" groups, which is why questions like "what went well?" tend to lead to more in-depth exploration. The most enlightening moments have occurred when asked "how did it feel to be the client?" One plausible reason is that the experiences of "performing" the technique versus being the client typically are very different, which may create a moment of cognitive dissonance during which students become increasingly open to new perspectives. The question provides a window of opportunity for a valuable teachable moment, and therefore is deconstructed and emphasized via purposeful leading questions to which the answers often highlight inconsistencies for the student. Once the themes across student reports become repetitive, the discussion has reached what discourse researchers call "saturation." It is at this juncture that critical reflection turns to *articulating learning*.

To borrow from music theory, *articulating learning* is much like a coda in a musical piece, which directs the musician to return to a previous portion of the song. It is the point of review. The instructor might ask the question, "What does all of this mean? What can we take away from this?" The mastery articulated is not limited to what the student learned about the technique(s), but also what they comprehended about the limits of their subjective experience. Sometimes a session that felt successful to the social worker may have been frustrating to the client, or when we have felt discouraged the client has felt inspired.

Outcomes

Class discussions and student evaluations showed that students generally appeared to benefit from the project. For the first few trials, students were asked in class whether they felt a "very low," "competent," or "very high" sense of competence with the clinical practice skills from each of the models in this assignment. Students who were comfortable enough to share generally expressed feeling "very low" in their sense of competence. However, during the course wrap-up discussion, students were asked again how they would rate their sense of competence, and the majority stated "very high."

The approach eventually was added to the syllabus as a graded assignment, and therefore comments were collected on student evaluations, providing useful information as to why they felt this approach was helpful. Below are a few examples.

> "I learned the most during the demonstration with my professor for several reasons. The first being that my nerves were up as they would be once we start out in the profession for the first year or so and I needed to act under pressure. Secondly, I knew a great deal about each of my classmates where I did not know nearly as much about my professor so I was able to get to know my client and ask questions to better understand the situation."

"The professor stepping in as the client was helpful because it replicated a true client therapy session, and all of the feelings are similar to when working with a client. I had no idea what the professor was going to say his problem was and this required using the skills taught in class, and having the ability to respond quickly."

"This strategy offered us the opportunity to work with multiple peers and the professor, as well as not feel pressure from having other students watch. This intimate type of approach was also helpful because there was room to give and receive constructive criticism ... I felt like this approach was the most accurate simulation of what a real therapeutic session would be like."

"I had the same feelings when working with the professor as I would working with a client for the first time."

"This exercise was also beneficial in my work with clients during my practicum and it has allowed me to strengthen my counseling skills outside of the classroom."

"I was able to gain feedback and it seemed as though I was with an actual client because of the pressure I felt."

While students appeared to benefit from the approach, these comments should not be interpreted as, and are not purported to be, scientific inquiry of the effectiveness of the model, but rather as the experience of a small graduate class of students.

Conclusion

The Teacher As Client Therapy [TACT] simulation model for experiential learning is an approach that affords an instructor the opportunity to work with students individually, serving in the role of the student's client, followed by immediate supervision and consultation. This model appears to be a promising approach for increasing student feelings of competence in practicing social work techniques, as noted in student evaluations. Participants noted that the approach offers benefits greater than simulated interviews with classmates, video-taped mock interviews, or one-way mirror observations. Some reported that the clinical approximation offered opportunities to discover "blind spots" and to trouble-shoot. As a faculty member, the construct offered increased opportunities to evaluate student competence, in both application and cognitive understanding, which was further reinforced using the DEAL model for critical reflection. Instructors interested in adopting this paradigm may refer to this article as a general guide, or tailor their approach to incorporate any preferred practice model or technique (such as task-centered, motivational interviewing, mindfulness) in place of (or in addition to) those presented. While the online version is presented here as a "bug fix" for off-campus programs, it also could serve as a nice addition to a hybrid or fully online program.

Disclosure statement

No potential conflict of interest was reported by the author.

References

Ash, S. L., & Clayton, P. H. (2009). Generating, deepening, and documenting learning: The power of critical reflection in applied learning. *Journal of Applied Learning in Higher Education*, *1*(1), 25–48.

Council in Social Work Education [CSWE]. (2018, April). *Envisioning the future of social work: Report of the CSWE futures task force*. Author. Retrieved from https://cswe.org/About-CSWE/Governance/Boardof-Directors/2018-19-Strategic-Planning-Process/CSWE-FTF-Four-Futures-for-Social-Work-FINAL-2.aspx

de Shazer, S., & Dolan, Y. (2012). *More than miracles: The state of the art of solution-focused brief therapy*. Philadelphia, PA: Taylor & Francis.

Greenwald, R. (2013). *Progressive counting within a phase model of trauma-informed treatment*. New York and London: Routledge.

Linsk, N. L., & Tunney, K. (1997). Learning to care: Use of practice simulation to train health social workers. *Journal of Social Work Education*, *33*(3), 473–489. doi:10.1080/10437797.1997.10778887

Mooradian, J. (2007). Simulated family therapy interviews in clinical social work education. *Journal of Teaching in Social Work*, *27*, 89–104. doi:10.1300/J067v27n01_06

Mooradian, J. (2008). Using simulated sessions to enhance social work education. *Journal of Social Work Education*, *44*(3), 21–36. doi:10.5175/JSWE.2008.200700026

Richmond, M. E. (1917). *Social diagnosis*. New York, NY: Russell Sage Foundation.

White, M. (2007). *Maps of narrative practice*. New York, NY: W.W. Norton.

VoiceThread as a Tool in Online BSW Education

Janet M. Joiner and Debra Patterson

ABSTRACT

This paper presents pilot study results with 59 students enrolled in online Bachelor of Social Work courses that used VoiceThread (VT), an asynchronous communication platform. This study explored benefits and limitations associated with using VT to complete assignments, learn course content, and engage classmates. Students completed an online survey related to their VT experiences, with results indicating VT was effective in helping students engage with classmates and professors, learn course content, and improve presentation skills. Implications for using VT to facilitate learning in online courses is discussed. However, further research is needed to support the use of VT in online courses.

Student interest in Bachelor of Social Work (BSW) degree programs which offer contemporary education, and that are delivered in a user-friendly, convenient, and accessible format, are changing the landscape of traditional social work education (Neuman, 2006). To keep pace with student needs for flexibility and convenience, online learning is becoming commonplace in social work education. Moreover, studies have indicated that online courses tend to be equally effective as face-to-face ones (Madoc-Jones & Parrott, 2005; Webber, Currin, Groves, Hay, & Fernando, 2010). Yet, student engagement with online courses has been a challenge for many due to their lack of proficiency with using informational and communication technologies (ICT), lower levels of socialization with peers (Neuman, 2006), and decreased levels of faculty-student interaction (Gross & Meriwether, 2016).

ICT is an assortment of digital tools used to develop new knowledge, warehouse data and other forms of eclectic content, distribute information, and facilitate engagement with others (Perron, Taylor, Glass, & Margerum-Leys, 2010). To address student engagement concerns in online BSW education, fortunately an asynchronous, cloud-based, audio-video recording platform called VoiceThread (VT) can be used. VT, a type of ICT, is a collaborative, interactive tool that allows faculty and students to engage with course material in an online environment. VT permits users to create accounts and connect with others by uploading PowerPoint slides that contain content, including video, pictures, images, and text (Fox, 2017). VT permits users to create accounts and arrange settings as open or closed systems. Users with open systems allow other VT users to access their sites freely and view and post video, text, or audio responses. Users opting for closed stations restrict access to certain users, usually by web link. VT also allows users to employ a variety of electronic devices, including desktop and laptop computers, tablet devices, and smart phones. Users can develop original content, share information, collaborate with their virtual communities, and store content.

Literature review

Connectivism (Siemens, 2004) has been embraced by many educators as a theory that can be used to strengthen student interaction and learning in online settings. Siemens (2004) introduced several principles of connectivism, including:

- Learning and knowledge rests in diversity of opinions
- Learning is a process of connecting specialized nodes or information sources
- Learning may reside in non-human appliances
- Capacity to know more is more critical than what is currently known
- Nurturing and maintaining connections is needed to facilitate continual learning
- Ability to see connections between fields, ideas, and concepts is a core skill
- Currency (accurate, up-to-date knowledge) is the intent of all connectivist learning activities
- Decision-making is itself a learning process. Choosing what to learn and the meaning of incoming information are seen through the lens of a shifting reality. While there is a right answer now, it may be wrong tomorrow due to alterations in the information climate affecting the decision. (p. 4)

Constructing online learning exercises and activities that encourage students to form relationships and associations with each other is a feature of connectivism (Bell, 2011). Through such relationships and interactions with others, learning can be stimulated and the transfer of new knowledge attained.

Connectivism theory was used to help guide the development of VT learning opportunities, deliver lecture content, and facilitate student engagement with one another and with the course instructor. The theory has helped faculty understand the changing technological landscape in higher education and the influence of ICT in courses.

The Council on Social Work Education (CSWE, 2015) recommended that BSW programs incorporate new knowledge, technology, and ideas that may have a bearing on contemporary and future social work education, practice, and research. The use of asynchronous recording platforms for online courses has been increasing worldwide; however, some social work educators have not fully embraced using technological advances with students (Brady, McLeod, & Young, 2015). Though some faculty believe ICT presents considerable challenges, others indicate that the quality of teaching and learning is greatly enhanced (Gose, 2017).

McAllister (2013) compared four BSW courses that were taught both online and face-to-face by the same instructors. Student grades or performance did not differ, although students thought developing online relationships with their instructors and classmates was more difficult. Fortunately, we believe that asynchronous tools (such as VT) can foster relationships while helping students develop professional competence (Young, McLeod, & Brady, 2018).

VT may be particularly beneficial for baccalaureate students who are beginning to develop a professional presentation of self, client interviewing skills, problem-solving strategies, and similar competencies, such as gathering and disseminating information (Chan & Pallapu, 2012; Fox, 2017). The purpose of this pilot study was to explore student perspectives on the use of VT in three online BSW courses.

Voicethread in the classroom

Creating spontaneous opportunities for student engagement can be challenging (Kirby & Hulan, 2016). However, an emerging learning theory, connectivism, could serve as an instructional framework for faculty who are interested in using an ICT, such as VT, with their students. Connectivism is based on the premise that students who use ICT to develop learning communities and/or study groups can engage with classmates and contribute to the educational process, instead of passively consuming course content (Dunaway, 2011).

Several studies (Chan & Pallapu, 2012; Ching & Hsu, 2013; Fox, 2017; Gonzalez & Moore, 2018) focused on the effectiveness of using VT with college students. The research explored VT use in online courses, including business, education, and nursing. Research by Chan and Pallapu (2012) explored online interactions of students enrolled in an undergraduate business policy course. The authors reported that VT could be used effectively to help students to learn course content and participate in educational activities. Ching and Hsu (2013) used VT with graduate-level students enrolled in online courses. Students in their study reported that VT was easy to use and the audio and video functions of VT helped them engage with their peers.

VT has also been deployed to enhance teaching and learning with nursing students. Research by Fox (2017) indicated that nursing students preferred to use VT rather than traditional text-based online discussion boards. These students reported that VT helped them to feel as if they were in class, engaging with peers and the instructor. Gonzalez and Moore (2018) studied VT use with graduate students enrolled in online thesis writing courses. Results from their research was encouraging, with students reporting positive experiences based on their ability to receive constructive feedback from their instructors using the VT tool. Each of these studies supported the use of VT as an effective modality for delivering academic content and encouraging interactions among students. Nevertheless, while VT has been used widely in higher education, with a variety of academic majors, research highlighting the use of this tool in social work education was not found.

Contemporary learners often use ICT to feel connected, while accessing news and other information (Fang, Mishna, Zhang, Van Wert, & Bogo, 2014). VT can be used on-the-go. In this way, VT can help bring online academic material to life and provide students with flexibility around other obligations (Fox, 2017). BSW students also can benefit from VT because they can use both Android and Apple mobile devices to access course materials through VT. Users can upload and edit PowerPoint presentations to their VT accounts and distribute links to faculty or students that would allow them to both view and comment on their presentations.

Although VT is becoming popular, research has not been identified that explored its effectiveness with BSW students. That would be the focus of our study.

Current project

The University of Detroit Mercy's Department of Social Work piloted three 15-week, fully online BSW courses during fall semester 2017, with all course content delivered asynchronously using VT. Students did not have the option to register for a hybrid and/or traditional face-to-face section because study courses were only offered online. None of the 73 students who enrolled in these three online courses objected to using VT. However, some students required additional support to complete assignments as they were not fully proficient using ICT. Additionally, a small number did not have access to a computer or mobile device with an embedded webcam. Some of these students visited the campus library to complete course assignments. (The reasons why certain students elected not to participate in the current study were not explored.)

Description of courses

The online courses included Introduction to Social Work (ISW), Social Welfare and Social Justice (SWSJ), and Human Behavior in the Social Environment I (HBSE I). To assist students in adjusting to their online courses and VT, the first assignment in each course involved posting a VT introductory video about themselves on the course Blackboard Learn (BbL) site. This assignment was developed to stimulate learning and featured students sharing basic information about themselves (e.g., name, year in college, career interest) to allow classmates and the instructor to get to know them.

ISW exposed students to the history of the profession, foundational knowledge, skills, and values, as well as career opportunities. Two VT assignments accounted for 40% of each student's final course grade. Assignments included a Social Problems PowerPoint Presentation, which was the benchmark assignment for the course. Students were expected to have a clear introduction to their topic and were encouraged to be creative in their presentation of information. The second assignment, a VoiceThread Social Issue News Article and Write-Up, required students to select a newsworthy article on a topic of personal interest. They then were expected to create a video summary of the article using no more than five PowerPoint slides. An open time frame was provided to help students increase their self-regulation abilities, strengthen verbal communication skills, as well as integrate and clarify content in the absence of strict time limits.

SWSJ focused on social welfare programs in the United States. from a political, philosophical, and historical perspective, and how these programs relate to social justice. In SWSJ and HBSE, VT-based assignments accounted for 30% of a student's final course grade and included weekly Self-Reflections, worth 1 point each, using the video function of VT. VT Self-Reflections were based on course weekly readings, instructor PowerPoint lecture content, supplemental YouTube videos, and online engagement with the course instructor and other students.

HBSE I provided a basic understanding of human behavior from a multicultural perspective, emphasizing conception through childhood, as well as biological, psychological, and social functioning. Here students were expected to share their perceptions of the most important elements that they had learned during a specific week, how they engaged with their classmates and instructor, and if they conducted online searches for additional resource information to support their learning. Finally, students were expected to share supplementary information they believed to be relevant and helpful.

Operational costs

The university did not hold a VT license, and the university's Instructional Technology (IT) Department/Instructional Design Studio was unable to offer technical assistance to faculty interested in using VT. The course instructor was reimbursed (99) for the annual VT single instructor license. Students registered for free VT accounts, allowing them to engage and post assignments using the link provided by their instructor.

Instructor training

The course instructors had experience using VT with students enrolled in a fully online BSW program at a different university. Additionally, instructors participated in a free synchronous workshop offered by VT on their website. (VT offers free on-demand video-recorded workshops on their website and YouTube.) The instructors used VT to video and/or audio record lecture content which students could access at their convenience. They also used VT to provide students with feedback regarding their VT posts.

Student training

Students were invited to participate in an orientation to prepare them for successful online education and the use of VT. A traditional face-to-face orientation was used because some students lacked experience with online courses and were not familiar with VT. The 90-minute introduction demonstrated using VT for their assignments, and these assignments were explained in detail, with students encouraged to ask questions. Editing and submitting recorded assignments were demonstrated. The orientation included multiple topics, including professional presentation of self when using VT and using ethical behaviors during online engagement. Students were encouraged to bring a laptop or mobile device to the orientation and to install VT accounts using their university email address.

Privacy

To ensure protection of student records, guidelines for the Family Educational Rights and Privacy Act (FERPA, 1974) were followed. Instructors used highest-level privacy settings to ensure content could be viewed only by students enrolled in the course, and student grades were not posted or discussed on VT. At the end of the semester, course instructors deleted all VT posts to maintain student privacy.

Methods

Study setting

The setting for this descriptive pilot study is a private, urban, Jesuit university located in the midwestern United States. The BSW program has an ethnically diverse student population of less than 100 students with 55% of study participants identifying as African American/Black, 31% as Caucasian, and 14% as another race (e.g., Latino/a, Native American or Multiracial). Course enrollment ranged from 15 to 20 students.

Procedures

A quantitative and qualitative survey was used to collect data on student perceptions of the use of VT in the selected online courses. Students were asked to complete an online survey during the fifth week of the 2017 fall semester using a unique link created by Survey Monkey. They were sent an announcement through BbL to introduce the purpose of the study, details about the survey (including the link), and their rights as study participants. As required by the university's institutional review board, students provided informed consent to participate in the study by emailing their agreement to participate to the principal investigator (PI). Thus, participation was confidential, not anonymous. Students were not offered credit or any other reward in exchange for their participation.

Participants

Students from the three online courses were asked to participate in the study. Students could take these classes sequentially or in the same semester. Fifty-nine (81%) of the students completed the electronic survey, including 14 (61%) enrolled in ISW, 21(88%) in SWSJ, and 24 (92%) in HBSE I. Of the 59 students who completed the survey, 36 (61%) were enrolled in one online class, 16 in two online classes (27%), and 7 (12%) in all three online classes. Because identifying information was not collected, it is unknown if students enrolled in multiple classes responded to the survey more than once. Of those who indicated they were enrolled in multiple courses, only two had the same demographic data. However, these two surveys contained vastly different open-ended responses and ratings. Thus, it is unlikely that a student completed a survey more than once.

Students ranged in age from 18 to more than 55 years of age, with the largest group (n = 20, 33.9%) between 18 and 24 years of age, followed by students from 35 to 44 years of age (n = 15, 25.3%). Seven (11.9%) students were age 55 years or over. Fifty (85%) students were female and nine (15%) were male, and forty-two (71%) were enrolled full-time and 17 (29%) part-time. Students were from diverse racial/ ethnic groups, which were similar to those enrolled in the three classes, and in the social work program at the university. Students were asked to report all device(s) they used to record their VT assignments and were given a list of possible devices and asked to select all that apply. Due to the potential for multiple responses, the total percentage exceeded 100%. The students reported using personal computers (n = 50, 84.7%), smart phones/cell phones (n = 17, 28.8%), electronic tablets (n = 4, 6.8%), and the campus library system (n = 2, 3.4%). [See Table 1.]

Table 1. Demographic characteristics (N = 59).

Demographic Characteristics	Number	Percent
Age		
18 to 24	20	33.9
25 to 34	8	13.6
35 to 44	15	25.3
45 to 54	9	15.3
55 and over	7	11.9
Gender		
Male	9	84.7
Female	50	15.3
Race/Ethnicity		
African American/Black	40	67.8
Caucasian/White	10	16.9
Hispanic	6	10.2
Middle Eastern	2	3.4
Multiple Ethnicity	1	1.7
Student Status		
Full-time	42	71.2
Part-time	17	28.8
Course Participation	Number	Percent
Course Enrollment		
One Online Course	36	61.1
Two Online Courses	16	27.1
Three Online courses	7	11.8
Devices used with VT		
Home computer/Laptop	50	84.7
Campus library computer	2	3.4
Smart phone	18	30.5
Tablet	4	6.8

Measurement

The survey was created to examine student perceptions of VT use in online BSW courses. They were asked to rate the helpfulness of the orientation to the course and the VT video recording of the course syllabus in understanding class expectations via a 5-point Likert style scale ranging from extremely helpful to either "did not attend" or "did not view." Three questions assessed student perceptions of VT via ratings on a four-point scale from 1 for "not well at all" to 4 for "extremely well." In addition to these five key questions, the survey also asked students to indicate how VT impacted their workload, providing three response categories: 1 = too light; 2 = about right; and 3 = too heavy. Students were also asked to respond to open-ended questions that inquired about: (a) how VT helped them in the online course; (b) benefits they experienced using VT; and (c) limitations they experienced using VT. The survey collected basic demographics about the students (e.g., race, age, and gender) and their student status (full-time, part-time). Additionally, the survey obtained data on types of devices students used when recording their VT responses.

Data analysis

The small sample size limited data analysis to descriptive and parametric statistics using IBM-SPSS Version 25. Frequency counts and percentages were obtained for categorical variables, with descriptive statistics used for continuous variables. Spearman's rho correlations tested the relationship between age and perceptions of VT. Mann-Whitney U tests for two independent samples examined differences in student perceptions of VT by gender, race, and student status.

An inductive approach was used to analyze the open-ended responses which were read repeatedly to capture a holistic view of student perceptions of VT. Next, responses were reviewed word-by-word to develop initial codes. These codes were sorted into meaningful clusters related to domains of the five close-ended items.

Results

Students were requested to rate the helpfulness of the Orientation to Online Course training. Of the 40 (68%) students who attended the orientation, 27 (68%) indicated it was very or extremely helpful, but three (7%) did not find it to be at all helpful. Further, thirty-six (61.1%) students indicated viewing the VT video recording of the course syllabus was very or extremely helpful in understanding class expectations.

In each of the online courses, students were required to create weekly VT videos to demonstrate knowledge of course content and to create opportunities for interaction among their colleagues. Twenty-five (42%) stated that VT helped them get to know their classmates very or extremely well and 15 (25.4%) shared that VT clearly provided opportunities to communicate with their classmates. Some students indicated:

- VT is also a great way to interact with classmates and the professor.
- VT helped them understand views from other classmates in a way that would be lost through discussion boards.

When asked how well the VT videos helped them learn course content, 29 (49%) students indicated VT videos helped them learn the content very to extremely well, while 7 (12%) reported the VT videos did not help them to do so at all. In commenting about how VT helped them, some students wrote that VT was useful by:

- Explaining what I have learned, and to be able to hear myself explaining it.
- Helping me understand the course content better. VoiceThread makes students accountable for actually learning the work; no more hiding silently in class.

Table 2. Student perceptions of VT helpfulness.

Perceptions of VT Helpfulness	M	SD	Min	Max
Orientation	3.05	1.01	1	4
VT Video Recording of Syllabus	2.94	0.95	1	4
Acquainted with Classmates	2.33	0.92	1	4
Learning Content	2.87	0.95	1	4
Presentation Skills	2.92	0.93	1	4

• Assisting me in understanding the chapters better because they are being talked about by the professor instead of my having to read the book alone. And, with VoiceThread I can get a second opinion about the chapters by my peers without being lectured in a class.

Students were asked to rate the helpfulness of VT in improving their presentation skills. Thirty-nine (66%) students indicated VT was very to extremely helpful with developing their presentation skills. [See Table 2.] Students provided additional information on how VT aided them with communication and presentation skills, commenting that VT helped:

• Conduct myself in a professional manner by respecting those who are using voice thread as well. It also allows me to self-reflect on my strengths and weakness regarding public speaking.
• Be more vocal about my opinions and helped me become more comfortable in class discussions.
• To get over my fear of speaking in front of people.

Responses to these key items were correlated with students' ages to determine if VT was better accepted by younger students. The results of the Spearman's rho correlations provided one statistically significant correlation ($rs = - .31, p = .019$), indicating that younger students found VT more helpful in improving presentation skills than older students. [See Table 3.] The responses to the key items were also compared by gender, race, and student status using Mann-Whitney U tests for two independent samples. No statistically significant results were found, providing support that students viewed VT similarly regardless of gender, race, or student status. [See Table 4.]

Table 3. Spearman rho correlations: selected variables by age.

Variable	N	r	p
How helpful did you find the orientation to Online SW courses meeting?	59	−.09	.508
How helpful was viewing the VoiceThread video recording of the course syllabus in helping you understand class expectations?	59	−.04	.745
How well does using VoiceThread help you get to know your classmates?	59	.02	.905
How well does posting your VoiceThread videos help you learn course content?	59	−.10	.475
How helpful is VoiceThread in improving your presentation skills?	59	−.31	.019

Table 4. Mann-Whitney test for independent samples: selected variables by gender, race, and student status.

Variable	Mean Rank			
Gender	Female (n = 50)	Male (n = 9)	Z	p
How helpful did you find the orientation to Online SW courses meeting?	30.0	30.0	.00	1.000
How helpful was viewing the VoiceThread video recording of the course syllabus in helping you understand class expectations?	30.24	28.67	-.27	.790
How well does using VoiceThread help you get to know your classmates?	29.99	30.06	-.01	.991
How well does posting your VoiceThread videos help you learn course content?	30.06	29.67	-.07	.947
How helpful is VoiceThread in improving your presentation skills?	30.90	25.00	-1.00	.319
Race	African American (n = 40)	Other Ethnic Groups (n = 19)		
How helpful did you find the orientation to Online SW courses meeting?	31.01	27.87	-.68	.498
How helpful was viewing the VoiceThread video recording of the course syllabus in helping you understand class expectations?	32.73	24.26	-1.86	.063
How well does using VoiceThread help you get to know your classmates?	28.84	32.45	-.80	.426
How well does posting your VoiceThread videos help you learn course content?	29.88	30.26	-.09	.932
How helpful is VoiceThread in improving your presentation skills?	28.58	33.00	-.97	.332
Student Status	Full-time (n = 42)	Part-time (n = 17)		
How helpful did you find the orientation to Online SW courses meeting?	29.65	30.85	-.25	.802
How helpful was viewing the VoiceThread video recording of the course syllabus in helping you understand class expectations?	28.45	33.82	-1.14	.253
How well does using VoiceThread help you get to know your classmates?	30.55	28.65	-.41	.685
How well does posting your VoiceThread videos help you learn course content?	29.07	32.29	-.69	.493
How helpful is VoiceThread in improving your presentation skills?	29.49	31.26	-.38	.706

The students also were asked how using VT influenced their workload, offering three response options: too heavy, about right, and too light. Forty-three (73.0%) indicated using VT made their workload about right and 16 (27%) stated that using VT made their workload too heavy.

Students were asked to list benefits or limitations they experienced in using VT. Five core benefits were identified: (1) A few students noted that VT helped them engage with other students by understanding their class-mates' opinions as well as sharing their own. (2) Several noted that VT fostered their growth, including enhancing their presentation skills, with some commenting that VT helped them overcome anxiety related to pre-sentations. (3) Some students noted that VT helped them retain more information from assignments. (4) Other students noted that VT helped them develop technology skills, such as learning to navigate the computer and communicating through technology. (5) Finally, a number of students mentioned the convenience of VT and as the flexibility of posting content at a time that worked best for them.

However, an analysis of student comments identified several limitations. One student mentioned poor VT video quality, another shared that the VT app did not work well, and one indicated that using VT caused too much pressure. An additional student remarked, "using VT does not really help in understanding the information right away." Although student comments related to early VT experiences were generally positive, the Principal Investigator identified an additional concern. IT and campus library staff were unable to provide support to students or to faculty using VT because of the nature of the pilot project. In the future, this issue might be addressed if additional academic departments were informed of the benefits from using VT in college courses. The PI was available to provide inservice training to library staff on VT, so students using the tool in the future on campus might now be in a position to receive additional support.

Discussion

The purpose of this pilot study was to explore benefits and limitations associated with the use of VT with students enrolled in online BSW courses. Study findings revealed most students viewed their new experience favorably. Providing a face-to-face orientation for students that focused on mastering the VT tool was perceived to be helpful by nearly all students who attended. Ensuring that students understand how to use ICT (like VT) effectively we found can promote critical thinking and problem-solving skills, as well as help students to interact with both faculty and classmates. One study by Young and colleagues (2018) found that social work faculty who used ICT reported enhanced instruction and increased student interaction which was demonstrated in new and challenging ways. Results from the current study supported this finding, with students stating that posting VT self-reflections helped them learn course content and better know their classmates.

Baker and Iverson Hitchcock (2017) asserted that many BSW students use a variety of mobile devices in their daily lives, but needed education on using them appropriately in professional settings. Results from our study support this finding, as most students indicated they had access to a variety of electronic devices to complete VT assignments, but lacked adequate skills related to online professional presentation of self. We found that completion of weekly self-reflections, along with feedback from course instructors, helped students improve presentation and communication skills.

For the majority of students, incorporating VT into online courses offered multiple advantages without increasing class workload. Benefits of VT included convenience, since VT could be accessed wherever an Internet connection was available and students thus were able to use a variety of mobile devices to complete assignments.

Implications for social work education

BSW educators are beginning to incorporate innovative ways to enhance teaching and learning. VT is one application that can likely benefit both students and faculty. Online modules (or traditional face-to-face orientation programs) can be offered to help students become adept at using VT. Faculty teaching online courses may similarly benefit from training to use VT. Faculty, as well, must be knowledgeable about FERPA (1974) policy to protect student privacy, especially when students are posting video course content.

Faculty using tools like VT in their online classes should monitor student posts. This monitoring could include regularly posting encouraging feedback to students, responding to their posts in a timely manner, offering additional instruction as needed, redirecting or deleting inappropriate posts, and sharing sensitive constructive feedback with students privately.

Limitations

The following limitations are acknowledged for this study. The sample was small and homogeneous with respect to participant demographics, resulting in nonsignificant relationships with regard to student perceptions of VT use. Implications for future research could explore how a larger sample and diverse demographics could influence engagement with ICT, specifically VT. Due to the small size of the social work program, the three courses included in this study were offered only online. Findings might be different in baccalaureate programs where students could select their preferred educational platform. For example, students who preferred online courses might have more positive perceptions of VT than those enrolled in traditional face-to-face and/or hybrid courses.

Conclusions

Findings from the current study suggest VT was a viable tool for engaging students in online BSW classes, helping students bridge communication gaps, having an active voice, and building ICT competency. VT also helped faculty get to know their students and to strengthen their online presence in courses. Future research also is needed to explore instructional methods that are most effective in helping students master course content on VT, perhaps including faculty developed video-lectures, supplemental digital materials from textbook publishers, and/or videos generated from Internet sources. With additional research, it is anticipated that VT technology can be used to help effectively prepare our students for competent practice in the digital age.

Disclosure statement

No potential conflict of interest was reported by the authors.

References

Baker, L. R., & Iverson Hitchcock, L. (2017). Using Pinterest in undergraduate social work education: Assignment development and pilot survey results. *Journal of Social Work Education*, *53*(3), 535–545. doi:10.1080/10437797.2016.1272515

Bell, F. (2011). Connectivism: Its place in theory-informed research and innovation in technology-enabled learning. *The International Review of Research in Open and Distributed Learning*, *12*(3), 98–118. doi:10.19173/irrodl.v12i3.902

Brady, S. R., McLeod, D., & Young, J. A. (2015). Developing ethical guidelines for creating social media technology policy in social work classrooms. *Advances in Social Work*, *16*(1), 43–54. Retrieved from http://advancesinsocialwork.iupui.edu/index.php/advancesinsocial work/article/view/17977/19919

Chan, M., & Pallapu, P. (2012). An exploratory study on the use of VoiceThread in a business policy course. *Journal of Online Learning and Teaching*, *8*(3), 223–237. Retrieved from http://jolt.merlot.org/vol8no3/chan_0912.htm

Ching, Y.-H., & Hsu, Y.-C. (2013). Collaborative learning using VoiceThread in an online graduate course. *Knowledge Management & ELearning*, *5*(3), 298–314. Retrieved from http://www.kmel-journal.org/ojs/index.php/online-publication/article/viewFile/267/189

Council on Social Work Education. (2015). *Educational Policy and Accreditation Standards*. Retrieved from https://cswe.org/Accreditation/Standards-and-Policies/2015-EPAS

Dunaway, M. K. (2011). Connectivism. *Reference Services Review*, *39*(4), 675–685. doi:10.1108/009073211111

Family Educational Rights and Privacy Act [FERPA]. (1974) *(20 U.S.C. § 1232g; 34 CFR Part 99)*. Retrieved from https://www2.ed.gov/policy/gen/guid/fpco/ferpa/index.html

Fang, L., Mishna, F., Zhang, V. F., Van Wert, M., & Bogo, M. (2014). Social media and social work education: Understanding and dealing with the new digital world. *Social Work in Health Care*, *53*, 800–814. doi:10.1080/00981389.2014.943455

Fox, O. H. (2017). Using VoiceThread to promote collaborative learning in on-line clinical nurse leader courses. *Journal of Professional Nursing*, *33*(1), 20–26. doi:10.1016/j.profnurs.2016.08.009

Gonzalez, M., & Moore, N. S. (2018). Supporting graduate student writers with voicethread. *Journal of Educational Technology Systems*, *46*(4), 485–504. doi:10.1177/0047239517749245

Gose, B. (2017). A new generation of digital distraction. *The Chronicle of Higher Education*, *64*(4). Retrieved from https://www.chronicle.com/article/Gen-Z-Changes-the-Debate-About/241163

Gross, L., & Meriwether, J. L. (2016). Student engagement through digital data. *New Directions for Student Services*, *2016*(155), 75–89. doi:10.1002/ss.20184

Kirby, E. G., & Hulan, N. (2016). Student perceptions of self and community within an online environment: The use of VoiceThread to foster community. *Journal of Teaching and Learning with Technology*, *5*(1), 87–99. doi:10.14434/jotlt.v5n1.19411

Madoc-Jones, I., & Parrott, L. (2005). Virtual social work education: Theory and experience. *Social Work Education*, *24*, 755–768. doi:10.1080/02615470500238678

McAllister, C. (2013). A process evaluation of an online BSW program: Getting the student perspective. *Journal of Teaching in Social Work*, *33*(4–5), 514–530. doi:10.1080/08841233.2013.838200

Neuman, K. (2006). Using distance education to connect diverse communities, colleges, and students. *Journal of Baccalaureate Social Work*, *11*(2), 16–27. doi:10.18084/1084-7219.11.2.16

Perron, B. E., Taylor, H. O., Glass, J. E., & Margerum-Leys, J. (2010). Information and communication technologies in social work. *Advances in Social Work*, *11*(2), 67. Retrieved from https://www.ncbi.nlm.nih.gov/pmc/articles/PMC3117433/

Siemens, G. (2004, December). *Connectivism: A theory for the digital age*. Retrieved from http://devrijeruimte.org/content/artikelen/Connectivism.pdf

Webber, M., Currin, L., Groves, N., Hay, D., & Fernando, N. (2010). Social workers can e-learn: Evaluation of a pilot post-qualifying e-learning course in research methods and critical appraisal skills for social workers. *Social Work Education*, *29*(1), 48–66. doi:10.1080/02615470902838745

Young, J. A., McLeod, D. A., & Brady, S. R. (2018). The ethics challenge: 21st century social work education, social media, and digital literacies. *The Journal of Social Work Values and Ethics*, *15*, 1–22. Retrieved from http://jswve.org/download/15-1/15-1-Articles/13-The-Ethics-Challenge-15-1.pdf

Exploring Online and Blended Course Delivery in Social Group Work

Irene Carter, Thecla Damianakis, Sharon Munro, Hannah Skinner, Sumaiya Matin, and Tanya Nash Andrews

ABSTRACT

Agency group work has increased, but opportunities for social work group practice in educational settings have not kept pace. One option in response is technology-based learning, and students appear to have positive perceptions of online group project work. Online courses appear to have outcomes comparable to those that occur with in-person groups but require careful monitoring of group processes and group-based technologies. The authors discuss the factors involved in developing and implementing online and blended course delivery in teaching group work.

Introduction

There has been a tremendous increase in the use of online modalities in modern higher education (Callister & Love, 2016; Cohen, Simon, McLaughlin, Muskat, & White, 2016). Social work education has joined this trend (Fulton, Walsh, Azulai, Gulbrandsen, & Tong, 2015; Holmes, Tracy, Painter, Oestreich, & Park, 2015; Kurzman, 2013). O'Farrell and Bates (2009) noted that students are embracing electronic media and resources such as websites, electronic journals, and e-mail to advance their group projects.

There is sparse information, however, regarding online methodologies for teaching group work (Muskat & Mesbur, 2011). Nonetheless, the use of learning management systems, such as Blackboard, have been widely accepted as vehicles to deliver online social work education. Learning management systems allow instructors to organize course materials. They also provide opportunities for distance interaction among students, facilitated through discussion boards, where students can participate individually or collaboratively by posting responses to instructors' or students' inquiries (Holmes et al., 2015). Some benefits of online discussion groups that have been noted in the literature include increased accessibility (Fulton et al., 2015), convenience and flexibility

(Carter, Matin, & Wilson, 2013), greater speed and efficiency in student–instructor communication (Cohen et al., 2016), adaptability to differing learning styles, a wider variety of delivery methods (Nelson & Duncan, 2015), and cost-effectiveness (Cohen et al., 2016; Hunter, 2011). Discussion groups can supplement in-class material and provide opportunities for active learning through student interaction with classmates while encouraging the development of critical thinking (Saade, Morin, & Thomas, 2012).

Challenges noted in the use of technology for group work education include a lack of student participation (Chang & Kang, 2016), difficulty with technology, inadequate resources, misunderstandings about course expectations (Blissenden, Clarke, & Strevens, 2012), nontraditional course delivery that is not in person (Carter, Munro, & Matin, 2013), high workloads for students and instructors (Dykman & Davis, 2008), and time constraints (Ekmecki, 2013). Evidence indicates that blended learning, which combines both online and in-person instruction within a single course (Graham, 2013), can be equally if not more effective than traditional instruction alone (Cummings, Foels, & Chaffin, 2013). Indeed, including modalities such as discussion boards and online chat rooms in regular social work courses allows students to integrate knowledge about group processes in both online and in-person settings (Oliveira, Tinoca, & Pereira, 2011).

In this article, group strategies for online and blended groups that are consistent with the Standards for Social Work Practice with Groups (Association for the Advancement of Social Work with Groups [AASWG], 2006) are discussed, illustrating the importance of incorporating key concepts of group work in online and blended courses. The facilitation of group development processes includes establishing course structure and goals to increase clarity and discourage destructive group dynamics, such as the *free rider effect* and *sucker effect*; facilitating group norms, group cohesion, and social connectedness; monitoring group conflict; addressing power dynamics; and understanding the impact on student–instructor relationships. Recommendations subsequently are made for supporting faculty in implementing online social work groups.

Literature review

Fostering critical thinking in online group work

Debates have persisted about the role of instructors in higher education and whether that role consists of simply communicating knowledge to students or ensuring that students have the capacity to comprehend, analyze, and find solutions for societal issues (Lim, 2011). It is argued that the development of critical-thinking skills is a vital component of social work education because it is essential to being an effective practitioner (Samson, 2016). Social work practice requires that professionals be able to analyze, interpret, assess, communicate, evaluate, and intervene among multiple sources of knowledge and sources of information in a manner that respects the dignity and diversity of the people served (Deal & Pittman, 2009). Therefore, it is essential that online, blended, and traditional courses in social work programs foster critical thinking.

Although the connection between teaching critical thinking online and social work courses has been established in the literature (Maidment, 2005), research outlining *how* to foster or teach critical thinking in an online environment is limited. It has been suggested that teaching critical thinking is more challenging in an online environment than a traditional in-person classroom. This proposition may be the result of the use of computers to facilitate online education in lower levels of learning through multiple choice and true-or-false examinations largely testing the memorization of facts. Therefore, technology traditionally has not been used in education to teach higher level skills, such as critical thinking.

In modern online and blended education, instructors have considerably more options to foster critical thinking, particularly within a group context. For example, blended and online learning environments allow for ongoing discussions, as they are not constrained by in-person class start and end times. This reality allows students to participate within online discussions continuously, espousing deeper learning when compared to an in-person timed discussion, and has subsequently been found to encourage critical thinking (Saade et al., 2012). Threaded discussions have been found to prompt more diverse responses, whereas nonthreaded discussions can yield repetitive answers (Vonderwell, Liang, & Alderman, 2007). Overall, higher level learning skills, such as critical thinking, require open-ended queries that can be responded to at length and with the freedom of straying from predetermined answers, such as those in multiple-choice questions (Saadé & Huang, 2009). Open-ended questions and answers can be delivered through blogs, discussion boards, wikis, and e-mail within online education modalities to encourage both group and individual thinking. During electronic discussions, multiple perspectives also may exist as opposed to the single view of an instructor that is communicated via traditional, vertical teaching methods (Ogunleye, 2010).

The importance of active online instructors in modeling critical thinking also has been identified in the literature (Domakin, 2013). For example, Hung and Chou (2015) noted that online instructors should encourage critical thinking by providing students with feedback on discussion posts, probing students with questions regarding their responses, sharing their personal opinions, and challenging students to consider new concepts and perspectives. Instructors can determine when to engage actively in group discussions and when to provide space for students to challenge one another, as their online interactions develop.

Establishing course structure

The group work component of social work education becomes increasingly significant when structuring an online course or program. A review of the literature indicates that multiple universities use the Blackboard Learning System to facilitate online courses, particularly online group work (Chang & Kang, 2016; Moore et al., 2015; Secret, Bentley, & Kadolph, 2016). Blackboard is a learning management system that permits instructors to organize and post class materials for student access and assessment while allowing students to submit assignments and engage in discussion boards, blogs, and wikis (Holmes et al., 2015). Along with Blackboard, Google programs are commonly used throughout online group courses to facilitate collaborative work (Chang & Kang, 2016; Holmes et al., 2015; Morgan, Williams, Cameron, & Wade, 2014). In Google Documents and Google Presentation, individual students can log in to their group's particular piece of work (i.e., a group essay, PowerPoint presentation, or sharing board) and add individual contributions, which will be apparent to other group members when they sign in to that area. Google programs provide collaborative online technology that facilitate distance work and allow instructors to view group progress and track individual contributions (Holmes et al., 2015).

In preparing an online social work course that involves group work, one essential factor for effective instruction is clarity and transparency in group tasks, time lines, and expectations in the syllabus. Given the lack of in-person communication with the instructor, the clarity and transparency of expectations are important so that students can concentrate their efforts on collaboration within their groups rather than trying to understand ambiguous expectations set by the instructor (Morgan et al., 2014).

Another factor that instructors must consider (when organizing the delivery of an online course with integrated group work) is leadership within the created student groups. Although the instructor determines leadership expectations, it is recommended that student groups have the freedom to determine the type of leadership that will be used within their own group (Chang & Kang, 2016). For example, group members can choose to distribute the leadership among multiple group participants, have one specified group leader throughout the life of the group, or alternate leadership among group members (Morgan et al., 2014). All styles of leadership have been found to be successful within online groups as long as they have been established democratically among members (Chang & Kang, 2016).

Individual student evaluation is vital in the planning of an online course. It is recommended that instructors use individual marking schemes for online group work courses instead of assigning group marks (Chang & Kang, 2016; Morgan et al., 2014). Individual evaluation has been found to result in an increase in student group productivity and motivation because it eliminates the *free-rider effect*, where one or more students complete little to no group work, as well as the *sucker effect*, where a few students complete all of the group work. Instructors can implement individual evaluation within the group context by organizing the course syllabus to include individually completed assignments, followed by self and peer evaluations by the students. To prevent the free-rider and sucker effects, instructors must once again be clear in their communication of the syllabus expectations to ensure that they understand the inclusion of individual evaluations, thereby discouraging destructive group behavior prior to it arising. An open discussion at the start of the course about the negative consequences of free-riding may further help to reduce the likelihood of its occurrence.

Facilitating group norms, group cohesion, and social connectedness

The importance of social connectedness and group cohesion is a consistent theme from multiple academic enquiries. Goldingay and Land's (2014) study on social presence in online social work education confirms that relationships among peers have a significant influence on student motivation. Hence, the creation of an environment that encourages student-to-student interaction will likely result in a beneficial online learning environment (Goldingay & Land, 2014). The lack of nonverbal cues in distance learning settings understandably may make it more difficult for students to achieve a sense of social connectedness with one another (Slagter van Tryon & Bishop, 2009). Therefore, it is often the responsibility of the instructor to employ a variety of teaching strategies that will reinforce positive group norms and foster feelings of cohesion to counter the distant nature of the online modality (Goldingay & Land, 2014). Group work activities can help students to feel connected and to have faith in group work activities because such activities encourage "ongoing social interactions and collaborative functioning" (Slagter van Tryon & Bishop, 2009, p. 291). Slagter van Tryon and Bishop (2009) additionally recommend that instructors provide frequent opportunities for students to interact while being actively involved in managing communication issues. For example, the selection of a common experience for students to simulate as a group, such as grief, will allow the participants to relate by sharing the thoughts and feelings about a past experience involving significant loss perhaps of a family member, friend, or pet due to death. The faculty member can use the strategy of having students share a story of their loss and employ discussion by encouraging them to respond to each story presented by their colleagues. This exercise should be preceded by guidelines to ensure sensitivity and followed by a PowerPoint lecture on grief, describing various forms of grief, and individual reactions to it. To prepare the students for a taped, simulated group session involving a particular story of grief, the teacher could have each group in the class read a story about loss and mourning, such as the short book *Tuesdays with Morrie: An Old Man, a Young Man, and Life's Greatest Lesson* (Albom, 1997). This book tells of the friendship between Mitch Albom—the young man—and Morrie Schwartz, his friend and former professor who is slowly dying of Lou Gehrig's disease, depicting an effort to look for meaning in life through loss and grief. Summaries of each group's reactions to the story of Mitch and Morrie could then be posted to the course site. Following videotaped, simulated group sessions on one of Mitch Albom's losses, summaries of the various student group experiences could be posted to the course website for further discussion about concepts regarding loss, grief, and mourning.

Online group work discussions require specific guidelines and should reflect Standards for Social Groupwork, such as those developed by AASWG (2006; Muskat & Mesbur, 2011). There should be clear expectations about the purpose and use of online discussions; the development of explicit group norms; agreement on content and timing of postings; the development of norms around interpersonal safety; details about what is considered to be appropriate online disclosure, attention to confidentiality; a focus on group stages; proper introductions; monitoring of conflict; preparation for endings; enhancement of the development of mutual aid; instructor (leader) involvement in monitoring (and leading) group discussions; and attendance expectations. Although social connectedness is ideal among students, instructor involvement is necessary to encourage commitment to these norms. For example, Marks, Sibley, and Arbaugh (2005) noted that students may be dividing work in ways that limit interaction among members. In that case, instructor input regarding role and assignment allocations will be likely beneficial in ensuring equal participation and group cohesion opportunities.

Instructor monitoring of group conflict

Although social connectedness is a necessary component of online education, it can cause conflict (Xie, Miller, & Allison, 2013). Although disagreement also can occur frequently within traditional in-person educational environments, it can be amplified in online learning environments (Xie et al., 2013). The instructor's knowledge about group work and its potential for causing interpersonal group conflict can be helpful in anticipating comparable reactions in student groups within an online format. Conflict within online environments also is increasingly common because students are often communicating solely through text-based media and therefore extralinguistic cues, such as tone of voice, observations of nonverbal communication, and the ability to experience the energy and atmosphere surrounding interactions, are not possible (Xie et al., 2013).

Conflict also can result from factors that are not necessarily present in in-person settings. Xie et al. (2013) discussed the different rules and norms that students experience and follow in online settings, such as exerting more control over the learning environment than the instructor. Within the online setting, participants must "accept responsibility for one another's learning, … [which] creates emotional tension for students and may threaten their perceived belongingness to the learning community, which can cause social conflict" (Xie et al., 2013, p. 405). Online disinhibition, or behavior that might appear in online communications that would be less likely to occur during in-person conversations, is also a common cause for conflict in online education. The anonymity of the distance venue may cause students to be more outspoken (and to initiate conflict situations) even though they may be more reserved in offline environments (Xie et al., 2013). This reality may prove to be particularly true for online group work education, where discussion posts and posted communications are increasingly subjective and often related to social justice and self-reflection (Sharpe, Benfield, Lessner, & DeCicco, 2005). Although these interactions provide opportunities to learn about interpersonal skills, they also can lead to misunderstandings, contrasting opinions, feelings of increased vulnerability, and conflict (Domakin, 2013). In the story of Mitch and Morrie in *Tuesdays with Morrie* (Albom, 1997), there are likely to be varying student opinions as well as conflictual attitudes about dying and terminal illness. To ensure sensitivity to the feelings of others while respecting individual opinions, it is essential that the instructor provide guidance with examples of how to respect autonomy while remaining sensitive to the varying feelings and opinions of other group members. Differences voiced by students provide the teacher with opportunities to demonstrate to students how to make use of social work ethics and the *Standards for Social Work Practice with Groups* (AASWG, 2006) to assist with managing and negotiating differences in an acceptable, professional manner.

It is not known if an online modality is effective for delivering experiential or skills-based learning to manage stress, negotiate issues, solve problems, and manage conflict, but all of these are critical social work skills for students to master in group work courses. Callister and Love (2016) found that students learning online did not develop negotiating skills as well as their counterparts in traditional in-person learning environments. Although there is little evidence surrounding how to teach students, these crucial social work skills through the online modality, the presence of field work in all professional social work programs, both online and in-person, would assist in the development of this expertise, which is crucial for effective group work practice.

Xie et al. (2013) suggested that instructors can manage conflict in an online learning environment by (a) the use of internal normalization, which involves intentionally ignoring inappropriate or harsh comments to diffuse or avoid conflict situations, thereby allowing students to resolve conflicts themselves, and (b) the deployment of external intervention, wherein the instructor reminds students about the significance of their choice of language as well as the importance of asking for clarification to avoid misunderstandings. As groups move into the working phase of group development, which is often when group members test one another, experience conflict, and make adjustments (Toseland & Rivas, 2012), it is helpful for instructors to anticipate conflict as part of the group process and to stay continuously engaged rather than acting as passive facilitators.

Addressing power dynamics in online groups

Student-to-student

With in-person classrooms, student discussions can be negatively affected when participants monitor and censor verbal or nonverbal communications. This experience can result in prejudicial judgments being made in which privileged students often are validated more frequently than students who are part of traditionally oppressed groups. Although small groups in online and blended learning contexts also experience power dynamics between group members, online exchanges can decrease power hierarchies (Bertera & Littlefield, 2003). Students within online education environments have equal opportunities to share and to participate in online exchanges. Students can exchange information and opinions through social networking sites such as blogs, podcasts, and social media (Kilpeläinen, Päykkönen, & Sankala, 2011) while engaging in more formal exchanges through designated learning management systems by using formats such as discussion boards. This gives them opportunities for reflection, problem solving, and helping one another. Knowledge is transmitted horizontally and in an equitable environment as students collaborate and eliminate power differentials (Maidment, 2005; Ogunleye, 2010), which can prove to be an empowering experience. For example, Fulton et al. (2015) pointed out that online education provides equal access to resources for those with disabilities that may not always exist in a traditional in-person, on-campus format. It has also been noted that students who tend to be introverted, shy, or more reflective in their thinking may benefit from an online format because it provides opportunities to express viewpoints within the freedom of asynchronous communication and gives participants time for reflection prior to engaging in discussions (Cohen et al., 2016; Ogunleye, 2010).

The inclusive nature of online education closely mirrors social work values and group practices and therefore is compatible with social work education and ethics. Online education requires that students embody certain social work and group values and that they have equitable access to adequate technology to facilitate inclusive practices (Maidment, 2005). For example, Quinney and Fowler (2013) described a social work course that used online education to break down the power hierarchies between the students and service users by including service users in online discussions. This demonstrates that if expectations and processes of the online course or program include equitable practices, it is possible for instructors to provide an online environment that will be more inclusive in nature. Reamer (2013) also looked at the ethical issues related to online courses and noted the importance of ensuring that they are properly developed, and for the right reasons, rather than revenue generation. He also emphasized the need to ensure that the clinical component of an online program is well organized and administered so that students enrolled in such courses have the same opportunities as their in-class equivalents to develop strong clinical skills. Attention, as well, is needed to prevent plagiarism and to ensure that confidentiality and student privacy are respected throughout the online process. Such preparation will help students to be autonomous and to take on more responsibility and control in their education (Jones, 2015; Ogunleye, 2010).

Student-to-instructor

Students experience more autonomy in online and blended educational environments since they can *choose* to respond to messages, make comments, and engage in the learning process. This makes them active learners with greater control over their education (Jones, 2015; Ogunleye, 2010). This modality levels the typical instructor-student power hierarchy by reducing the vertical, instructor-to-student information exchanges and encourages the horizontal mode of sharing and collectively generating information.

Online communities, however, can present a challenging transition for instructors as these communities tend to promote a peer-to-peer learning model which reduces the instructor's control over the learning environment and may result in instructors feeling that they are not being well-utilized and/ or have less authority with their students (McShane, 2004). Allen and Seaman (2013) have also found that instructors often have to put more effort into learning about online education and its effects on their students. Moreover, as they adjust to a new way of learning and collaborating, students often find group assignments particularly complex (Land & Bayne, 2006). They have to adapt to unfamiliar group dynamics, develop online communication skills, understand the new roles that take place in virtual groups, and know how to balance individual presence online (Fulton et al., 2015; Land & Bayne, 2006).

Online education often allows for increased freedom and extended communication, as students and instructors are no longer confined by class start and end times, which raises the issue of boundaries (McShane, 2004). Cohen et al. (2016) noted that students generally participate in the online learning management systems at a time that is convenient for them, and therefore they may share information at different times of the day. Given that there are no longer predetermined hours dedicated to the course, this reality can result in extended work hours for instructors, with students expecting immediate feedback and instructors feeling pressure to respond (Cohen et al., 2016). In response, instructors may need to reinforce more contained boundaries within the scheduled class times or add synchronous communication opportunities (McAllister, 2013). Scheduled videoconferencing sessions, chat rooms, implementation of a blended model, and incorporation of some in-person class sessions can allow students to ask questions and receive immediate assistance that is not always feasible via asynchronous communication (McAllister, 2013). When considering online social work course delivery, Levin, Whitsett, and Wood (2013) recommended a balance between asynchronous learning activities and synchronous meetings; generally, a balance of 50% synchronous and 50% asynchronous (Flynn, Maiden, Smith, Wiley, & Wood, 2013; Levin et al., 2013). The incorporation of both communication styles allows for the flexibility of asynchronous content (i.e., viewing case vignettes, participating in discussion boards, etc.), often used to prepare for the scheduled synchronous videoconferencing meetings, which promote a trust-building, intimate environment traditional to social work education (Levin et al., 2013). Instructors may also think that they have to be more careful when providing feedback to students because their communications can be documented and permanently recorded within an online modality as opposed to spontaneous in-person conversations (Cohen et al., 2016). Although students must assume more control over their education in online learning environments, the instructor's presence remains a valuable one (Fulton et al., 2015). Students tend to be more motivated to learn in online environments when instructors are active participants. Instructors can also model leadership qualities, demonstrate effective online group interactions, and use probing questions to encourage students to engage in analysis and critical thinking (Fulton et al., 2015; Marks et al., 2005).

The importance of getting the student perspective and feedback about online courses has been noted (McAllister, 2013). In McAllister's study, four equivalent BSW courses—both online and face-to-face—were evaluated. McAllister (2013) noted that although the online courses provided much more flexibility, particularly for students with tight time schedules and little if any ability to travel to campus, there were also drawbacks that needed to be addressed. Students indicated that "online learning provides fewer opportunities for in-the-moment communication and spontaneous exchanges among students and faculty" (p. 527). McAllister also found that students in the online courses were not making more contact with instructors through any other means except in the blended classes where students had monthly meetings with their instructors. She therefore recommended that "faculty teaching online may want to proactively establish synchronous meeting times with their online students, by phone, videoconference, or face-to-face, to initiate a connection to each student" (p. 527).

Recommendations

There are many similarities between the work involved in facilitating online groups within a social work education environment and that done for in-person settings, which should make the experience less daunting. However, the process of transitioning from in-person group facilitation in traditional physical classrooms to the online version can be intimidating for faculty. Yet because this process requires dedication, openness to change, collaboration, and consideration of contrasting perspectives should not deter higher education institutions from undertaking the task. If the transition is implemented effectively, group learning via an online modality can create a vibrant, interactive environment that is a core part of the learning process (Morgan et al., 2014). In this context, the following recommendations should be considered when transitioning from in-person educational environments to online facilitation of social work courses, and ultimately to full programs.

Support for instructors

Adequate instructor support is essential for the smooth transition from in-person to online education, particularly when incorporating the group work method into an online course. Nevertheless, it often is lacking in higher education institutions (Dawson & Fenster, 2015). Morgan et al. (2014) found that guidance for facilitators is essential for both the development and implementation of online courses, particularly in the area of technological support. Therefore, additional resources are required for instructors including training opportunities, both online and in person, in areas and programs that will assist in course development. Turnitin, the aforementioned Google Programs, and narrated PowerPoint Presentations have been identified as key to facilitating online social work courses that incorporate group work (Dawson & Fenster, 2015). Informal support for instructors should not be underestimated, as it has proven beneficial in facilitating online education. Bailey and Johnson (2014) suggested the creation of an online *lounge* style discussion board for instructors to gain informal support and advice from their colleagues about the concerns, challenges, and trials of online group work instruction, and Dawson and Fenster (2015) emphasized the importance of collectivity and shared discussions during the transition and implementation phases.

Departmental support

Departmental committees are essential in the transition from in-person environments to online education (Dawson & Fenster, 2015; Moore et al., 2015). Both ad hoc and extended committees can be established to organize and delegate tasks associated with the transition, implementation, and accountability issues connected with distance education. Moore et al. (2015) specifically recommended the creation of ad hoc committees that can be responsible for gathering information required to begin the transition, such as admissions criteria, availability of funds, and curriculum development. Extended committees can further the work of the ad hoc committees by training faculty, instructors, and field staff; developing appropriate evaluation formats; ensuring that guidelines are ethical; and attending to any technological concerns that may arise. As noted earlier, it is important to include all faculty (even those who may be less interested in online education) in the ongoing discussions and decisions to allow full participation and to ensure that all viewpoints are considered (Dawson & Fenster, 2015).

Included faculty must also expand further than direct instructors to include field faculty and instructors, as well. Field work is crucial in social work education, and therefore a review of the organization and supervision of student internships must be a priority. Because online students are more geographically dispersed, field work internships will also likely reflect this location distribution (Levin et al., 2013). Hence, institutions must consider expanding their faculty and implementing an external field instructor model, where hired regional field faculty complete in-person, on-site field supervision or engage in virtual supervision and communication through the chosen learning management systems and videoconferencing technology (Flynn et al., 2013).

Progress from individual courses to full online program

Moore et al. (2015) outlined the process of transforming a full MSW program into an online modality. They chose the initial courses for transition carefully. The practice courses, advanced research course, and diversity course were deemed to be too interactive and therefore were not initially chosen for online delivery (Moore et al., 2015). By carefully selecting the initial courses for online delivery and avoiding ones that were uncertain prospects for an online environment, faculty members were better able to determine whether online courses would be successful without compromising the education of the social work students. However, we have argued in this article that key concepts from group work may serve as important facilitative guides and support online learning environments when implementing online practice courses in social work with groups. Thus a group work course may be an excellent one to prioritize for experiential learning in an online format.

McAllister (2013) proposed a unique online social work course evaluation that considers grades, as well as student experiences and course satisfaction. By allowing the same professor to instruct both the in-person and online version of the same social work course in the same academic year, the online course could be effectively assessed through the students' completion of online, anonymous surveys, and the comparison of student grades. Incorporating evaluation throughout the course implementation process will allow faculty to identify concerns prior to the transformation to a full online or blended MSW program while prioritizing the qualitative learning experience for students.

Alignment with university vision

One factor that must be addressed within the transition period from in-person to online social work education is alignment with the university vision and its previously established policies, mission, and learning outcomes (Dawson & Fenster, 2015; Moore et al., 2015). Therefore, prior to a transition, faculty must ensure that the online program uses appropriate, adequate online teaching strategies for social work education to create ethical, competent social workers to work online. Reamer (2013) examined the types of complex ethical issues that can arise in online courses. He stated that the key ones that need to be addressed include "student access; course and degree program quality and integrity; gatekeeping and academic honesty; and privacy and surveillance" (p. 380).

Library resources and services

Academic libraries and librarians are an integral part of online courses and provide a wealth of services and resources to support them (Gore, 2014; Thomsett-Scott & May, 2009). It has been noted that in the virtual environment, the library can appear to be invisible, so it is important that instructors be aware of library services and resources and promote them to their students (Cahoy & Moyo, 2005). Librarians collaborate with faculty and other related campus departments to develop curricula, provide research assistance and support materials, and teach information literacy skills (Becker, 2014; Cahoy & Moyo, 2005; Shell et al., 2010; Wu, 2013). Access to online resources and services through libraries is essential so that students can effectively locate, use, and critically evaluate the materials that they need for their coursework (Association of College & Research Libraries, 2016). Interlibrary loan services enable students to access materials that their home institution libraries do not possess in their collections. There are also important copyright and licensing issues that need to be taken into consideration with online courses, and academic libraries can assist with copyright clearance (Shell et al., 2010; Wu, 2013). For all of the preceding reasons, academic libraries and librarians need to be involved in all stages of online course development (Shell et al., 2010).

Conclusion

The implementation of online social work group courses requires the establishment of course structure; the facilitation of group norms, group cohesion, and social connectedness; the monitoring of group conflict; and the addressing of power dynamics. Although the traditional instructor–student power hierarchy is reduced in online social work education, and student authority increased, instructor presence and active involvement is crucial. Online courses also require collaboration between instructors and academic libraries and other related academic units on campus.

The overarching goal in transition to online social work education is to ensure that students have the skills and abilities to work with underserviced populations, which includes individuals in rural and remote areas and those who cannot attend in-person groups or sessions due to physical, emotional, or transportation challenges (Nelson & Duncan, 2015). Careful attention to the experiences and suggestions reported here should help to ensure that the transition to online social work delivery will prepare students to become highly competent and ethical social work practitioners for our technology-driven future (Damianakis, Climans, & Marziali, 2008; Damianakis, Tough, Marziali, & Dawson, 2015; Dergal, Damianakis, & Marziali, 2006).

Disclosure statement

No potential conflict of interest was reported by the authors.

References

Albom, M. (1997). *Tuesdays with Morrie: An old man, a young man, and life's greatest lesson.* New York, NY: Doubleday.

Allen, I. E., & Seaman, J. (2013). Changing course: Ten years of tracking online education in the United States. *The Online Learning Consortium.* Retrieved from http://onlinelearning consortium.org/publications/survey/changing_course_2012

Association for the Advancement of Social Work with Groups [AASWG]. (2006). *Standards for social work practice with groups* (2nd ed.). Alexandria, VA: AASWG Inc. Retrieved from www.aaswg.org

Association of College & Research Libraries. (2016). *Framework for information literacy for higher education.* Retrieved from http://www.ala.org/acrl/standards/ilframework

Bailey, K. R., & Johnson, E. J. (2014). Internet-based technologies in social work education: Experiences, perspectives and use. *Caribbean Teaching Scholar, 4*(1), 23–37.

Becker, B. W. (2014). A simple solution to embedding library content into every online course. *Behavioral & Social Sciences Librarian, 33*(3), 170–173. doi:10.1080/01639269.2014.934094

Bertera, E. M., & Littlefield, M. B. (2003). Evaluation of electronic discussion forums in social work diversity education: A comparison of anonymous and identified participation. *Journal of Technology in Human Services, 21*(4), 53–71. doi:10.1300/J017v21n04_04

Blissenden, M., Clarke, S., & Strevens, C. (2012). Developing online legal communities. *International Journal of Law and Management, 54*(2), 153–164. doi:10.1108/17542431211208568

Cahoy, E. S., & Moyo, L. M. (2005). Faculty perspectives on e-learners' library research needs. *Journal of Library and Information Services in Distance Learning, 2*(4), 1–17. doi:10.1300/J192v02n04_01

Callister, R. R., & Love, M. S. (2016). A comparison of learning outcomes in skills-based courses: Online versus face-to-face formats. *Decision Sciences Journal of Innovative Education, 14*(2), 243–256. doi:10.1111/dsji.12093

Carter, I., Matin, S., & Wilson, A. (2013). Promoting professional involvement in the development and maintenance of support groups for persons with autism. *Professional Development: the International Journal of Continuing Social Work Education, 16*(1), 4–17.

Carter, I., Munro, S., & Matin, S. (2013). Exploring autonomy in group work practice with persons with intellectual disabilities. *Social Work with Groups, 36*(2–3), 236–248. doi:10.1080/01609513.2012.762618

Chang, B., & Kang, H. (2016). Challenges facing group work online. *Distance Education,* 1–16. doi:10.1080/01587919.2016.1154781

Cohen, M. B., Simon, S., McLaughlin, D., Muskat, B., & White, M. (2016). Challenges and opportunities for applying group work principles to enhance online learning in social work. In M. Gianino & D. McLaughlin (Eds.), *Revitalizing our social group work heritage: A bridge to the future (Proceedings of the XXXV international symposium of the international association for social work with groups, Boston, Massachusetts, USA, June 6th-9th, 2013)*(pp. 21–41). Boston, MA: Whiting & Birch.

Cummings, S., Foels, L., & Chaffin, K. (2013). Comparative analysis of distance education and classroom-based formats for a clinical social work practice course. *Social Work Education, 32*(1), 68–80. doi:10.1080/02615479.2011.648179

Damianakis, T., Climans, R., & Marziali, E. (2008). Social workers experiences of virtual psychotherapeutic support groups of family caregivers for Alzheimer's, Parkinson's, Stroke, Fronto temporal dementia and traumatic brain injury. *Social Work with Groups, 31*(2), 99–116. doi:10.1080/01609510801960833

Damianakis, T., Tough, A., Marziali, E., & Dawson, D. (2015). Therapy online: A web-based video support group for family caregivers of survivors with traumatic brain injury. *The Journal of Head Trauma Rehabilitation,* 1–9. doi:10.1097/HTR.0000000000000178

Dawson, B. A., & Fenster, J. (2015). Web-based social work courses: Guidelines for developing and implementing an online environment. *Journal of Teaching in Social Work, 35*(4), 365–377. doi:10.1080/08841233.2015.1068905

Deal, K. D., & Pittman, J. (2009). Examining predictors of social work students' critical thinking skills. *Advances in Social Work, 10*(1), 87–102.

Dergal, J., Damianakis, T., & Marziali, E. (2006). Clinical practice standards and ethical issues applied to a virtual group intervention for spousal caregivers of people with Alzheimer's. *Social Work in Health Care, 44*(1–3), 225–243. doi:10.1300/J010v44n03_07

Domakin, A. (2013). Can online discussions help student social workers learn when studying communication? *Social Work Education, 32*(1), 81–99. doi:10.1080/02615479.2011.639356

Dykman, C. A., & Davis, C. K. (2008). Online education forum: Part two – teaching online versus teaching conventionally. *Journal of Information Systems Education, 19*(2), 157–164.

Ekmecki, O. (2013). Being there: Establishing instructor presence in an online learning environment. *Higher Education Studies, 3*(1), 29–38. doi:10.5539/hes.v3n1p29

Flynn, M., Maiden, R. J., Smith, W., Wiley, J., & Wood, G. (2013). Launching the virtual academic center: Issues and challenges in innovation. *Journal of Teaching in Social Work, 33*(4–5), 339–356. doi:10.1080/08841233.2013.843364

Fulton, A. E., Walsh, C. A., Azulai, A., Gulbrandsen, C., & Tong, H. (2015). Collaborative online teaching: A model for gerontological social work education. *International Journal of E-Learning & Distance Education, 30*(1), 1-15.

Goldingay, S., & Land, C. (2014). Emotion: The 'e' in engagement in online distance education in social work. *Journal of Open, Flexible and Distance Learning, 18*(1), 58–72.

Gore, H. (2014). Massive open online courses (MOOCs) and their impact on academic library services: Exploring the issues and challenges. *New Review of Academic Librarianship, 20*(1), 4–28. doi:10.1080/13614533.2013.851609

Graham, C. R. (2013). Emerging practice and research in blended learning. In M. G. Moore (Ed.), *Handbook of distance education* (pp. 333–350). New York, N.Y: Routledge.

Holmes, M., Tracy, E. M., Painter, L. L., Oestreich, T., & Park, H. (2015). Moving from flipcharts to the flipped classroom: Using technology driven teaching methods to promote active learning in foundation and advanced masters social work courses. *Clinical Social Work Journal, 43*(2), 215–224. doi:10.1007/s10615-015-0521-x

Hung, M. L., & Chou, C. (2015). Students' perceptions of instructors' roles in blended and online learning environments: A comparative study. *Computers and Education, 81*, 315–325. doi:10.1016/j.compedu.2014.10.022

Hunter, D. Y. (2011). Who holds the pen? strategies to student satisfaction scores in online learning environments. *The Business Review, Cambridge, 18*(2), 75–81.

Jones, S. H. (2015). Benefits and challenges of online education for clinical social work: Three examples. *Clinical Social Work Journal, 43*(2), 225–235. doi:10.1007/s10615-014-0508-z

Kilpeläinen, A., Päykkönen, K., & Sankala, J. (2011). The use of social media to improve social work education in remote areas. *Journal of Technology in Human Services, 29*(1), 1–12. doi:10.1080/15228835.2011.572609

Kurzman, P. A. (2013). The evolution of distance learning and online education. *Journal of Teaching in Social Work, 33*(4–5), 331.338. doi:10.1080/08841233.2013.843346

Land, R., & Bayne, S. (2006). Issues in cyberspace education. In M. Savin-Barden & K. Wilkie (Eds.), *Problem-based learning online* (pp. 14–23). New York, NY: Open University Press.

Levin, S., Whitsett, D., & Wood, G. (2013). Teaching MSW social work practice in a blended online learning environment. *Journal of Teaching in Social Work, 33*(4–5), 408–420. doi:10.1080/08841233.2013.829168

Lim, L. (2011). Beyond logic and argument analysis: Critical thinking, everyday problems and democratic deliberation in Cambridge international examinations' thinking skills curriculum. *Journal of Curriculum Studies, 43*, 783–807. doi:10.1080/00220272.2011.590231

Maidment, J. (2005). Teaching social work online: Dilemmas and debates. *Social Work Education: The International Journal, 24*(2), 185–195. doi:10.1080/0261547052000333126

Marks, R. B., Sibley, S. D., & Arbaugh, J. B. (2005). A structural equation model of predictors for effective online learning. *Journal of Management Education, 29*(4), 531–563. doi:10.1177/1052562904271199

McAllister, C. (2013). A process evaluation of an online BSW program: Getting the student perspective. *Journal of Teaching in Social Work, 33*(4–5), 514–530. doi:10.1080/08841233.2013.838200

McShane, K. (2004). Integrating face-to-face and online teaching: Academics' role concept and teaching choices. *Teaching in Higher Education*, 9(1), 3–16. doi:10/1080.1356251032000155795

Moore, S. E., Golder, S., Sterrett, E., Faul, A. C., Yankeelov, P., Weathers Mathis, L., & Barbee, A. P. (2015). Social work online education: A model for getting started and staying connected. *Journal of Social Work Education*, 51(3), 505–518. doi:10.1080/10437797.2015.1043200

Morgan, K., Williams, K. C., Cameron, B. A., & Wade, C. E. (2014). Faculty perceptions of online group work. *The Quarterly Review of Distance Education*, 15(4), 37–41.

Muskat, B., & Mesbur, E. S. (2011). Adaptations for teaching social work with groups in the age of technology. *Groupwork*, 21(1), 88–109. doi:10.1921/095182411X578829

Nelson, E. L., & Duncan, A. B. (2015). Cognitive behavioral therapy using televideo. *Cognitive and Behavioral Practice*, 22(3), 269–280. doi:10.1016/j.cbpra.2015.03.001

O'Farrell, M., & Bates, J. (2009). Student information behaviours during group projects: A study of LIS students in University College Dublin, Ireland. *Aslib Proceedings*, 61(3), 302–315. doi:10.1108/00012530910959835

Ogunleye, A. O. (2010). Evaluating an online learning programme from students' perspectives. *Journal of College Teaching and Learning*, 7(1), 79–89.

Oliveira, I., Tinoca, L., & Pereira, A. (2011). Online group work patterns: How to promote a successful collaboration. *Computers & Education*, 57(1), 1348–1357. doi:10.1016/j.compedu.2011.01.017

Quinney, L., & Fowler, P. (2013). Facilitating shared online group learning between carer, service users and social work students. *Social Work Education*, 32(8), 1021–1031. doi:10.1080/02615479.2012.734801

Reamer, F. G. (2013). Distance and online social work education: Novel ethical challenges. *Journal of Teaching in Social Work*, 33(4–5), 369–384. doi:10.1080/08841233.2013.828669

Saadé, R., & Huang, Q. (2009). Meaningful learning in discussion forums: Towards discourse analysis. *Issues in Informing Science and Information Technology*, 6, 87–99. doi:10.28945/1044

Saade, R. G., Morin, D., & Thomas, J. D. E. (2012). Critical thinking in e-learning environments. *Computers in Human Behaviour*, 28(5), 1608–1617. doi:10.1016/j.chb.2012.03.025

Samson, P. L. (2016). Critical thinking in social work education: A research synthesis. *Journal of Social Work Education*, 52(2), 147–156. doi:10.1080/10437797.2016.1151270

Secret, M., Bentley, K. J., & Kadolph, J. C. (2016). Student voices speak quality assurance: Continual improvement in online social work education. *Journal of Social Work Education*, 52(1), 30–42. doi:10.1080/10437797.2016.1112630

Sharpe, R., Benfield, G., Lessner, E., & DeCicco, E. (2005). *Final report: Scoping study for the pedagogy strand of the JISC learning programme*. Retrieved from http://www.jisc.ac.uk/uploaded_documents/scoping%20study%20final%20report%20v4.1.doc

Shell, B., Duvernay, J., Ewbank, A. D., Konomos, P., Leaming, A., & Sylvester, G. (2010). A comprehensive plan for library support of online and extended education. *Journal of Library Administration*, 50(7–8), 951–971. doi:10.1080/01930826.2010.488996

Slagter van Tryon, P. J., & Bishop, M. J. (2009). Theoretical foundations for enhancing social connectedness in online learning environments. *Distance Education*, 30(3), 291–315. doi:10.1080/01587910903236312

Thomsett-Scott, B., & May, F. (2009). How may we help you? online education faculty tell us what they need from libraries and librarians. *Journal of Library Administration*, 49(1–2), 111–135. doi:10.1080/01930820802312888

Toseland, R. W., & Rivas, R. (2012). *An introduction to group work practice* (7th ed.). Needham Heights, MA: Allyn & Bacon.

Vonderwell, S., Liang, X., & Alderman, K. (2007). Asynchronous discussions and assessment in online learning. *Journal of Research on Technology in Education*, *39*(3), 309–328. doi:10.1080/15391523.2007.10782485

Wu, K. (2013). Academic libraries in the age of MOOCs. *Reference Services Review*, *41*(3), 576–587. doi:10.1108/RSR-03-2013-0015

Xie, K., Miller, N. C., & Allison, J. R. (2013). Toward a social conflict evolution model: Examining the adverse power of conflictual social interaction in online learning. *Computers & Education*, *63*(1), 404–415. doi:10.1016/j.compedu.2013.01.003

Converting a Face-To-Face Introductory Research Methods Course to an Online Format: Pedagogical Issues and Technological Tools

Mary Secret, Christopher Jennings Ward, and Ananda Newmark

ABSTRACT

This paper presents a step-by-step conversion of a face-to-face (F2F) entry level social work research methods course to a computer-mediated format. An overview of teaching practices and the important pedagogical foundations associated with this curricular effort are discussed followed by an introduction to the electronic platform utilized in the course. Five new teaching practices that guide the F2F-to-online course conversion of this introductory research methods course are presented with corresponding teaching activities and technological tools. A conversion matrix aligns the teaching practices, classroom activities, and provides references for the identified tools.

Faculty invest a significant amount of time and energy in developing syllabi, creating classroom lectures, exercises and materials, and perfecting teaching techniques for traditional, face-to-face (F2F) classroom settings to meet student learning needs and help achieve course objectives. Whether apprehensive or eager, instructors willing to move from the traditional to the electronic classroom can benefit from maximizing the curricular investments they have made in their (F2F) courses. However, "classroom and online environments are both equally complex, subtle and hard to define, so transferring from one mode into the other is fraught with pitfalls, especially for faculty with little experience of online course formats" (Young & Perovic, 2016, p. 390). Faculty are more likely to risk innovative teaching strategies when the newer strategies can be connected to existing classroom practices and experiences (Oleson & Hora, 2014); thus, the transition to online teaching can be facilitated if instructors can build upon a baseline of effective F2F teaching practices. Using an MSW foundational introductory research methods course as an exemplar, this article presents a step-by-step approach for converting a F2F course for use in an online computer-mediated learning environment. The conversion is anchored by five teaching practices identified by the authors as specific to the course objectives for this intro-ductory research methods course. These practices, however, are not intended to be generalized to all research methods courses or other social work offerings.

Derived from the literature on research methods pedagogy, from several years' experience of teaching introductory research methods, and from a Delphi method exploration of teaching practices conducted with social work educators in programs across the country, the teaching practices and tools presented in this paper illustrate how similar classroom activities can be delivered in either a F2F or an electronic format. Importantly, the redesign of this online option considers the technological aspects of the course and selection of technical tools as secondary to (and derived from) teaching practices that are associated with the F2F delivery.

Following an overview of general teaching practices, pedagogy, and Learning Management Systems (LMS), the authors present the five specific teaching practices and illustrate how the F2F classroom-based activities can be converted to similar online protocols with the careful selection of techni-cal tools. Noting the generic term associated with a particular technological tool (i.e., web-conferencing) as distinct from brand names by which the tool is marketed (i.e., 'Google Hangout'), a 'conversion matrix' summarizes the alignment of the teaching practices, the curricular activities for both F2F and online formats, and the several technology tools and provides the references for more familiar hardware and software.

Teaching practices overview

Several lists of best-practices in teaching have been generated and applied to a variety of educational settings (Fook, 2012; Johnson, 2014b; Sweet, Blythe, & Carpenter, 2018). Themes that have emerged from some of the more commonly recognized lists (for both F2F and online formats) include peer-to-peer interaction, student engagement in learning, emphasis on practice and student effort consistent with high expectations, personalization to the individual student, variation in classroom activities and experiences, and emphasis on a higher-order thought process that includes reflection and focus on real-world problems (Miller, 2014). [See Miller (2014) for the identification and description of the specific lists.] Not surprising, many of these themes are captured in the teaching practices discussed later in this paper as being germane to both online and F2F learning environments.

As one of many experts in the field, Miller asserts that there is sufficient overlap between the best-practices lists for F2F and online teaching to conclude that "good teaching is good teaching, regardless of technology" (Miller, 2014, p. 23). Similarly, the commonalities and overlap of teaching strategies used effectively at both the undergraduate and the graduate level seem to outweigh the few differences (Fook, 2012; Lumpkin, Achen, & Dodd, 2015; Ilic, 2009). Nonetheless, Paynter and Barnes (2015) warn that, although there are many similarities in teaching practices at the graduate and under-graduate level, "undergraduate students may need to focus on the lower levels of Bloom's Taxonomy, often cultivating information for the first time at the knowledge level, while graduate students should be expected to take this information and apply and expand it and relate it to other areas" (p. 68).

The link between critical thinking, evidence-based teaching practices, and student learning outcomes is well established (Bidabadi, Isfahani, Rouhollahi, & Khalili, 2016; Ennis, 2018; Miller, 2014; Samson, 2016; Sheffield, 2018). "Evidence-based methods are often presented with research that shows impressive results, including demonstrable gains in student learning; extra benefits for first generation and underrepresented students; improvements in attitudes toward the subject matter; or improved academic persistence and success" (Horii, 2018, p. 3).

In addition to cognitive science and evidence-based methods (Weinstein, Madan, & Sumeracki, 2018), other factors that influence teaching choices include those embedded in the institutional culture, infrastructure, and system of rewards and supports of the host university (Smith, 2012) as well as certain characteristics of the instructor such as prior experience as a learner, existing skill set, knowledge of the subject matter, student course evaluations, previous and current teaching experiences, and belief systems (Cameron, 2017; Oleson & Hora, 2014). In particular, preconceived beliefs and attitudes about the effectiveness of online education will likely influence an instructor's willingness to consider online teaching and the achievement of successful teaching outcomes (Miller, 2014).

The most prominent premise iterated throughout the literature on teach-ing practices is that the choice of teaching practice derives from (and must correspond with) the objectives of the course (George, 2009; Horii, 2018).

> Teaching methods are tools; they are means to achieving teaching objectives. There are no good or bad teaching methods; there are only appropriate teaching methods for specific teaching objectives. In order to decide which teaching method or methods to use for a given course or lesson, a faculty member needs to ask what are objectives for the course or lesson and what teaching methods may help achieve the objectives (Teaching Guide, n.d., p. 1).

The teaching practices discussed in this article are situated in a curriculum design model articulated by George (2009) that highlights the important relationship and distinction between teaching, which is what instructors do, and learning which is what students do. George (2009) stresses that the decisions about how and what to teach should be guided by the learning needs of students in meeting course outcomes. In this exemplar introductory level social work research methods course, the authors defer to the Council on Social Work Education's 2015

Educational Policy and Accreditation Standards (EPAS), Social Work Competency #4 – to Engage In Practice-informed Research and Research-informed Practice – as the overall anticipated course outcome (CSWE, 2015). A two-part iterative question ensues – "what type of learning experiences do students need to achieve basic research competency?" and "what does the research methods instructor need to do to facilitate student achievement of the competency at the foundational level?" The authors suggest the following teaching practices as especially suited for an introductory research methods course: help students distinguish the essential from the less essential content; reinforce engaged learning by student-to-student interactive experiences; provide ongoing formative assessment of student learning strengths and weaknesses; test for "walking knowledge" of introductory research methods content; and, guide the application of course material to real-world settings.

The recognition and implementation of these 'teaching practices' ensures that the focus of the course, whether it be F2F or online, will be anchored in the learning needs of the students. Despite the fact that "proficiency in technological tools that the world offers now and in the future are a responsibility that professors owe to their students, themselves and society" (Stillar, 2012, p. 149), instructors must avoid preoccupation with either the allure or the dread of the myriad of available technological tools. Keengwe, Onchwari and Agamba's (2013) assertion, 'pedagogy above technology' (p. 892) demands that technological tools be appropriately integrated to facilitate, and not divert, the student learning experience (Chickering & Ehrmann, 1996; Churches, 2009; Shattuck et al., n.d.). The conversion matrix reinforces this important connection between pedagogy and technological tools.

Pedagogical foundation

The acceleration of digital technologies has co-occurred with, and indeed has both inspired and been fueled by, constructivist learning theory (Anderson & Dron, 2011; McCombs, 2015; Parker, Maor, & Herrington, 2013; Stillar, 2012). Learning activities which are based on constructivist theory allow students to form their own representations of knowledge and to independently explore an information space to obtain content, higher level concepts and 'learn how to learn' (Keengwe et al., 2013, p. 888). Understanding and using course content is dependent not only on the instructor's presentation of the material, but on the students' prior learning experiences and existing knowledge base, as well as from their own exploration of resources that they access on the internet (Keengwe et al., 2013; McCombs, 2015). Furthermore, mastery of course content is demonstrated not merely by students reiterating that content but by their ability to meaningfully engage with and apply content to solve complex problems and to subsequently reflect on their learning experiences (Anderson & Dron, 2011; Keengwe et al., 2013).

In general, the conversion from F2F to online formats accentuates the shift to a constructivist model from an instructivist approach (Keengwe et al., 2013; Shattuck et al., n.d.), and from instructor-centered to learner-centered. For example, the physical layout of the traditional classroom positions the instructor, standing in front of the class to deliver lectures or lead class discussions on course material, at the center of the educational experience as the transmitter of knowledge. Students are subsequently asked to complete assignments or tests, documenting their grasp of the material. In contrast, the instructor's presence in the online classroom is embedded in the online course website or LMS interface, discussed in detail below.

However, the experiences of the authors, as well as others, in teaching introductory research methods courses (Hardway & Stroud, 2014; Schulze, 2009; Secret, Bryant, & Cummings, 2017) suggest that these courses present special challenges for those educators singularly dependent upon constructivist learning approaches. For introductory level research courses, students must have an accurate grasp of basic research methods concepts, achieved more effectively via didactic, instructivist methods, as a precursor to the constructivist learning experiences. The use of a mixed method teaching approach, similar to what was used in this course – specifically, teacher-centered didactic methods integrated with student-centered, more constructivist approaches – has been found to be effective for all levels of education (Barraket, 2005; Bidabadi et al., 2016).

Bloom's Taxonomy of Learning (Anderson & Krathwohl, 2001) provides an ideal framework to marry the instructivist and constructivist approaches used in this course. Bloom's taxonomy is a hierarchical categorization of six cognitive processes presented in order from the simplest, lower order thinking, to the most complex, higher-order levels of thinking and learning, to wit: remembering (to recall facts or basic concepts or retrieve previous learned information); understanding (the comprehension of ideas and concepts and ability to restate in one's own words); applying (use information in new situations; take classroom learning to settings outside of the classroom); analyzing (make connections among ideas, to separate material or concepts into component parts); evaluating (to make judgments or justify a position about the value of specific information); and creating (to produce original work) (Anderson & Krathwohl, 2001; Preville, n.d.). Recognized as an effective, empirically supported conceptual framework for teaching research methods (Strayhorn, 2009), Bloom's taxonomy is the foremost strategy suggested to help students learn 'deeply' (Sweet et al., 2018). It is used extensively, from elementary school level to post-secondary level, to guide structured learning activities and student assessment (Stanny, 2016). Most importantly, the "taxonomy is not about the tools and technologies – as these are just the medium; instead, it is about using these tools to achieve, recall, understand, apply, analyze, evaluate and create new knowledge" (Churches, 2009, p. 3). [An extensive list of books and articles about

Bloom's Taxonomy can be found at Questia. Also, see Bloom's Digital Taxonomy (Churches, 2009) for a detailed description of the electronic tools associated with each level of the taxonomy.]

The learning management system

Many of the technology tools identified in the following sections are embedded in or accessed through software system generically known as 'e-learning platforms' or Learning Management Systems (LMS). The LMS can best be visualized as an electronic campus, or a multi-faceted learning environment, which creates and organizes online spaces to deliver most activities associated with teaching and learning in any number of educational venues. The type, structure, and components of the LMS learning spaces, under vendor brand names such as Blackboard, Moodle, Canvas, Edmodo, etc., generally are chosen, administered, and financed by the educational institution. Common features of most LMS platforms include: electronic storage spaces where course content, like syllabi, course readings, PowerPoint slides, and other course documents, can be uploaded by the instructor and accessed by the students; interactive spaces, such as discussion boards and what is known as 'WIKI' pages, for student-to-student and student-to-instructor exchange of ideas and collaboration; assignment spaces that instructors create for students to take tests or upload papers and other written assignments; a grade center, which is linked to the assignment spaces, where instructors can post student grades; a communication space where students and instructors can use email, face-to-face web-conferencing, as well as access various internet linkages; a tracking system that records student activity, often referred to as analytics; and a help space where students and instructors can find detailed information about the LMS features and components (Benta, Bologa, Dzitac, & Dzitac, 2015; Chapman, 2009; Farmakis & Kaulbach, 2013). LMS is restricted to students enrolled in the course, or other users permitted by the instructor, but open source platforms, such as WordPress, have similar content and management features as the LMS but are accessible to anyone using the Internet and thus can be used as an alternative to the more protected LMS (Croteau, 2015). [Blackboard was the vendor LMS used at the university where these research methods F2F to online conversion occurred.]

Teaching practices for an introductory research methods course

Identify essential from less essential content

The first teaching practice, "help students identify the essential from the less essential content", is associated with the lower order thinking skills of remembering and understanding identified in Bloom's taxonomy. Research content, a "combination of theoretical/conceptual understanding and practical skills acquisition" (Ehiyazaryan-White, 2012, p. 3), often is perceived by students as unfamiliar and confusing, hence students often need help prioritizing essential information to avoid becoming 'lost in the weeds' (Howard & Brady, 2015). Because "too many topics work against student learning, making it necessary for educators to make difficult decisions about what will or will not be included in a course" (Principles of Teaching, 2015, p. 1), cognitive load theory is a useful theoretical grounding for this teaching practice. Based on the premise that working memory has a limited capacity to retain new information, and that instruction which exceeds working memory hampers educational achievement, cognitive load theory has long been used to guide instructional design that focuses on presenting complex material in ways that build schematic learning, that is, by linking concrete examples to abstract concepts, and assimilating new knowledge into existing knowledge and familiar contexts (Hollender, Hofmann, Deneke, & Schmitz, 2010; Jong, 2010; Shattuck et al., n.d.).

Helping students distinguish essential from less-essential information begins with the selection of the course textbooks, reading materials and other resources that prescribe the content that students will need to remember and understand. Two important points are noted regarding choosing research methods texts: (a) attention to cognitive load theory by ensuring that the text and other reading material are clearly highlighted and summarized at frequent intervals throughout the chapters, and that there are abundant examples (particularly related to social work practice) to clarify complex concepts and terms; (b) availability of an online 'Student Study Guide' and other textbook ancillaries, including electronic chapter quizzes, review questions, flashcards, PowerPoint lecture slides, and references for Internet resources that are used to help deliver course content. The text itself does not need to be available electronically (although more and more are), yet electronic supplementary resources specifically linked to the text can help bring student attention to the most salient points for both online and F2F learners.

Educators also help students distinguish essential from less essential material through lectures and structured class discussions. Converting lectures to electronic format, by creating screencasts from existing F2F lecture notes and PowerPoint slides, maximizes the efforts put into an F2F class. Screencasts are video recordings of the computer screen, usually accompanied by audio narration by the instructor (Technology Dictionary, 2017). In contrast to live lectures in F2F classes, screencasts offer students the advantage of being able to listen to lectures multiple times and the flexibility of listening to them at more convenient times. Screencasts are especially adept at presenting information visuospatially, which, by tapping several sensory modalities, can increase working memory (Jong, 2010). With an appropriate screencast program, instructors can sit in their offices, or anywhere else, upload their lecture, graphics, and whatever additional material they want to share with students, onto their computer and then narrate the important points, similar to speaking to a 'live' class. Helpfully, several Internet resources provide 'tips' on how to create effective screencasts (Ruffini, 2012). Screencasting capabilities, of course, often are dependent on the technological resources and choices made by host institutions which fortunately are increasingly providing technological support for classroom instructors to create and upload screencasts through specialized instructional designers.

Screencasts are most often associated with asynchronous learning, that is, learning which occurs at different times and in different places. While the capability for synchronous learning, learning that is time specific, for the online classroom increasingly is available via web-conferencing tools, the asynchronous format currently is more common. Web-conferencing is the umbrella term for technologies that allow two or more individuals from different locations to see and talk with each other over the internet (Technology Dictionary, 2017). Even in full-time online courses, instructors and students can arrange to 'meet' online and interact in real time. These synchronous videos or conferencing tools support any number of learning practices but they are especially useful in helping instructors clarify complex research concepts for either individuals or groups of students, solidifying Bloom's lower level of thinking skills. Although some web-conferencing tools, such as 'Collaborate' or 'Zoom,' are located in various institutionalized LMSs, many (such as 'Google Hangouts,' 'Skype', or 'Go to Meeting') are publicly available. [See Conversion Matrix, Table 1.]

Reinforce engaged learning by student-to-student interactive experiences

The "reinforce engaged learning by student-to-student interactive experiences" teaching practice occurs most readily through collaborative learning projects in which students work together to achieve shared learning goals (Loes & Pascarella, 2017). Collaborative learning has a long history in instructional design, dating from the works of educational pioneers Piaget and Vygotsky, and later supported by Chickering and Gamson's (1987) principles of good educational practices which identified " developing reciprocity and cooperation among students" (p.1) as a key ingredient to achieving effective learning outcomes. The benefits of collaborative learning include increased cognitive motivation, academic achievement, critical thinking skills and openness to diversity (Loes & Pascarella, 2017; Shattuck et al., n.d.). The potential of such learning communities to meet the challenges of research methods courses has been recognized (Kilburn, Nind, & Wiles, 2014), most notably in the online literature (Bates, Rodriguez, & Drysdale, 2007; Pfeffer & Rogalin, 2012; Sabey & Horrocks, 2011).

In this exemplar research methods course, the student-to-student collaborative learning experience is rooted in the development of a group research proposal, an

Table 1. Conversion matrix.

Teaching Practices	Curricular Activities		Branded Tools
	F2F	Hybrid, Fully Online, or Web-based Tool	

Help students identify the essential from the less essential content.	• Textbook selection
	• Class lectures
	• Structured class discussions
		(1) Textbook selection with ancillaries
		(2) Screencasts
		(3) Web conferencing
			The top 3 per tools were selected from the Top 200 Tools for Learning (2017) listing
			(1) Review of current and popular publishing companies (i.e.: Pearson, Cengage, McGraw Hill, etc., …) of traditional and/or open source textbooks to ensure supportive, ancillary resources is recommended prior to selecting a text
			(2) Screencasts
			  (a) Camtasia: https://www.techsmith.com/video-editor.
			  (b) Screencast-O-Matic: www.screencastomatic.com html
			  (c) Screenflow: https://www.telestream.net/screenflow/
			(3) Web Conferencing
			  (a) Skype: http://www.skype.net/
			  (b) Zoom: http://zoom.us/
			  (c) Google Hangouts: https://hangouts.google.com/

Reinforce Engaged Learning by Instructor-to -Student and Student-to Student Interactive Experiences	• Small group work collaboration
	• Report group work back to instructor and entire class for discussion and feedback
		(1) Web conferencing
		(2) Messaging applications
		(3) Discussion boards
			(1) Web Conferencing
			  (a) Skype: http://www.skype.net/
			  (b) Zoom: http://zoom.us/
			  (c) Google Hangouts: https://hangouts.google.com/
			(2) Messaging Applications
			  (a) Skype: http://www.skype.net/
			  (b) WhatsApp: http://www.whatsapp.com/
			  (c) Google Hangouts: https://hangouts.google.com/
			(3) Discussion Boards in top three LMS systems::
			  (a) Moodle: http://www.moodle.org/
			    (a) Discussion board feature- Called "Forum"
			  (b) Canvas: http://www.instructure.com/
			    (1) (b) Discussion board feature-Called "Discussions"
			  (c) Blackboard Learn: http://blackboard.com/
			    (i) Discussion board feature-Called "Discussion board"

(Continued)

Table 1. (Continued).

Teaching Practices	Curricular Activities		Branded Tools
Ongoing Formative Assessment of Student Strengths and Weakness	Informal observation of students' facial expressions, mannerisms, and classroom discussion via: • 'One minute' paper, • Impromptu multiple-choice and fill-in-the-blank content specific questions, often using personal response systems known as 'clickers', • research project step-by-step worksheets	(1) Course textbook electronic quiz capacity (2) LMS mediated tools Student Journaling, Discussion boards, and Worksheets	(1) Explore textbooks for student assessment packages/ tools (2) Learning management systems (LMS) provide a host of technological tools to facilitate each of the identified, online curricular activities. Examples of these tools are: (a) Wiki feature (b) Journaling feature (c) Discussion board feature Top three LMS systems: (1) Moodle: http://www.moodle.org/ (a) Wiki feature-Called "Wiki module" (b) Journaling feature- Called"Journal module" (c) Discussion board feature- Called "Forum" (2) Canvas: http://www.instructure.com/ (a) Wiki feature-Called "Wiki Page" (b) Journaling feature- Called "Assignments" (Does not use due date function) (c) Discussion board feature- Called "Discussions" (3) Blackboard Learn: http://blackboard.com/ (a) Wiki feature- "Wiki" (b) Journaling feature- "Journals" (c) Discussion board feature-Called "Discussion board"

(Continued)

Table 1. (Continued).

Teaching Practices	Curricular Activities	Branded Tools
Test for "walking knowledge"	In class closed/open book exam, quiz, test, etc …	(1) Tests and Assignments via LMS System Moodle: http://www.moodle.org/ (a) Assignment features-
	(1) Tests and assignments via LMSs (LMS system) (2) Lockdown browser (LMS component)	(i) Timed exams-Called "Quiz" Canvas: http://www.instructure.com/ (b) Assignment features
		(i) Timed exams-Called "Quiz" Blackboard Learn: http://blackboard.com/ (c) Assignment features-
		(i) Timed exams-Called "Test" (2) Lockdown Browser
		(a) Respondus (available with Blackboard, Canvas, Brightspace, Moodle, and Schoology): http:respondus.com
		(b) WebAssign LockDown Browser (Cengage Publishing): https://www.webassign.com/instructors/features/secure-testing/lockdown-browser/
		(c) Pearson LockDown Browser: https://www.webassign.com/instructors/features/secure-testing/lockdown-browser/
Guide the application of course material to real world settings	Assignments, research worksheets, research proposal (group work) to facilitate active learning	Cloud Computing Platforms
	Cloud Computing Platforms to facilitate a group work (Group assignments, Worksheets and Research Proposal) and instructor access for supervision and feedback	(1) Google Suite: https://gsuite.google.com/ (2) Dropbox: http://www.dropbox.com/ (3) OneDrive: http://www.onedrive.com/

Table 1. The technological tools that are identified and used in the conversion matrix were selected by using the top three listed tools (as identified by each 'teaching practice') per the Top 200 Tools for Learning 2017 (reference correctly: http://c4lpt.co.uk/top100tools/) and then organized by teaching practices throughout the matrix. The Top 200 Tools for Learning 2017 is compiled by Jane Hart at the Center for Learning and Performance Technologies and from the votes of over 2100 learning professionals in over 50 countries. This matrix does not endorse any one particular software or product, rather identifies examples of technological tools that may be used in organizing your online teaching activities. As with many technologies, there are free versions of software that often have basic functionality without all of the "bells and whistles" as well as premium versions that are often available for purchase and include all of the software's functionality and can be downloaded and installed on desktops, laptops, and/or mobile computing devices.

assignment that requires students to consider and apply, as a group, all material covered in the course to produce an original research proposal as a final assignment. Although collaborative learning can be associated with all levels of Bloom's taxonomy, it is most clearly recognized as supporting the higher-order levels of evaluating and creating in the context of this course. At the evaluation level, the group effort to develop the proposal forces group members to justify their positions and the suggestions they bring to the group process; and, at the creation level, a new product, a research proposal unique to the needs and interests of the group members, emerges from this collaboration.

The proposal assignment is a semester-long, team-based and graded activity, with 2–4 student members per research team. Students choose their own group members, based on research interests, at the beginning of the course, develop a contract that details who is responsible for which sections of the research proposal, work together throughout the semester, preparing and submitting a research proposal, and complete both a group and an individual assessment and reflection at the end of the semester that considers their and their group members' contributions to the final product.

Because F2F students are expected to schedule group time to work on the proposal outside of scheduled class time, converting this teaching practice to the online setting is straightforward. Students use e-mail as the initial means of communication; they then rely on google hangouts or web conferencing (described above) for synchronous collaborative learning, and the LMS sites such as Discussion Board Forums and WIKIs for asynchronous learning. "A discussion board (known also by names such as *discussion group, discussion forum, message board,* and *online forum*) is a general term for any online "bulletin board" whereby anyone with access to the board can leave and expect to see responses to messages" (Discussion Board, 2011, p. 1). In the online course, at the beginning of the semester, the instructor initiates an all-class discussion board in the LMS for students to share research interests and thereby form their small groups. Once the research proposal groups are formed, the instructor establishes a separate LMS discussion board and a 'WIKI' space for each group project which allows ongoing student-to-student and student-to-instructor communication about the specific research proposal throughout the semester. 'WIKIs' are a designated page or blank space on the LMS site that students can write on, or upload images or links. "WIKIs allow students to contribute and modify course-related material in a collaborative area". Students can create new content or edit existing content as well as view revisions and provide comments. The group contract as well as the final research proposal are uploaded via the LMS assignment area. [See conversion matrix for more detail on these electronic tools in Table 1.]

Provide ongoing formative assessment of student strength and weakness

The iterative nature of the research process, the unfamiliarity of research concepts and terminology, and the cumulative knowledge-building aspect of learning research methods require that instructors assess the strengths and weaknesses of students on an ongoing basis to ensure that a proper learning scaffolding is in place (Girod & Wojcikiewicz, 2009; Johnson, 2014a; Schulze, 2009; Shepard, 2005). Continuous assessment and feedback from the instructor ensures students that they are accurately absorbing the domain-relevant content that forms the building blocks for the application of this knowledge in the development of their research proposal. It is critical to "address misconceptions and misunderstandings, and correct mistakes" (Vai & Sosulski, 2016, p. 153) that are part of the learning process for many introductory research methods students before they finalize their research proposal. Thus, "ongoing formative assessment of student strengths and weaknesses" is the third teaching practice. In contrast to summative assessment, which is concerned with evaluative judgements about student learning outcomes that often occur at the end of the course (e.g., the final research proposal assignment or final exam), formative assessment gathers information about the progression and quality of student learning during the course and makes appropriate instruction modifications (Angelo & Cross, 1998; Whys and Hows of Assessment, 2015). Increasingly recognized as an effective mechanism to promote deep learning, as well as being an antecedent to higher learning skills (Gikandi, Morrow, & Davis, 2011; Kealey, 2010), formative assessment is associated with 'comprehension', level 2 of Bloom's taxonomy of learning, which is concerned with how students grasp meaning, interpret facts, and explain, rephrase and summarize content (Anderson & Krathwohl, 2001).

Instructors in F2F classes often conduct formative assessments intuitively and informally by observation of students' facial expressions, mannerisms, and classroom interactions, or by more structured approaches systematically embedded into course instruction (Angelo & Cross, 1998; Kealey, 2010). In this F2F research class, three major techniques are used to gather information about student learning: (a) the 'one minute' paper which asks students to recall the most challenging and the most understood concepts; (b) impromptu multiple-choice and fill-in-the-blank content specific questions, often using personal response systems known as 'clickers'; and (c) research proposal worksheets that move students through the research process in a step-by-step basis toward the development of a final research proposal. Five research proposal worksheets, one for each major step of the research proposal development process (i.e., developing the research question, reviewing the literature, choosing a research design, identifying/creating measures, and planning the sampling and data collection approach), are completed jointly by the members of each group at various points throughout the semester. The worksheets are discussed with students during class time and followed up with written feedback. Instructor approval on one worksheet is required for students to proceed to the next step in the research process, thus ensuring that appropriate scaffolding is in place as the students move through the learning process (Shepard, 2005). The worksheets reveal powerful insights about a student's grasp of the material at each step of the research process, allowing the instructor to correct misinformation, misconceptions or errors in interpretation before they can jeopardize a student's ability to produce an acceptable final research proposal.

Ample opportunities exist to transfer these teaching techniques to the online classroom setting. The use of the course textbook's electronic quiz capacity, coupled with the 'journal' feature of the LMS, converts the F2F 'one minute' paper and the multiple-choice and fill-in-the-blank content specific quizzes to the online format. For example, students log onto the course text 'Student Study Site' and complete the chapter self-assessment quizzes on a weekly basis. They take the quiz as many times as necessary to answer 80% of the questions correctly. Students then use the individual 'journal' feature available through the LMS – a designated online space where students create meaning and internalize learning as they engage in personalized one-on-one conversations with the instructor (Getting Started With Blackboard Learn Interactive Tools, 2012, p. 1) – to share their experiences about the quiz and seek additional clarification of the course material. Because the electronic journal allows confidential communication between student and instructor, it combats student reluctance to ask questions for fear of appearing less knowledgeable than their classmates and thereby offers them a safe environment to express themselves and receive individualized feedback. These quiz and journal activities are considered class participation and account for 10% of the total course grade, similar to class participation in the F2F class.

The research proposal worksheets are converted to the online setting through the LMS 'WIKI' feature described above. For this exemplar course, the instructor creates a designated WIKI space for each proposal group and uploads the five proposal worksheets into the WIKI space. The instructor is able to enter the site online and, paralleling the process in the F2F class, comment on the students' work at any time, correcting erroneous information and providing guidance as students move through the proposal development process. [See the conversion matrix for information about these and other electronic tools in Table 1.]

Test for "walking knowledge"

Testing contributes to student learning by helping students retain and hold information in long-term memory for future use (Karpicke & Roediger, 2008;

Lee & Ahn, 2017; Miller, 2014). The "test for walking knowledge" practice is a closed-book midterm exam that represents what is considered to be the de facto agenda of the most critical knowledge associated with the initial learning of research methods in an introductory level course. Any course test is an act of communication about what the discipline values and considers important to the particular area of study (Boud, 2000). The midterm exam is an intentional teaching strategy to ensure that students have built and integrated a repertoire of the most important knowledge and skills covered in most social science research courses (Patterson, 2010; Rubin, 2009). This practice is termed 'test for walking knowledge' because it provides the scaffolding, or foundational knowledge, that can be quickly recalled and easily transferable by students as they finalize their research proposal. In this sense, 'testing for walking knowledge' is one of Bloom's lower order thinking skills, used to better equip students to meet the challenge of developing the final research proposal associated with the higher-order thinking skills of application and evaluation. This practice is also termed 'test for walking knowledge' because it is structured to help students develop sustainable knowledge about research methods that they can carry with them into the practice world upon graduation and that will contribute to lifelong learning (Boud & Falchikov, 2006).

The midterm test for walking knowledge has several components, all of which are linked to best practices identified in the scholarship of teaching and learning. First, the instructor incorporates cognitive load theory by allowing students the opportunity to develop and bring into the classroom a one page 'cheat/review sheet', of any type of information they choose, to reference during the closed-book exam (Karpicke & Roediger III, 2008; Miller, 2014). Students reported that the 'cheat/review sheet' not only reduced test anxiety but was an excellent tool that helped them prepare for the exam and provided some level of "confidence that new learning tasks can be mastered", an important element in any activity associated with sustainable knowledge (Boud, 2000, p. 161). Second, the exam is a balance of direct recall items, comprehension items, and a series of brief case study vignettes, followed by multiple choice, short answer and short essay responses that require students to begin applying the material to practice settings. Thus, the exam captures learning at the first three levels of Bloom's taxonomy and identifies gaps in students' knowledge that can be addressed during the 2nd half of the semester. Third, the graded exam is returned to students and reviewed in class to correct any misinformation and to strengthen students' 'walking knowledge' base (Vai & Sosulski, 2016). Fourth, students who scored below 80% were given the option to provide (for extra credit) a corrected explanation of any question they got wrong on the exam (Weimer, 2010).

Converting the midterm exam to an online format makes use of the assignment feature in LMS which allows instructors to upload existing tests or to create a wide variety of new ones, such as multiple choice, fill-in-the-blank, matching, short answer, and essay, directly in the LMS. The content of this online midterm is the same as that for the F2F class with the advantage of automatic online grading provided through the LMS. However, unless students are required to take the online test in a proctored facility, there is no way to completely eliminate the possibility of student cheating in an online closed-book testing situation, which is the preferred administration for walking knowledge practice testing. Fortunately, there are several online strategies to approximate the F2F closed-book nature of the midterm: (a) including a question at the end of the exam where students answer 'yes' or 'no' that they had completed the exam without any additional resources (except the cheat/review sheet); (b) using what is generically termed as a 'lockdown' browser, an online software program that interfaces with the particular LMS used to administer the exam and locks down the online testing environment on the electronic device that the student is using for the exam, preventing students from accessing e-mail, the internet, or other applications on the device while they are completing the exam; and (c) using the LMS test options to force completion within one sitting and within 2.5 hours, the same conditions imposed on students in the F2F class. These options limit the opportunities for students to access other individuals or materials for help with the answers to the exam. However, in any online assessment situation, nothing will prevent a student who wants to cheat from accessing other electronic devices that are not 'locked down' (or other resources) to find answers to the exam questions.

The LMS testing option also allows students to view the correct answer for each question as they record the answer for that question, or immediately upon the completion of the exam, or at a later date, at the instructor's discretion, providing as much or as little explanation for each of the answers as desired. Students who want to take advantage of the extra credit assignment submit it through the regular assignment feature of the LMS. [The conversion matrix in Table 1 provides more information about the different types of lockdown browsers, being mindful that the marketing choice for the browser tool generally rests with the university administration.]

Guide the application material to real-world settings

The final teaching practice is to, "guide the application of course material to real-world settings". This practice, reflective of the principles of engaged learning discussed above, is associated with the third level of Bloom's taxonomy – application – to use information in new situations and take classroom learning to settings outside of the classroom. Active learning is broadly defined as " ... any teaching method which gets students actively involved, as opposed to instructional approaches that rely on didactic modes of knowledge transmission" (Keyser, 2000, p. 35). This process may take the form of engaging students in practical or problem-based tasks in which they are encouraged to practice, experiment and engage with the topic. Students " ... must talk about what they are learning, write about it, relate it to past experiences and apply it to their daily lives. They must make what they learn part of themselves" (Chickering & Gamson, 1987, p. 4). In this exemplar research methods course, active learning through the application level of Bloom's taxonomy is operationalized by the creation of a research proposal, which represents an assignment that compels the use higher-order thinking skills by requiring students to apply textbook concepts to situations that are tethered to real-world circumstances, contexts, and environments in which they will be/are practicing (Kilburn et al., 2014).

A research proposal assignment represents an excellent cumulative product for assessing student competency, as required by the Council on Social Work Education (CSWE) Educational Policy and Accreditation Standards (EPAS) for baccalaureate and masters of social work programs (Council on Social Work Education (CSWE), 2015). Hardway and Stroud (2014) suggest that using student choice to increase students' knowledge of research methodology improves their attitudes toward research and promotes acquisition of professional skills. They further posit that " ... students learn best when they are actively engaged in the process and are most intrinsically motivated when they feel they have autonomy over their learning" (p. 381). Thus, in this exemplar introductory research class, students can choose to address one of the major research roles for clinical or macro social work practice: (1) knowledge-building and theory testing or (2) evaluating practice with individuals, couples, families, communities, and other groups. Because students also choose their topic, and their project group members, the proposals are easily linked to or based in students' past experiences or current work or practicum placements.

Several of the prior teaching practices converge in this application of course material to real-world settings: distinguishing the essential from the non-essential is the critical first step in identifying the core concepts and methods that need to be applied in the development of a research proposal; students work collaboratively on their research proposal worksheets and submit the proposal as a group to facilitate engaged learning; formative assessment guides and reinforces student learning to yield an acceptable research proposal; and, through testing for 'walking' knowledge, students internalize the most important research methods for application in their research. The host of technological tools categorized as "cloud computing platforms" increases the ability of students to collaborate on their proposal using cloud sharing options through the Internet. For example, Google Suite is a packaged, Internet-based application that can be downloaded and used for cooperative editing of documents, spreadsheets, and presentations in real time. Google Docs, Google Sheets, and Google Slides are three examples of software from Google Suite that can be opened, shared, and edited by multiple individuals simultaneously, and users are able to see character-by-character changes as they make edits by applying what they have learned in the course.

Conclusion

This article presents, and encourages, an approach for instructors to consider as they convert social work courses from a F2F format to the online environment. The authors assert that basic, but interrelated, pedagogical practices need to guide the design of any course, regardless of delivery format, and illustrate how a modified constructivist approach, coupled with Bloom's Taxonomy of learning, inspires five specific teaching practices that can anchor the conversion of an introductory social work research course. One of the challenges instructors face in moving course content to the online environment is gaining familiarity with (and being able to make judicious selections from) an ever-increasing quagmire of technology tools and market providers that support, rather than obfuscate, course learning goals. A conversion matrix can help simplify what could otherwise be an onerous, and off-putting task, by extracting from this quagmire the most essential technology tools that match specific teaching practices and thus facilitate the conversion from a F2F to an online format.

References

Anderson, L., & Krathwohl, D. (2001). *A taxonomy for learning, teaching, and assessing: A revision of Bloom's taxonomy of educational objectives (Complete ed.)*. New York, NY: Longman.

Anderson, T., & Dron, J. (2011). Three generations of distance education pedagogy. *International Review of Research in Open and Distance Learning, 12*(3), 80–97. doi:10.19173/irrodl.v12i3.890

Angelo, T., & Cross, K. P. (1998). *Classroom assessment techniques: A handbook for college teachers*. San Francisco, CA: Jossey-Bass.

Barraket, J. (2005). Teaching research method using a student-centred approach? Critical reflections on practice. *Journal of University Teaching & Learning Practice, 2*(2). Retrieved from http://ro.uow.edu.au/jutlp/vol2/iss2/3

Bates, S. C., Rodríguez, M. M. D., & Drysdale, M. J. (2007). Supporting and encouraging behavioral research among distance education students. *CUR Quarterly, 28*(1), 18–22.

Benta, D., Bologa, S., Dzitac, S., & Dzitac, I. (2015). University level learning and teaching via e-learning platforms. *Procedia Computer Science, 55,* 1366–1373. doi:10.1016/j.procs.2015.07.123

Bidabadi, S. N., Isfahani, A. N., Rouhollahi, A., & Khalili, R. (2016). Effective teaching methods in higher education: Requirements and barriers. *Journal of Advances in Medical Education and Profession, 4*(4), 170–178.

Boud, D. (2000). Sustainable assessment: Rethinking assessment for the learning society. *Studies in Continuing Education, 22*(2), 151–167. doi:10.1080/713695728

Boud, D., & Falchikov, N. (2006). Aligning assessment with long-term Learning. *Assessment & Evaluation in Higher Education, 31*(4), 399–413. doi:10.1080/02602930600679050

Cameron, L. (2017). How learning designs, teaching methods and activities differ by discipline in Australian universities. *Journal Of Learning Design, 10*(2), 69–84. doi:10.5204/jld.v10i2.289

Chapman, D. (2009). Introduction to learning management systems. In C. Howard, J. Boettcher, L. Justice, K. Schenk, P. Rogers, & G. Berg (Eds.), *Encyclopedia of Distance Learning* (pp. 1149–1155). Hershey, PA: IGI Global. doi:10.4018/978-1-59140-555-9.ch171

Chickering, A., & Ehrmann, S. C. (1996). Implementing the seven principles: Technology as lever. *AAHE Bulletin,* 3–6.

Chickering, A. W., & Gamson, Z. F. (1987). Seven principles for good practice in undergraduate education. *AAHE Bulletin, 39*(7), 3–7.

Churches, A. (2009). *Bloom's digital taxonomy.* Retrieved from https://www.uab.edu/elearning/images/facultytoolkit/bloom_digital_taxonomy_v3_01web.pdf.

Council on Social Work Education (CSWE). (2015). *Educational policy and accreditation standards for baccalaureate and master's of social work programs 2015.* Retrieved from https://www.cswe.org/Accreditation/Standards-and-Policies/EPAS-Handbook

Croteau, D. (2015, August 25). *Blackboard, WordPress, or Both?* Retrieved from https://davidrcroteau.net/blog-post/blackboard-wordpress-or-both.

Discussion Board. (2011). Retrieved from https://whatis.techtarget.com/definition/discussion-board-discussion-group-message-board-online-forum

Ehiyazaryan-White, E. (2012). Developing open academic practices in research methods teaching within a Higher Education in Further Education context. *Journal of Interactive Media in Education, 2,*1–13.

Ennis, R. H. (2018). Critical thinking across the curriculum: A vision. *Topoi: An International Review Of Philosophy, 37*(1), 165–184. doi:10.1007/s11245-016-9401-4

Farmakis, H., & Kaulbach, M. (2013). Teaching online? A guide on how to get started. *The International Journal of Organizational Innovation, 3*(2), 34–40.

Fook, C. (2012). Best practices of teaching in higher education in United States: A case study. *Procedia - Social and Behavioral Sciences, 46,* 4817–4821. doi:10.1016/j.sbspro.2012.06.341

George, J. W. (2009). Classical curriculum design. Arts and humanities in higher education: An international journal of theory. *Research And Practice, 8*(2), 160–179.

Getting Started With Blackboard Learn Interactive Tools. (2012). *In Blackboard.* Retrieved from http://ondemand.blackboard.com/r91/documents/getting_started_with_interactive_tools.pdf 10.1094/PDIS-11-11-0999-PDN

Gikandi, J. W., Morrow, D., & Davis, N. E. (2011). Online formative assessment in higher education: A review of the literature. *Computers & Education, 57*(4), 2333–2351. doi:10.1016/j.compedu.2011.06.004

Girod, M., & Wojcikiewicz, S. (2009). Comparing distance vs. campus-based delivery of research methods courses. *Educational Research Quarterly, 33*(2), 47–56.

Guide, T. (n.d.). *Selecting appropriate teaching methods*. UB Center for Educational Innovation. Retrieved from https://www.buffalo.edu/ubcei/resources/.../selecting-appropriate-teaching-methods.html

Hardway, C. L., & Stroud, M. (2014). Using student choice to increase students' knowledge of research methodology, improve their attitudes toward research, and promote acquisition of professional skills. *International Journal of Teaching and Learning in Higher Education, 26* (3), 381–392.

Hollender, N., Hofmann, C., Deneke, M., & Schmitz, B. (2010). Integrating cognitive load theory and concepts of human-computer interaction. *Computers in Human Behavior, 26* (6), 1278–1288. doi:10.1016/j.chb.2010.05.031

Horii, C. V. (2018, May). Wise instructional choices in an evidence-driven era. *NEA Higher Education Advocate, 36*(3), 6–9.

Howard, C., & Brady, M. (2015). Teaching social research methods after the critical turn: Challenges and benefits of a constructivist pedagogy. *International Journal of Social Research Methodology, 18*(5), 511–525. doi:10.1080/13645579.2015.1062625

Ilic, D. (2009). Teaching evidence-based practice: Perspectives from the undergraduate and post-graduate viewpoint. *Annals of the Academy of Medicine, 38*(6), 559–563.

Johnson, B. A. (2014a). Transformation of online teaching practices through implementation of appreciative inquiry. *Online Learning, 18*(3), 1–23. doi:10.24059/olj.v18i3.428

Johnson, S. (2014b). Applying the seven principles of good practice: Technology as a lever–In an online research course. *Journal Of Interactive Online Learning, 13*(2), 41–50.

Jong, T. (2010). Cognitive load theory, educational research, and instructional design: Some food for thought. *Instructional Science, 38*(2), 105–134. doi:10.1007/s11251-009-9110-0

Karpicke, J. D., & Roediger III, H. L. (2008). The critical importance of retrieval for learning. *Science, 319*(5865), 966–968. doi:10.1126/science.1152408

Kealey, E. (2010). Assessment and evaluation in social work education: Formative and summative approaches. *Journal of Teaching in Social Work, 30*(1), 64–74. doi:10.1080/08841230903479557

Keengwe, J., Onchwari, G., & Agamba, J. (2013). Promoting effective e-learning practices through the constructivist pedagogy. *Education and Information Technologies, 19*(4), 887–898. doi:10.1007/s10639-013-9260-1

Keyser, M. (2000). Active learning and cooperative learning: Understanding the difference and using both styles effectively. *Research Strategies, 17*(1), 35–44. doi:10.1016/S0734-3310(00)00022-7

Kilburn, D., Nind, M., & Wiles, R. (2014). Learning as researchers and teachers: The development of a pedagogical culture for social science research methods?. *British Journal of Educational Studies, 62*(2), 191–207. doi:10.1080/00071005.2014.918576

Lee, H. S., & Ahn, D. (2017, May 25). Testing prepares students to learn better: The forward effect of testing in category learning. *Journal of Educational Psychology*. Advance online publication. doi:10.1037/edu0000211

Loes, C. N., & Pascarella, E. T. (2017). Collaborative learning and critical thinking: Testing the link. *Journal Of Higher Education, 88*(5), 726–753. doi:10.1080/00221546.2017.1291257

Lumpkin, A., Achen, R., & Dodd, R. (2015). Focusing teaching on students: Examining student perceptions of learning strategies. *Quest (00336297), 67*(4), 352–366. doi:10.1080/00336297.2015.1082143

McCombs, B. (2015). Learner-centered online instruction. *New Directions for Teaching and Learning, 144*, 57–71. doi:10.1002/tl.20163

Miller, M. D. (2014). *Minds on line: Teaching effectively with technology*. Cambridge, Mass: Harvard University Press.

Oleson, A., & Hora, M. (2014). Teaching the way they were taught? Revisiting the sources of teaching knowledge and the role of prior experience in shaping faculty teaching practices. *Higher Education (00181560), 68*(1), 29–45. doi:10.1007/s10734-013-9678-9

Parker, J., Maor, D., & Herrington, J. (2013). Authentic online learning: Aligning learner needs, pedagogy and technology. *Issues in Educational Research, 23*(2), 227–241.

Patterson, G. T. (2010). A composite review of social work research textbooks. *Journal of Teaching in Social Work, 30*(2), 237–246. doi:10.1080/08841230903482486

Paynter, K., & Barnes, J. (2015). Teaching undergraduate students versus graduate students online: Similarities, differences, and instructional approaches. In D. Rutledge & D. Slykhuis (Eds.), *Proceedings of SITE 2015–Society for information technology & teacher education international conference* (pp. 67–71). Las Vegas, NV, United States: Association for the Advancement of Computing in Education (AACE). Retrieved from https://www.learnte chlib.org/primary/p/149968/

Pfeffer, C. A., & Rogalin, C. L. (2012). Three strategies for teaching research methods: A case study. *Teaching Sociology, 40*(4), 368–376. doi:10.1177/0092055X12446783

Preville, P. (n.d.). *The professor's guide to using Bloom's Taxonomy: How to put America's most influential pedagogical model to work in your college classroom.* Retrieved from https://tophat.com/wp-content/uploads/Blooms_taxonomy_FINAL.pdf

Principles of Teaching. (2015). *Eberly center for teaching excellence & educational innovation.* Pittsburgh, PA: Carnegie Mellon University. Retrieved from https://www.cmu.edu/teach ing/principles/teaching.html

Reiff, M., & Ballin, A. (2016). Adult graduate student voices: Good and bad learning experiences. *Adult Learning, 27*(2), 76–83. doi:10.1177/1045159516629927

Rubin, A. (2009). Teaching social work research methods. In E. Mullen (Ed.), *Oxford bibliographies in social work.* New York, NY: Oxford University Press. Retrieved from http://www.oxfordbibliographies.com/view/document/obo-9780195389678/obo-9780195389678-0008.xml

Ruffini, M., (2012). Screencasting to engage learning. *Educause Review Online.* Retrieved from http://er.educause.edu/articles/2012/11/screencasting-to-engage-learning. 10.1094/PDIS-11-11-0999-PDN

Sabey, A., & Horrocks, S. (2011). From soap opera to research methods teaching: Developing an interactive website/DVD to teach research in health and social care. *Electronic Journal of e-Learning, 9*(1), 98–104.

Samson, P. L. (2016). Critical thinking in social work education: A research synthesis. *Journal Of Social Work Education, 52*(2), 147–156. doi:10.1080/10437797.2016.1151270

Schulze, S. (2009). Teaching research methods in a distance education context: Concerns and challenges. *South African Journal Of Higher Education, 23*(5), 992–1008. doi:10.4314/sajhe.v23i5.48812

Secret, M., Bryant, N., & Cummings, C. (2017). Teaching an interdisciplinary graduate level methods course in an openly-networked connected learning environment: A Glass half full. *Journal of Educators Online, 14*(2), 90–106. doi:10.9743/jeo

Shattuck, K. I., Frese, J., Lalla, S., Mikalson, J., Simunich, B., & Wang, L. (n.d.). *Results of review of the 2011-2013 research literature (Rep.).* Retrieved from https://www.qualitymatters.org/sites/default/files/research-docs-pdfs/2013-Literature-Review-Summary-Report.pdf

Sheffield, C. B. (2018). Promoting critical thinking in higher education: My experiences as the inaugural Eugene H. Fram chair in applied critical thinking at rochester institute of technology. *Topoi, 37*(1), 155–163. doi:10.1007/s11245-016-9392-1

Shepard, L. A. (2005). Linking formative assessment to scaffolding. *Educational Leadership, 63*(3), 66–70.

Smith, K. (2012). Lessons learnt from literature on the diffusion of innovative learning and teaching practices in higher education. *Innovations In Education And Teaching International, 49*(2), 173–182. doi:10.1080/14703297.2012.677599

Stanny, C. J. (2016). Reevaluating bloom's taxonomy: What measurable verbs can and cannot say about student learning. *Education Sciences, 6*(37), 1–12. doi:10.3390/educsci6040037

Stillar, B. (2012). 21st century learning: How college classroom interaction will change in the decades ahead. *International Journal of Technology, Knowledge & Society, 8*(1), 143–151. doi:10.18848/1832-3669/CGP/v08i01/56266

Strayhorn, T. (2009). The (in)effectiveness of various approaches to teaching research methods. In M. Garner, C. Wagner, & B. Kawulich (Eds.), *Teaching research methods in the social sciences* (pp. 119–130). Farnham, UK: Ashgate Publishing Group.

Sweet, C., Blythe, H., & Carpenter, R. (2018). Innovating academic leadership. *National Teaching & Learning Forum,27*, (3), 9–11. doi:10.1002/ntlf.30153

Technology Dictionary. (2017). *In Technopedia.* Retrieved from https://www.techopedia.com/dictionary.

Vai, M., & Sosulski, K. (2016). *Essentials of online course design: A standards-based guide* (2nd ed.). New York, NY: Routledge.

Weimer, M. (2010). A course redesign that contributed to student success. In *Course design and development ideas that work* (pp. 4–5). Madison, WI: Magna Publications. Retrieved from https://www.facultyfocus.com/free-reports/course-design-and-development-ideas-that-work/

Weinstein, Y., Madan, C. R., & Sumeracki, M. A. (2018). Teaching the science of learning. *Cognitive Research: Principles and Implications, 3*(2). doi:10.1186/s41235-018-0099-2

Whys and Hows of Assessment. 2015. *In Eberly Center for Teaching Excellence & Educational Innovation.* Pittsburgh, PA: Carnegie Mellon University. Retrieved from https://www.cmu.edu/teaching/assessment/basics/formative-summative.html

Young, C., & Perovic, N. (2016). Rapid and creative course design: As easy as ABC? *Procedia - Social and Behavioral Sciences, 228*, 390–395. doi:10.1016/j.sbspro.2016.07.058

Using a Virtual Agency to Teach Research

Raymond Sanchez Mayers, Rachel Schwartz, Laura Curran, and Fontaine H. Fulghum

ABSTRACT
Use of instructional technology in social work has grown rapidly in recent years. Despite this increase, there is limited empirical investigation of its impact. In this paper we describe the use of a virtual agency for the teaching of research methods and program evaluation at a school of social work. Evaluation of the virtual agency showed that students in general were satisfied with its use and that higher satisfaction led to higher satisfaction with the overall course. The authors also discuss some of the strengths and weaknesses of using a virtual agency for teaching research and program evaluation.

Introduction

Instructional technology and media have been used pedagogically, including social work education, for several decades (Shorkey & Uebel, 2014). Starting in the 1950s with tape recording, to the 1960s with videotape technology, to the 1980s and the advent of computer and internet-based technologies, social work education has been using, although not always embracing, new technologies. In the 1990s, widespread use of personal computers, electronic mailing systems, email, and internet chat rooms proliferated. The use of television to provide instruction also came into being, followed by hybrid programs, distance education, and fully online social work programs.

Some of the new technology being used in online and even on-the-ground (OTG) programs involves instructional applications that simulate reality, or realistic social work situations. Practice simulations, through live role plays (and more recently through structured clinical examinations) have long constituted a central or "signature" component of social work teaching and assessment (Bogo, Rawlings, Katz, & Logie, 2014; Golde, 2007; Sunarich & Rowan, 2017). Social work educators increasingly have attempted to adapt such simulations to a virtual context with the proliferation of online classes and programs. Recent innovations in this area, for instance, include the development of a mobile digital application for teaching interviewing skills (Turner, Landmann, & Kirkland, 2019), the use of video conferencing in

Color versions of one or more of the figures in the article can be found online at www.tandfonline.com/wtsw

online courses to conduct role plays (Fitch, Canda, Cary, & Freese, 2016), and the deployment of social media tools (Stanley-Clarke, English, & Yeung, 2018).

Relatedly, the usages of virtual worlds and virtual reality (VR) have been adapted in various educational settings. A virtual world may be described as a place that exists, " … entirely in networked environments in which people co-exist, communicate and interact through their avatars. These worlds are dynamic and interactive environments that support a broad range of social, entertainment, educational, and productive activities that are loosely based on activities in the physical world" (Gu & Maher, 2014, p. 6). In this context, an avatar has been described as a " … personalizable 3-D representation of the self" (Lee, 2014, p. 95).

Virtual worlds and other computer assisted technologies have been used in health care training for physicians, nurses, and pharmacists, as well as for treatment, assessment, and evaluation (Ghanbarzadeh, Ghapanchi, Blumenstein, & Talaei-Khoei, 2014). For example, educational websites have been created in psychiatric training (Torous et al., 2015), and 3-D interactive virtual human bodies have been created for use in medical training (News Medical Life Sciences, 2012). Virtual reality technologies also have been used with prison inmates for formal education, job training, and psychological rehabilitation (Farley, 2018). Importantly, research has found positive overall learning outcomes associated with VR technologies (Farra, Miller, Timm, & Schafer, 2012; Merchant, Goetz, Cifuentes, Keeney-Kennicutt, & Davis, 2014).

Nevertheless, the application of virtual worlds in social work education is a relatively recent phenomenon. They have been used, for example, to research how social work practitioners make judgements in child welfare (Wastell et al., 2011) and to teach case management skills, permitting students to practice conducting intakes with avatars (Levine & Adams, 2013). Other educators have used a virtual world called "Second Life" to teach social work students interviewing skills using a *chatbot*, an automated avatar programmed to answer student questions (Tandy, Vernon, & Lynch, 2017). One social work program adapted Second Life to teach direct practice skills by setting up a virtual home visit in which the student participated (Wilson, Brown, Wood, & Farkas, 2013). Second Life has been found to be a beneficial tool for social work to teach values, skills and knowledge, as well as to allow students to feel more emotionally connected to the content (Reinsmith-Jones, Kibbe, Crayton, & Campbell, 2015).

As detailed above, the pedagogical literature on instructional technologies in social work, (and simulations in particular) has largely discussed their use in relation to the development of direct practice skills. Yet, their application is not limited to the direct practice realm. For instance, one social work program set up an asynchronous virtual field agency in which students could practice leadership and administrative skills. According to Williams-Gray (2014), "The virtual agency … becomes a simulated field site that supports students as critical thinkers engaged in both justification and discovery." (p. 116). This paper similarly will examine use of a virtual field agency to teach research skills in a MSW program. While the virtual agency (VA) detailed below does not rely on some of the more sophisticated VR technologies, it nevertheless includes aspects of simulation and exemplifies the growing influence and promise of instructional technologies and virtual pedagogy in social work education.

The virtual agency

The virtual agency to be described here was imbedded as part of a requirement for a second-year MSW research course focusing on evaluating practice at the micro and mezzo (agency) level. The course is the second of two required research courses in the curriculum. Among its goals, based on the Council of Social Work Education's (2015) standards, are that students will be able to: Select and use appropriate methods for evaluation of outcomes; apply critical thinking to the analysis and interpretation of evaluation data; and both translate and present evaluation data to various stakeholders/audiences. In order to reach these goals, students have to complete two major assignments. The first is a single-system assignment completed individually with an actual participant; the second involves a program evaluation carried out using an actual agency or simulated agency. For this task, students work in teams to develop evaluation questions, conduct literature reviews on their chosen topic, gather and analyze data, and write an evaluation report whose findings are presented to the entire class at the end of the semester. The program evaluation assignment is the same whether the student uses an actual or virtual agency, and whether the student is in an online or OTG class.

The virtual agency was developed to address the learning needs of students who were not concurrently enrolled in the course and a field placement practicum (While concurrent enrollment is typical, a significant minority of students may opt for atypical course sequencing). While the original intent was for only students without placements to use the virtual agency, all students were permitted to do so, whether they had a field placement or not. Therefore, out of a desire for students to have hands-on experience with program evaluation, a 2-D (rather than an immersive 3-D) virtual agency was developed. While this virtual agency originally was conceived of for the fully online research course, it was quickly apparent that it could be easily translated as an online asset/supplement in OTG courses as well. We felt that offering the virtual agency to students enrolled in both online and OTG classes would positively impact access for students, offering alternative ways to complete assignments, and demonstrating the growing influence of virtual pedagogy in a traditional classroom.

The development of the virtual agency was guided by the *Cognitive-Affective Theory of Learning with Media (CATML)* (Moreno, 2006b), with its evidence-based principles that help educators maximize student learning, and related to Mayer's Cognitive Theory of Learning (CTLM) (Mayer, 2008). Moreno and Mayer, along with others, have conducted numerous studies on learning as it relates to multimedia, and have defined learning as involving a number of steps including outside stimuli (in this case some form of instructional technology) entering the student's sensory memory, with the student then attending to these stimuli within their working memory. Since working memory has limited capacity, students must select only a few pieces of information for further processing, and connect and organize this information with their prior knowledge. The information is believed then to be integrated into long-term memory where it will be available for retrieval. These processes are mediated by motivational factors as well as by individual cognitive styles and abilities (Moreno, 2006a, 2006b). Based on extensive research, principles derived from CATML that optimize student learning have been developed, and those most relevant to the virtual agency include: "*Interactivity*: Students learn better by manipulating the materials rather than by passively observing others manipulate the materials; and, *Reflection*: Students learn better when given opportunities to reflect during the meaning making process" (Moreno, 2006b, p. 65).

The research methods and program evaluation course taught was based on certain pedagogical assumptions, to include that students learn best by doing, and that actual application of theory and knowledge in a practice setting is the best way to learn (the *Interactivity Principle*). Additional suppositions are that students will learn better when able to integrate and write about the findings of their work (the *Reflexivity Principle*) (Moreno, 2006b) or that the field practicum is the perfect setting to apply these theories and new knowledge (Dietz, Westerfelt, & Barton, 2004).

The technology used here was a variant of a virtual world – it was a virtual organization. That is, it solely existed on the internet, had webpages, an organizational structure, leadership, a budget and was meant to simulate an actual human service agency. While the virtual agency created for this assignment is not a "traditional" virtual world so far that it does not include live simulations or role plays, it does provide a virtual setting which allows for exploration and imitation of a live prototypical situation, such as the gathering of data needed for a program evaluation. Human Services of Southern New Jersey, Inc. (2017) was created as a mythical multiservice agency. Some of its programs include drug abuse treatment, an after-school program for adolescent girls, and temporary housing assistance for homeless individuals and families. Each program has a separate web page with a description of its services and information about their outcomes. [See Figure 1 for an agency screenshot.]

In this virtual agency, a website was set up that appears to be that of an actual agency. It lists key staff, programs, governance, and budget. Students

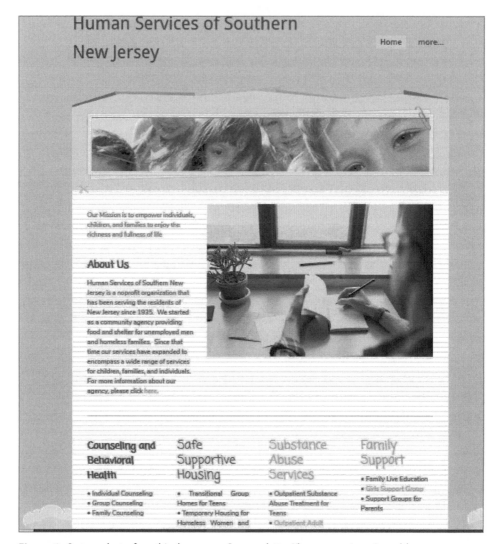

Figure 1. Screen shot of mythical agency. Source: http://humanservicesnj.weebly.com.

are able to click on a program, see a full description, and access (fictitious) client data in Excel spreadsheet format that can be downloaded and analyzed with any popular statistical software, such as SPSS, Stata, Winks. For the Research II course we use a very simple, user-friendly, and free open-source statistical program called Statistics Open for All (SOFA), which can readily be downloaded from the internet (Paton-Simpson & Associates, 2009). Although SOFA was first chosen to be used by online students, all could use it, and it has a much shorter learning curve than more sophisticated programs such as SPSS. Students in the online courses worked in virtual teams, that is, " … groups of people that strive towards a common goal, are distributed across locations, and communicate with each other through the use of information and communication technology (ICT) in a varying degree" (Alahuhta, Nordbäck, Sivunen, & Surakka, 2014, p. 2). Students in OTG courses worked in face-to-face teams, or by phone or Skype. As noted, the virtual agency website is similar to many seen on the internet, and the data available to students are based on an interdisciplinary set of research and intervention perspectives and hence conducive to the completion of a program evaluation paper.

For instance, the first program, *Girls Support Group*, uses simulated self-esteem data from 12-week after-school support groups for teenage girls. The data are in Excel spreadsheet format and contain pre-test and post-test information from the Rosenberg Self-Esteem Scale (Rosenberg, 1965). Students have to find literature about support groups for girls, of which there is an abundance, as well as learn about the Self-Esteem Scale. They then deploy a statistical package (such as SPSS or SOFA) to analyze the data, using a Paired-Samples t-Test to see if there are significant changes in the girls' levels of self-esteem.

The second program, *Outpatient Adult Substance Abuse Treatment*, uses simulated data from a group of males in treatment along with a comparison group of males who are on a waiting list. In this case, the data are from urine test results and students can compare the two groups using an Independent Samples t-Test. They should be able to find abundant literature on outpatient substance abuse treatment, as well as urine tests being used as an outcome measure of treatment effectiveness.

In describing the programs and their treatment approaches, students are able to use creativity and imagination. They are told they can feel free to add any material they wish to develop about the programs that has not been described on the website. This allowance has enabled students to be creative with aspects of the agency; for example, some teams choose treatment modalities such as mindfulness, cognitive behavioral therapy, and art therapy to describe treatment approaches, conduct literature reviews on these topics, and fold them into their papers.

Method

Initial assessment of the virtual agency focused on student feedback. In order to evaluate student reactions to the use of the virtual agency, questions were added to the regular University-wide evaluations that take place at the end of each semester. There were questions regarding decisions to use the virtual agency (no field or worksite, more convenient, easier), as well as queries related to satisfaction (with navigation, learning, usefulness, and ease). A qualitative open-ended question asking for general comments also was included. For purposes of analysis, a further variable was added from the evaluations, that of student ratings of the course (on a 1–5 scale). [See Table 1.]

Table 1. Evaluation questions regarding decisions to use the virtual agency.

	n	%
Had no field placement	65	14.74
Had no worksite	53	12.02
It seemed more convenient to use	212	48.07
It seemed easier than gathering my own data	111	25.17

Note. Total N = 441 multiple responses

All evaluations of the 49 Research II courses offered by the School's MSW program in summer 2017, fall 2017, and fall 2018 were obtained. Students in six of the courses did not use the Virtual Agency. We are not clear as to why, that is, whether students chose not to use it or whether instructors did not make it available to them. In all of the other courses, at least some students used the Virtual Agency in order to conduct the program evaluation assignment. All of the responses were anonymous, so no demographic data were available, just the semester the class took place, the campus if OTG, and whether the courses were online or OTG. Mean scores were obtained from each course evaluation. There were 633 responses to the evaluation from the 49 courses, 25 online and 24 OTG. The six courses which had no response to the questions about the Virtual Agency were excluded from further analysis. In fifty percent (50.1%, n = 312) of the courses, the Virtual Agency was used by at least some students. More online students (58.1%) used the Virtual Agency than OTG students (42.5%).

Grand means were obtained for each question and analyzed using Stata 15.1. Because of the high collinearity among navigation, learning, and usefulness, a new variable using these three variables (called "Satisfaction") was created to be used in analysis. Testing revealed a high level of reliability of the scale ($\alpha = .95$).

Results

While the virtual agency (VA) was initially set up to meet the needs of students lacking placements, it was found that field and worksites mainly were of concern to summer students as they did not have them available. For most other students, the main decisions for using the VA were based on expectations of convenience ("It seemed more convenient to use"), followed by ease ("It seemed easier than gathering my own data"). [See Table 1.]

In terms of actual experience, students reported relatively high levels of satisfaction with using the VA in terms of ease of navigation, usefulness, learning, and overall ease of use. The highest mean score was for ease of use. The t-test showed no significant differences in mean scores between OTG and online courses although online students rated the VA slightly higher in terms of ease of navigation, learning, and ease of use. However, there was a low to moderate effect size for usefulness ("The information on the website was useful to my program evaluation assignment"). That is, OTG students found the VA somewhat more useful than the online students ($d = 0.24$). [See Table 2.]

Ordinal logistic regressions were conducted on "Satisfaction" and found that students who perceived the VA as easier to use were much more likely to be satisfied with it. [See Table 3.] One student said, "I thought it was a great alternative to use for the assignment instead of my field placement. It was easy to navigate and the information transferred nicely into SOFA stats." Another stated, "It is way easier to select an agency that has all the information virtually accessible to us because using my own or a classmate's field placement would be way too hard and complicated (unrealistic) to gather the data needed for this project. I felt it would probably be impossible for students (at least for myself and my group), with very little experience in research, to be able to come up with all of that information." While not statistically significant, participants who had no field agency (typically summer students) were less likely to be satisfied with using the virtual agency. Further, students who rated the course more highly were also more satisfied with using the virtual agency This was reflected in the analysis of course ratings, as well.

Ratings for overall quality of the research course ("I rate the overall quality of the course as … " ranged from 1 = poor to 5 = excellent. The mean for quality was 4.13 with an S.D. of 0.37. An ordinal logistic regression on course ratings indicated that while students who were satisfied with use of the VA were over two times more likely to rate it higher, those who perceived it easier to use were less likely to rate the course as highly. [See Table 4.] This outcome may be due to a sense of frustration on the part of some students who did not have an actual agency, as revealed in some of the qualitative statements. One student commented, "While it was easier to use NJ Human Services data, it was less meaningful than if we had done our own papers (not group) with

Table 2. Experience with using the virtual agency.

	OTG	Online			
Measure	M (SD)	M (SD)	t (41)	p	Cohen's d
Easy to navigate	3.27 (0.477)	3.34 (0.38)	−0.53	0.59	−0.17
Useful to my program evaluation assignment	3.36 (0.35)	3.27 (0.43)	0.74	0.46	0.24
Helped me learn	3.21 (0.47)	3.24 (0.47)	−0.24	0.81	−0.08
Easier than collecting my own data	3.37 (0.45)	3.39 (0.47)	−0.13	0.89	−0.04

Table 3. Ordinal logistic regression of factors related to student satisfaction with using the virtual agency.

Predictor	B	SE	p	OR	95% CI
Had no field site to use	−0.26	0.17	0.111	0.77	[.55, 1.06]
The Virtual Agency was easier to use	7.65	1.19	<.001	2093.89	[201.88, 21,718.09]
Student rating of course	1.88	0.81	0.021	6.52	[1.33, 32.00]

Note: CI = Confidence interval for odds ratio (OR)

Table 4. Ordinal logistic regression of factors related to course ratings.

Predictor	B	SE	OR	p	95% CI
Semester					
Fall 2017 (ref.)					
Summer 2017	2.55	1.34	12.82	0.058	[0.92, 179,22]
Fall 2018	1.23	0.67	3.43	0.066	[0.92, 12.81]
Had no field placement	−0.31	0.25	0.73	0.208	[0.45, 1.19]
More convenient to use VA	0.05	0.09	1.05	0.594	[0.88, 1.26]
Easier to use VA	−2.47	1.43	0.08	0.084	[0.01, 1.39]
Satisfaction with using VA	0.97	0.52	2.64	0.067	[0.936, 7.46]

Note: CI = Confidence interval for odds ratio (OR)
VA = Virtual Agency

some actual evaluation data from our field placement." Also, students who took the course in a shortened summer session, and were most likely to need to use the virtual agency to conduct a program evaluation, rated the overall quality of the course much higher than students in the regular fall semesters.

The range for Satisfaction was 6 to 12, with a mean of 9.85 and an S.D. of 1.22, indicating a moderately high level of satisfaction with the use of the VA. This outcome again was reflected in some of the participant statements such as, "The virtual agency has more data than my internship" and "I thought this element of the course was a BRILLIANT way to approach the need for data. I know my girls' placement was not very cooperative with requests like this, so it would have been really frustrating to try and use field-specific data. Loved that resource."

Although the VA was set up to be flexible, students had mixed feelings about this flexibility. Many liked it, with one stating, "There wasn't a lot of information about the programs, which was ok in one way because it allowed us to imagine/create the meat around the intervention". While we wanted to avoid putting too much information on the website for students to parrot, not all students liked this flexibility. One said, "While it was helpful, I wished it contained more information in regards to the agency".

Discussion

A limitation of this study is that we have relatively modest outcome data, although anecdotally instructors who taught the course found no difference in quality of work between students who used the VA and those who did not. Some negative aspects of using a virtual agency are that the availability of data means that students do not have the opportunity to engage in some aspects of research, such as designing a research protocol or data collection instrument, or of actually collecting data in an agency. Not doing the latter may be a deficiency of this option, even if having to work with others in an agency to gather data can be a messy, frustrating job. On the other hand, in having to actually gather data in an agency, students soon learn that the neat, linear approach to research portrayed in textbooks often is unlike the actual work of program evaluation. Some students were aware that collecting data can be a long, difficult process. One commented, "It helped me to focus on running statistics and doing more important, challenging work, rather than spending hours and hours collecting data. Analyzing the data is time consuming and challenging itself". Updates to the VA website may attempt to include ways for students to choose data to use, such as sampling techniques. This plan also speaks to some of the larger limitations of using simulations in social work education, even as they become increasingly popular (Bogo et al., 2014).

Another issue is that not all students have the same level of technological proficiency, and some have difficulty online with their computers or with websites. For example, one social work program used a virtual health center to teach social work students communication skills (Martin, 2017). Evaluation of the approach revealed intense dislike by students in using the virtual site. Martin (2017) concluded, "Main disadvantages of using the virtual health center related to the technology not working properly or being difficult to use, a steep learning curve, and a preference for face-to-face interaction" (p. 204). Some of these difficulties could prospectively be reduced by adequate provision and preparation of students with the relevant technology, good IT support, and means for students to meet virtually.

Among the positive aspects of using a virtual option is that the agency can be designed to be convenient and easy for students to use, requiring a minimal learning curve. The agency website, of course, is always available and can be accessed via the internet from anywhere. Data from agency programs can be downloaded and used with almost any statistical program since the datasets are in Excel spreadsheet format. As there is an abundance of literature on after-school girls' support groups as well as outpatient substance abuse treatment programs, participants will be able to locate articles easily for a literature review as part of their program evaluation papers. Further, students have been very creative in imagining the agency and its treatment approaches. Moreover, the virtual agency is particularly important for social work students who have no access to data from their workplace or from their internship. The virtual agency offers them an opportunity to simulate the conduct of a program evaluation with data based on published research literature.

Using the Virtual Agency for research is a means for students to be able to access data from an agency and use it to frame a program evaluation and make comments about the perceived success or failure of an intervention with clients. It is a positive learning experience for many and a way for them to see how to use agency data to evaluate the effectiveness of a program. Although some may feel that using the VA does not reflect real world settings, use of the VA allows students to develop a set of research skills, including framing evaluation questions, choosing important variables to study, analyzing data, and writing a program evaluation. Despite its limitations, this pedagogical paradigm may add to a growing body of literature on both the potential and constraints of simulation in social work education. Future research should continue to explore this area, as educators increasingly adopt such instructional methods.

Disclosure statement

No potential conflict of interest was reported by the authors.

References

Alahuhta, P., Nordbäck, E., Sivunen, A., & Surakka, T. (2014). Fostering team creativity in virtual worlds. *Journal of Virtual Worlds Research*, *7*(3), 1–22. doi:10.4101/jvwr.v7i3.7062

Bogo, M., Rawlings, M., Katz, E., & Logie, C. (2014). *Using simulation in assessment and teaching: OSCE adapted for social work*. Alexandria, VA: CSWE Press.

Council on Social Work Education. 2015. *Educational policy and accreditation standards for baccalaureate and master's social work programs*. Alexandria, VA: Author. Retrieved from https://www.cswe.org/getattachment/Accreditation/Accreditation-Process/2015-EPAS/2015EPAS_Web_FINAL.pdf.aspx

Dietz, T. J., Westerfelt, A., & Barton, T. R. (2004). Incorporating practice evaluation with the field practicum. *Journal of Baccalaureate Social Work*, *9*(2), 78–90. doi:10.18084/1084-7219.9.2.78

Farley, H. (2018). Using 3D worlds in prison: Driving, learning and escape. *Journal of Virtual Worlds Research*, *11*(1), 1–11. Retrieved from http://jvwresearch.org

Farra, S., Miller, E., Timm, N., & Schafer, J. (2012). Improved training for disasters using 3-D virtual reality simulation. *Western Journal of Nursing Research*, *35*(5), 655–671. doi:10.1177/0193945912471735

Fitch, D., Canda, K., Cary, S., & Freese, R. (2016). Facilitating social work role plays in online courses: The use of video conferencing. *Advances in Social Work*, *17*(1), 78–92. doi:10.18060/20874

Ghanbarzadeh, R., Ghapanchi, A. H., Blumenstein, M., & Talaei-Khoei, A. (2014). A decade of research on the use of three-dimensional virtual worlds in health care: A systematic literature review. *Journal of Medical Internet Research*, *16*(2), e47. doi:10.2196/jmir.3097

Golde, C. (2007). Signature pedagogies in doctoral education: Are they adaptable for the preparation of education researchers? *Educational Researcher*, *36*(6), 344–351. doi:10.3102/0013189X07308301

Gu, N., & Maher, M. L. (2014). *Designing adaptive virtual worlds*. Warsaw/Berlin: De Gruyter Open Ltd.

Human Services of Southern New Jersey, Inc. (2017). Retrieved from http://humanservicesnj.weebly.com

Lee, E. O. (2014). Use of avatars and a virtual community to increase cultural competence. *Journal of Technology in Human Services*, *32*(1/2), 93–107. doi:10.1080/15228835.2013.860364

Levine, L., & Adams, R. H. (2013). Introducing case management to students in a virtual world: An exploratory study. *Journal of Teaching in Social Work*, *33*(4/5), 552–565. doi:10.1080/08841233.2013.835766

Martin, J. (2017). Virtual worlds and social work education. *Australian Social Work*, *70*(2), 197–208. doi:10.1080/0312407X.2016.1238953

Mayer, R. E. (2008). Applying the science of learning: Evidence-based principles for the design of multimedia instruction. *American Psychologist*, *63*(8), 760–769. doi:10.1037/0003-066X.63.8.760

Merchant, Z., Goetz, E. T., Cifuentes, L., Keeney-Kennicutt, W., & Davis, T. J. (2014). Effectiveness of virtual reality-based instruction on students' learning outcomes in K-12 and higher education: A meta-analysis. *Computers & Education*, *70*, 29–40. doi:10.1016/j.compedu.2013.07.033

Moreno, R. (2006a). Does the modality principle hold for different media? A test of the method-affects-learning hypothesis. *Journal of Computer Assisted Learning, 22,* 149–158. doi:10.1111/j.1365-2729.2006.00170.x

Moreno, R. (2006b). Learning in high-tech and multimedia environments. *Current Directions in Psychological Science, 15*(2), 63–67. doi:10.1016/j.compedu.2013.07.033

News Medical Life Sciences. (2012, January 9). NYU medical students use online 3D interactive virtual human body. NYU School of Medicine. Retrieved from https://www.news-medical.net/news/20120109/NYU-medical-students-use-online-3D-interactive-virtual-human-body.aspx?utm_source=TrendMD&utm_medium=cpc&utm_campaign=AZoNetwork_TrendMD_1

Paton-Simpson & Associates. (2009). Statistics open for all (SOFA). [computer software]. Retrieved from http://sofastatistics.com.

Reinsmith-Jones, K., Kibbe, S., Crayton, T., & Campbell, E. (2015). Use of second life in social work education: Virtual world experiences and their effect on students. *Journal of Social Work Education, 51,* 90–108. doi:10.1080/10437797.2015.977167

Rosenberg, M. (1965). *Society and the adolescent self-image.* Princeton, NJ: Princeton University Press.

Shorkey, C. T., & Uebel, M. (2014). History and development of instructional technology and media in social work education. *Journal of Social Work Education, 50,* 247–261. doi:10.1080/10437797.2014.885248

Stanley-Clarke, N., English, A., & Yeung, P. (2018). Cutting the distance in distance education: Reflections on the use of e-technologies in a New Zealand social work program. *Journal of Teaching in Social Work, 38*(2), 137–150. doi:10.1080/08841233.2018.1433739

Sunarich, N., & Rowan, S. (2017). Social work simulation education in the field. *Field Educator, 7.1.* Retrieved from http://fieldeducator.simmons.edu/article/social-work-simulation-education-in-the-field/

Tandy, C., Vernon, R., & Lynch, D. (2017). Teaching note – Teaching student interviewing competencies through second life. *Journal of Social Work Education, 53*(1), 66–71. doi:10.1080/10437797.2016.1198292

Torous, J., O'Connor, R., Franzen, J., Snow, C., Boland, R., & Kitts, R. (2015). Creating a pilot educational psychiatry website: Opportunities, barriers, and next steps. *JMIR Medical Education, 1*(2), e14. doi:10.2196/mededu.4580

Turner, D., Landmann, M., & Kirkland, D. (2019). Making ideas "app"-en: The creation and evolution of a digital mobile resource to teach social work interviewing skills. *Social Work Education,* 1–12. doi:10.1080/02615479.2019.1611758

Wastell, D., Peckover, S., White, S., Broadhurst, K., Hall, C., & Pithouse, A. (2011). Social work in the laboratory: Using microworlds for practice research. *British Journal of Social Work, 41,* 744–760. doi:10.1093/bjsw/bcr014

Williams-Gray, B. (2014). Preparation for social service leadership: Field work and virtual organizations that promote critical thinking in administration practice. *Journal of Teaching in Social Work, 34*(2), 113–128. doi:10.1080/08841233.2014.892050

Wilson, A. B., Brown, S., Wood, Z. B., & Farkas, K. J. (2013). Teaching direct practice skills using web-based simulations: Home visiting in the virtual world. *Journal of Teaching in Social Work, 33*(4–5), 421–437. doi:10.1080/08841233.2013.833578

Part V

Tools for Assessment and Administration

Designing for Quality: Distance Education Rubrics for Online MSW Programs

Melissa B. Littlefield, Karen Rubinstein, and Cynthia Brown Laveist

ABSTRACT
There has been a rapid increase in the number of online MSW programs in the past decade without a commensurate body of literature on their administration. This article acquaints MSW program faculty and administrators with quality assurance rubrics, which are research-informed tools intended for use by distance education providers to develop, support and manage high quality online courses and programs. Graduate programs that are in the process of considering or actually designing an online delivery option, as well as those that are currently implementing online programs, may benefit from the use of such quality assurance rubrics.

During the past decade online MSW programs have proliferated. As of January, 2019, 78 MSW programs were listed on the CSWE website of online and hybrid MSW programs (CSWE, n.d.) versus only seven such MSW Programs listed in 2009 (Vernon, Vakalahi, Pierce, Pittman-Munke, & Frantz-Adkins, 2009). Though there is a long history of implementing brick and mortar courses (and to a lesser extent distance education programs) in social work education (Vernon et al., 2009), fully online MSW programs are a relatively new phenomenon. Nonetheless, it appears that MSW program faculty and administrators increasingly are finding themselves in the position of developing and implementing an online delivery option of their accredited degree programs. Yet, the rapid increase in the number of online programs has not been met with a commensurate amount of social work study of best practices for ensuring quality in their design and implementation. Rather, much of the existing literature on online social work education focuses primarily on delivering course content in an online format, including instructional methods. Considerably less attention has been given to the administration of these programs. While research on best practices for teaching social work online is essential to ensuring quality in social work programs, administrators also need pragmatic advice on planning, implementing, evaluating and continuously improving their programs as the state of the art in both knowledge of "what works" and educational technology improve. For example, as far back as 2005, research regarding online social work education had identified institutional aspects of program delivery that needed development and special attention (Maidment, 2005). Further, Reamer (2013) has raised important and often novel ethical issues around access for diverse students, program quality and integrity, gatekeeping and academic integrity, and privacy and surveillance, all of which require consideration.

Of particular interest to MSW program administrators is ensuring compliance of online MSW programs with CSWE Educational Policy and Accreditation Standards (EPAS). Thus, in addition to best practices for delivering the explicit curriculum online, administrators also need specific guidance for online education that attends to other areas of the EPAS including program mission and goals; the implicit curriculum (i.e, admissions, advisement, retention, termination, and student participation); faculty, administrative structure and resources; and full assessment of both explicit and implicit elements of the curriculum. Moore et al. (2015) addressed many of these areas in their description of the process by which they developed their online MSW program, and they offered lessons learned for those who might follow. While their work provides useful insights, it would appear that online program administrators could benefit from tools that could assist them in identifying and then developing the characteristics of quality online programs that align with CSWE policies for accreditation.

The purpose of this article is to acquaint MSW program faculty and administrators with a category of tools referred to as quality assurance rubrics and scorecards, which are intended for use by distance education providers across disciplines to develop, support and manage high quality online delivery. While not specific to social work education per se, quality assurance rubrics codify the specific aspects of online programs that will need to be developed, including those that pertain to the implicit curriculum, whether delivery will be synchronous, asynchronous, or hybrid. Additionally, quality scorecards may facilitate assessments of risk and return on investment based on the standards outlined in the scorecard(s) an institution adopts.

It should be noted that in the context of program evaluation, quality assurance is concerned with the integrity of program/course inputs, activities, and outputs and is thus congruent with the framework of formative evaluation. Quality assurance is connected to outcome evaluation in that 1) implementation of the standards is expected to achieve the desired program or course outcomes, and 2) quality assurance rubrics often include standards that address the establishment of a process for assessment of the overall course or program.

Quality assurance rubrics and scorecards in distance education

Distance education has long been a fixture of both K-12 and higher education, with the first iterations deploying the common technologies of their times. For example, early distance-based courses were conducted via mail, and even by radio in some countries. With the introduction of the Internet in the 1990s higher education institutions ventured into offering their first online courses. As their number increased, faculty and administrators raised concerns about defining and measuring their quality, and systematically evaluating them to promote continuous improvement over time. In response, faculty, nonprofit organizations, and for-profit Learning Management System (LMS) companies began research to determine the common practices used in successful online programs and to validate standards for quality that would cut across disciplines. Over the past 18 years this research has informed the creation of "quality assurance rubrics" and "scorecards", that is, sets of guidelines intended to encourage the application of consistent standards to program and course design and implementation, and to measure the achievement of the standards against a set of consistent criteria (Institute for Higher Education Policy, 2000; Roblyer & Wiencke (2003); Shattuck, 2015; Shelton, 2010). Early examples include the Quality Matters rubric, the University of California Chico's choice for quality instruction, and the Blackboard™ Exemplary Course Rubric (Shelton, 2010). More recent examples include the Online Learning Consortium (OLC) Quality Scorecard and the University of Central Florida's Teaching Online Preparation Toolkit (TOPkit). At present, there are numerous rubrics created by various institutions to guide program and course design. For example, a Google search at the time this article was written, using the search phrase "quality assurance rubrics online education," yielded "The Open SUNY Course Quality Review", "Quality Online Course Initiative Rubric" developed by the University of Illinois Online Network, and the "Online Course Design and Review Rubric" deployed by New Mexico State University, among others.

A seminal 2000 study published by the Institute for Higher Education Policy Study, titled "Quality on the Line: Benchmarks for Success in Internet Based Distance Education", has heavily influenced the development of quality assurance rubrics over the past decade. The study, funded by Blackboard, Inc., a leading learning management system (LMS) provider, and by the National Education Association, the major union representing educational professionals, consisted of a three-phase process in which quality standards were identified through a comprehensive literature review, followed by the selection of institutions of higher education that were considered to have expertise in online distance education, and subsequent visits to these institutions to determine the extent to which they actually integrated the standards identified in the literature in their programs. The result of the study was promulgation of 24 benchmarks (i.e., standards) considered essential to the quality of internet-based higher education (Institute for Higher Education Policy, 2000). The Blackboard Exemplary Course Rubric previously noted here resulted from this research and publication.

A decade later, Shelton (2010) conducted a Delphi study to develop a scorecard focusing on the administration of online programs. Forty-three expert online administrators participated in six rounds of panels to determine if the original 24 standards identified in the 2000 IHEP study, were still relevant and to expand the standards for program administration. This detailed examination resulted in the creation of a quality scorecard (currently referred to as the Online Learning Consortium Quality Scorecard), which contains 70 standards and a scoring mechanism for administrators to self-assess the sufficiency of their programs. This work was conducted under the auspices of the Sloan Consortium (funded by the Alfred P. Sloan Foundation) which became the Online Learning Consortium in 2014 and is now a member-supported, self-sustaining nonprofit (Online Learning Consortium, 2014).

With funding from the U.S. Department of Education Fund for the Improvement of Postsecondary Education (FIPSE), a group of distance educators in Maryland conducted yet another study from 2003–2006 in order to develop a research informed, replicable, and scalable program to ensure the quality of online programs. The central outcome was the Quality Matters Rubric and peer review process. At the conclusion of the grant period, Quality Matters was established as a nonprofit organization, sustaining itself thereafter through subscriptions and fee-based services (Shattuck, 2015). As of 2019, The Quality Matters community reports having over 1100 institutional members from higher education, K-12 secondary schools, educational publishing, and continuing education and professional development organizations. The Quality Matters Rubric is periodically updated by a panel of experts to incorporate current research and is currently in its 6th edition.

Quality assurance rubrics and scorecards can be understood as tools that facilitate a process of continuous course and program improvement. The concept was born out of the understanding that online distance education requires a different level and type of effort on the part of students and instructors in the teaching and learning endeavor, as well as distinct teaching tools to create the mechanisms and conditions for achieving learning outcomes (Institute for Higher Education Policy, 2000; Roblyer & Wiencke, 2003; Shattuck, 2015; Shelton, 2010). There would appear to be widespread recognition that despite several decades of experience, and the identification of various characteristics associated with effective online education, the state of knowledge is still relatively nascent. Hence, it will require ongoing study to validate the continuing relevance of standards as educational technology and online education instruction evolve. Indeed, Shelton (2010) has asserted that, as the nature of education has changed with the advent of "e-learning" (electronic learning), traditional measures of quality in education, such as "contact hours" and "physical attendance," must be replaced with measures of quality that are more meaningful in the new online learning environment.

Quality rubrics and scorecards typically are either implemented on the institutional or program level, centered on assessing the overall design and administration of online programs, or they are mainly focused on course design. Many institutions use a combination of several rubrics, as suits their needs and budget. Rubrics may be free of charge, under a Creative Commons license, or may be proprietary and require purchase. There is a great deal of content overlap among the proprietary and free rubrics related to course design. Table 1 below lists examples of open license and proprietary rubrics at the institution/program and course levels, that are widely used by online education programs across levels and disciplines. A brief discussion of each follows.

Online learning consortium (OLC) quality scorecard

The Online Learning Consortium (OLC) launched its Quality Scorecard in 2010. The genesis of the Scorecard occurred in 2000 when the Institution for Higher Education Policy (IHEP) conducted a case study, titled "Quality on the Line: Benchmarks for Success in Internet Education." The original IHEP standards later were validated in 2010. The purpose of the OLC Quality Scorecard is to "provide administrators with criteria for excellence in the administration of online programs" (Online Learning Consortium, 2019, para. 1).

The OLC Scorecard contains broad quality standards that may be applied to either large or small-scale online programs. Each of the following standards then is divided into several specific indicators. In total, there are 75 specific review standards subsumed under the nine following categories: Institutional Support, Technology Support, Course Development/ Instructional Design, Course Structure, Teaching and Learning, Social and Student Engagement, Faculty Support, Student Support, and Evaluation and Assessment.

Table 1. Proprietary and open license rubrics.

	Proprietary	Creative Commons Open License
Institutional/Programmatic	OLC Quality Scorecard	UCF-TOPkit
Course-Level	Quality Matters	Blackboard Exemplary Course Rubric

The strength of this scorecard is in the breadth and depth of its standards, which focus on every aspect of creating, managing and assessing an online program. The Scorecard's very specific standards allow administrators to examine policy and procedures at a high level, as well as to dive into the minutiae of course instructional design and delivery. It also includes criteria that allow administrators to examine "non-academic" standards around faculty support, student support, technology and security concerns, as well as faculty development. Finally, the "Evaluation and Assessment" standards focus not only on the existence of mechanisms for assessment and improvement but on plans for the online program as a whole. The OLC Scorecard is a tool that may also be implemented in planning for an online program as it identifies the necessary building blocks that are foundational to program success. Further, it enables administrators of existing programs to evaluate program strengths and opportunities for improvement. Each standard is scored on a scale of "Deficient", "Developing", "Accomplished" or "Exemplary." The Quality Scorecard rubric is intended for internal university use; OLC does not offer any form of public "credentialing" or peer review recognition for programs and courses developed using its rubric. The OLC Scorecard is available to institutions that subscribe to the nonprofit Online Learning Consortium and therefore is not a "free" or openly licensed rubric. OLC offers valuable professional development, yearly conferences, and services for both faculty and administrators.

TOPkit

The University of Central Florida's Teaching Online Preparation Toolkit (TOPkit) provides an extensive resource for preparing and maintaining online programs. The material on their TOPkit site is free and open for use by any college or university. UCF provides very useful resources, as well as an open Community of Practice. Users may share, copy and remix TOPkit resources for non-commercial purposes, as long as they properly attribute; and, if sharing or remixing, they use the same licensure.

TOPkit provides resources for planning, developing and evaluating online programs, including an interactive faculty development decision guide. On the programmatic level, the "Developing" section of TOPkit contains rubrics and checklists that may be used to plan and create new online programs. For example, the site contains Duke University's planning guide for online learning. While this document is not a rubric, it is a practical checklist that begins with programmatic-level concerns (starting with a Needs Analysis), and continues with checklists for course design and implementation. Finally, the document includes a section for adding online activities to a traditional course, and a detailed course design timeline based on the ADDIE instructional design model (2019, https://learninginnovation.duke.edu/pdf/onlinelearningguidecombined.pdf).

The benefit of using TOPkit is in its extensive supply of practical resources and its provision of an active Community of Practice. Institutions on a tight budget will find that the resources throughout TOPkit will provide sufficient information and guidance needed to put together a solid plan for creating and evaluating an online program. "The artifacts may be used in a variety of contexts such as self-assessment, instructional designer review, peer review, institutional online program effectiveness, and accreditation standards" (Bauer & Barrett-Greenly, n.d., para 2, retrieved from https://topkit.org/developing/checklists-rubrics/).

Quality matters rubric

The Quality Matters (QM) Rubric focuses solely on course design and does not consider broader "programmatic" or "institution-wide" standards, such as technology assistance, faculty development, or learner support outside of the course. Like OLC's Quality Scorecard, the Quality Matters rubric has its roots in serious research on best practices in online course design. Quality Matters began as part of the nonprofit organization, Maryland Online; however, it has since spun off to become a nonprofit organization itself. Quality Matters offers an exemplary rubric for curriculum design, as well as a system of course review. Courses that meet the QM rubric standards, and have passed through its review process, receive a widely recognized quality "seal" that may be publicly displayed. Quality Matters has a respected rubric for Higher Education and Continuing Studies courses (Maryland Online, 2016/2018a).

The QM Rubric focuses on quality online course development. There are eight general course design standards, each divided into several substandards, as well as 42 review standards which are rated on a scale of up to three points. Courses that achieve all of the mandatory "3-point" essential standards, along with an overall score of at least 85, are considered to have met QM quality course criteria (Maryland Online, 2016/2018b). The following are the eight General Standards on the QM rubric: Course Overview and Introduction, Learning Objectives (Competencies), Assessment and Measurement, Instructional Materials, Learning Activities and Learner Interaction, Course Technology, Learner Support, and Accessibility and Usability (Maryland Online, 2016/2018a).

Quality Matters developed an extensive, five stage, "Course Review Process" to accompany its rubric. This process allows institutions to conduct course reviews and quality benchmarking as an incremental process, allowing them to move from the first phase, "awareness of the QM Rubric," to establishing a peer review system that mirrors a "Full QM review," to the final stage of "Institutional Change." Quality Matters describes this final phase as, " … the organization has developed appropriate policies that extend the QM model into other key areas of teaching and learning – with QM Program Review, for example – and has committed resources to sustain and grow their quality assurance process" (Maryland Online, 2016/2018c, para. 7).

The benefit of using Quality Matters is that the rubric and review processes constitute internationally recognized standards of quality. For those who take advantage of QM professional development workshops, the rubric will be accompanied by detailed annotations that provide specific examples of how to meet each of the standards. The official "Full QM review" is fee for service; however, if they wish, universities can rely on using their own peer review process, as they move through the five phases of QM's "Course Review Process." Together, the rubric and review process create a robust system for creating and continuously improving online courses.

The QM rubric ideally should be adopted at the inception of an online program, since this will ensure course quality from the start. However, it may also be applied to evaluate and improve existing courses. Programs can move through "Course Review" at their own pace, and with their preferred level of support from Quality Matters.

Blackboard exemplary course program rubric

The Blackboard (Bb) Exemplary Course Program (ECP) Rubric is associated with Bb's Exemplary Course Program and is available for free on a Creates Commons Attribute 3 license. Institutions can freely use and repurpose all or parts of this rubric, as needed, as long as it is for non-commercial purposes. However, if an institution wants a course to receive "certified recognition" as an "Exemplary Course," it must be a member of the "Blackboard Community." Such certification is available for those institutions using the Blackboard or Moodle LMS. (Blackboard, Inc., n.d.).

As with Quality Matters, the ECP Rubric focuses solely on course design standards. Blackboard specifies that the "Rubric is reviewed and updated annually by clients and Blackboard experts who survey the current literature and base changes on the evolving field of best practices" (Woods, 2017, December 17, para. 2). Specifically, the standards fall into the four following categories, each with its own set of sub-standards:

(1) Course Design
(2) Interaction and Collaboration
(3) Assessment
(4) Learner Support

Review standards are weighted on a numerical scale of Exemplary (5–6 points), Accomplished (3–4 points), Promising (2 points), Incomplete (1 point), Not Evident (0 points).

The ECP Rubric standards match those of Quality Matters. Interestingly, the former contains student feedback standards not included in the QM rubric. For example, in the Learner Support category, a standard states that students can participate anonymously in course evaluation and that learners can give feedback to the instructor both during and after course delivery.

The benefit of the ECP rubric is that it is free for any institution to adopt, even if it is not a client of Blackboard. The rubric itself includes all of the same standards as with QM, as well as additional ones. The standards are written in a very detailed, yet concise, fashion; therefore, no additional annotations are needed to understand if a standard is met. Each of the five point range criteria clearly delineates what should be present in the course. The ECP rubric is an excellent choice for schools whose budget is very limited, and which need to implement a quality course design and review program.

As with QM, the ECP rubric is ideally adopted at the inception of course design; however, it also makes an excellent resource for improving existing courses If an institution is a Blackboard or Moodle client, it can join the Blackboard Community and take advantage of a range of free workshops and webinars on course design and delivery, and can also participate in the Exemplary Course Program. Blackboard also offers a fee-based consulting service for online courses. A copy of the ECP rubric may be found at https:// community.blackboard.com/docs/DOC-3505-blackboard-exemplary-course-program-rubric.

Quality assurance scorecards and the 2015 CSWE educational policy and accreditation standards

The EPAS broadly lay out the accreditation requirements for graduate programs; however, it may not be apparent to MSW administrators that which is necessary to implement these elements in an online context. Quality scorecards (including the OLC Scorecard and Quality Matters Course Rubric) align with aspects of CSWE Educational Policy and offer additional standards for assuring quality online programs. Thus, quality scorecards can serve as valuable supplements to the CSWE EPAS for online MSW administrators as they navigate development and implementation of their programs. Moreover, these administrators may have varying levels and types of support from their institutions in structuring and implementing their online programs. Therefore, a quality assurance rubric, such as OLC Quality Scorecard – which provides a comprehensive framework that specifies program and institutional level needs for quality distance education – can be an invaluable tool for assessing existing resources and processes that are available to support online MSW program options. Additionally, it can help determine those that need to be developed, including campus resources that may be called upon to support the online delivery option. Further, quality assurance rubrics can help programs plan for allocating resources for specific distance education needs and point to gaps in infrastructure, policies and processes at program and institutional levels. For example, which distance education supports can be assumed at the institutional level, versus which ones will need to be picked up by the program? For the purpose of further discussion we now will focus on the two rubrics adopted by the institution at which the authors of this article are employed. They are the "Online Learning Consortium Quality Scorecard for the Administration of Online Courses", which is an example of an institutional level scorecard, and the "Quality Matters Rubric", a course level illustration. These are both proprietary measures available as a benefit of the University's paid membership in the nonprofit organizations which developed them. The following section discusses how selected standards of the OLC Scorecard and Quality Matters Course Rubric align with CSWE Educational Policy.

Explicit curriculum – educational policy 1

Educational Policy 1 asserts that, in addition to addressing the purpose and espousing the values of the profession, an MSW program's mission and goals must be informed by program context. In particular, context is concerned with the needs and opportunities of the setting and program options (CSWE, 2015). The Institution-level OLC Scorecard directs MSW program administrators to consider how the benefits of online learning are related to the mission and goals of the university, school or department in which the program is situated. Its standards in the "institutional" category address issues around mission as well as strategic value and goals as MSW program administrators consider whether to offer an online delivery option. This naturally plays out in how an MSW program specifically crafts its online delivery option, including how much of the program will be offered online (e.g. will it be hybrid or fully online), and may also include considerations of which areas of specialized social work practice will be offered in an online program, if the online delivery option will only be available in specific geographic regions. For example, a strategic goal of our university and MSW department is to increase student enrollment. Further, our department mission is to prepare social workers for practice with urban African Americans. At the time of our online graduate program launch, there were no Historically Black Colleges and Universities (HBCU) offering an online MSW program. Therefore, our decision to initiate one was consistent with both our mission and strategic goals.

OLC "institutional" standards related to the program mission and goals also have implications for ethical issues raised by Frederic Reamer (2013). For example, if a program's mission and goals focus on social work for special populations, then it must be explicit about how the online program option will address inclusivity, and the needs of diverse students, consistent with its mission and goals of access for these student populations as well.

Explicit curriculum – educational policy 2

The explicit curriculum is the program's formal educational structure including the courses and field education deployed for each program option and may include forms of technology as a component of the curriculum. The present 2015 EPAS reasserts the shift (initiated with the 2008 EPAS) from curriculum design based on *what to teach* to a focus on learning outcomes (i.e., the competencies students must achieve). It specifies that programs use a curriculum design that begins with outcomes, expressed as competencies, and their component behaviors, and then design a learning experience that provides students with opportunities to demonstrate their achievement of these competencies. In keeping with this framework, assessment of student learning outcomes becomes crucial to providing evidence that programs are achieving their stated goals. (CSWE, 2015).

Quality scorecards offer a set of standards that provide a systematic approach and process by which programs can achieve a competency based curriculum design to comply with the current CSWE EPAS.

Essentially, quality scorecards take the approach that student learning outcomes (in the case of social work education, competencies as evidenced by behaviors and dimensions) drive the configuration of explicit curriculum content into courses, which have specific stated objectives derived from the competencies. This is congruent with expectations of the CSWE EPAS which stipulates that programs must operationalize the nine core competencies as behaviors and dimensions, which in turn will represent student learning outcomes. Programs then craft learning experiences designed to achieve the competencies through their explicit curriculum. The Quality Matters™ course rubric extends the conceptualization of Educational Policy 2.0, asserting that the key consideration in selecting course materials, learning activities, instructional technologies, and methods of assessment is their alignment with the course objectives. Further, quality scorecards emphasize that curriculum developers think through how to address social and environmental aspects of courses and include faculty presence as well as interaction and engagement among instructors and students, as these elements also are important to the acquisition of social work knowledge, attitudes, skills and cognitive processes, and the promotion of motivation and retention. Finally, assessment methods deployed should be designed so that students may demonstrate the specific dimensions of the given course competencies (i.e., knowledge, value, skill and cognitive process) expressed in the course objectives. The alignment of program and course objectives with the content and delivery of the learning experience, and the assessment of student learning outcomes, represents principles of sound instructional design that, while not unique to online programs and courses, certainly must undergird quality online and distance programs.

As is with the case with the EPAS, quality assurance scorecards and rubrics that focus on course development do not specify the methods by which their standards are to be achieved. Rather, they specify the components of solid online course design. This operational flexibility allows for programs with various missions and operating in differing contexts to meet their program goals and objectives. However, the OLC scorecard does include the standard that student-centered methods of instruction always be considered during the course development process.

Another limitation is that they do not provide specific standards or guidance to encourage diversity and inclusivity or to disrupt social and environmental dynamics that perpetuate mechanisms of oppression (such as silencing of people of color and women in discussion forums and group assignments). The exception is compliance with the Americans with Disabilities Act. QM's Standard 8, titled "Accessibility and Usability," focuses on designing physical and experiential aspects of the course that will accommodate differently abled students and faculty.

With regard to cultural competence and intersectionality, social work educators have used online discussion boards effectively to achieve EPAS expectations related to diversity (Bertera & Littlefield, 2003; Littlefield & Bertera, 2005). Moreover, Littlefield and Roberson (2005) have designed computer-mediated feminist learning experiences to support women's epistemological development in a social work course.

Implicit curriculum – educational policy 3

The implicit curriculum consists of the learning environment in which the explicit curriculum is carried out. It refers to a program's commitment to diversity, its student development policies and procedures, its faculty, and its administrative and governance structure. There is an emphasis on fairness and transparency in such policies and their implementation as well as adequate and fairly distributed resources. Moreover, the program's educational culture should reflect the mission, goals and context of the program and the values of the profession (CSWE, 2015).

In the experiences of the authors of this article, ensuring that student support services offered to on-campus students are also made available to online students requires intensive coordination and development efforts with other university offices. Online program administrators may find it useful to have the authority of an evidenced-based rubric, such as the OLC Scorecard, to advocate for parity in the provision of student support for online students.

The OLC Scorecard provides a great deal in the way of addressing the implicit curriculum for an online setting. Issues of diversity, in terms of providing a supportive and inclusive learning environment, specifically are addressed in its Course Development and Instructional Design standards including using "Web Content Accessibility Guidelines" for course content to accommodate persons with disabilities. Further, Course Structure standards call for alternate instructional strategies and special institutional resources for students with disabilities, and Student Support standards state that policies, procedures and resources are to be put in place for them. (Implementation of these diversity standards typically would require coordination with the university's office of student disability support services.) The OLC Scorecard, however, does not specifically address diverse identities other than persons with disabilities.

OLC Scorecard Student Support standards provide very specific direction around the type of information and support students need prior to and during their participation in an online educational program. These standards direct programs to assist students in determining whether they possess the self-motivation, commitment to online learning, and technological skills to perform effectively in an online format prior to admission. Online students are to have access to training and technical assistance to permit them to participate effectively in the program and to have equal access to academic, career and personal counseling, and non-instructional support services such as financial aid and registration. Additionally, standards indicate that students are to have opportunities to engage in an online community outside of courses and that efforts be made to minimize their isolation.

OLC Scorecard standards for Faculty Support stress that faculty should receive technical support in developing their courses and support in teaching online. With regard to administration and governance, OLC "Institutional" standards emphasize that institutions have governance and decision making structures and processes and adequate financial resources to support online program offerings as a strategic initiative in achieving the mission and goals of the institution. The scorecard also includes a standard that faculty should be involved in the development or decision-making around curriculum choices. However, it does not speak to issues regarding faculty participation in hiring and tenure policy of program personnel.

Assessment – educational policy 4

Assessment refers to the systematic gathering of data through multi-dimensional methods regarding student learning outcomes vis a vis social work competencies and collecting data about the implicit curriculum from program stakeholders. Programs develop an assessment plan in which designated faculty and field personnel assess competencies. The program reports outcomes and engages in a process of continuous program improvement based upon the findings of its assessment.

OLC Scorecard standards lay out a comprehensive set of program issues in the implicit curriculum to measure and monitor for continuous program improvement. These include student support services, recruitment and retention, compliance with accessibility standards, assessment of effectiveness of instruction, and stakeholder satisfaction. In addition, student learning outcomes at the course and program levels are to be reviewed regularly for continuous program improvement.

Conclusions and implications

The ideal design and implementation structure for online programs is holistic and one supported by the institution. It will include instructional design, faculty professional development, student support and program resources. In reality, however, the types and level of institutional support for online programs within a university will vary. Further, MSW program administrators will likely need to coordinate with various university offices to bring to bear the institutional resources requisite to support the online option.

Upon considering the adoption of any quality assurance rubrics, program administrators must weigh the scope and detail of each. Current and future goals, and the present state of their online program, should be considered in order to determine which rubric will best suit the institutional and program needs. A combination of tools is always an option.

It also bears noting that quality assurance scorecards and rubrics focus on the ideal. Programs must consider their staffing, institutional politics and present structures in order to determine if the standards of the rubric may ultimately be realistically achieved. That being said, the use of a recognized, research-based rubric may provide the external clout needed to make structural and attitudinal changes necessary to implement a program innovation.

Finally, this article has focused on online MSW programs, as that is the purview of the authors. However, online quality assurance rubrics are used across educational levels, from K-12 to higher education to continuing education. Moreover, there is significant overlap in CSWE accreditation standards for bachelors and masters programs and thus it stands to reason that much of the discussion in this paper would likely apply readily to bachelors and doctoral programs in social work, as well.

Disclosure statement

No potential conflict of interest was reported by the authors.

References

Bauer & Barrett-Greenly. (n.d.) *Checklists and rubrics, para 2*. Retrieved from https://topkit. org/developing/checklists-rubrics/

Bertera, E., & Littlefield, M. (2003). Evaluation of electronic discussion forums in social work diversity education: A comparison of anonymous and identified participation. *Journal of Technology in Human Services, 21*(4), 53–72. doi:10.1300/J017v21n04_04

Blackboard, Inc. (n.d.) *Exemplary course program*. Retrieved from https://community.black board.com/community/ecp/pages/program-volunteer-reviewer-information

CSWE. (2015). *Educational policy and accreditation standards educational policy and accreditation standards for baccalaureate and master's social work programs*. Retrieved from https://www.cswe.org/Accreditation/Standards-and-Policies/2015-EPAS

CSWE. (n.d.) *Online and distance education offerings by accredited programs*. Retrieved from https://cswe.org/Accreditation/Directory-of-Accredited-Programs/Online-and-Distance-Education

Institute for Higher Education Policy. (2000). *Quality on the line: Benchmarks for success in internet-based distance education*. Retrieved from http://www.ihep.org/sites/default/files/uploads/docs/pubs/qualityontheline.pdf

Littlefield, M. B., & Bertera, E. M. (2005). A discourse analysis of online dialogs in social work diversity courses: Topical themes, depth and tone. *Journal of Teaching in Social Work, 24* (3/4), 131–146. doi:10.1300/J067v24n03_09

Littlefield, M. B., & Roberson, K. C. (2005). Computer Technology for the Feminist Classroom. *Affilia, 20*(2), 186–202. doi:10.1177/0886109905274676

Maidment, J. (2005). Teaching social work online: Dilemmas and debates. *Social Work Education: The International Journal, 24*(2), 184–195. doi:10.1080/0261547052000333126

Maryland Online. (2016/2018a). *Why QM?* Retrieved from https://www.qualitymatters.org/why-quality-matters/

Maryland Online. (2016/2018b). *Course design rubric standards*. Retrieved from https://www.qualitymatters.org/qa-resources/rubric-standards/higher-ed-rubric

Maryland Online. (2016/2018c). *Why QM? Process*. Retrieved from https://www.qualitymatters.org/why-quality-matters/process

Moore, S. E., Golder, S., Sterrett, E., Faul, A. C., Yankeelov, P., Weathers Mathis, L., & Barbee, A. P. (2015). Social work online education: A model for getting started and staying connected. *Journal of Social Work Education, 51*, 508–518. doi:10.1080/10437797.2015.1043200

Online Learning Consortium. (2014, July 7). *The sloan consortium changes name to 'online learning consortium'* [Press Release] Retrieved from https://onlinelearningconsortium.org/consult/olc-quality-scorecard-history/

Online Learning Consortium. (2019). *OLC quality scorecard suite: A mandate for quality, para. 2*. Retrieved from https://onlinelearningconsortium.org/consult/olc-quality-scorecard-history/

Reamer, F. (2013). Distance and online social work education: Novel ethical challenges. *Journal of Teaching in Social Work, 43*(4/5), 369–384. doi:10.1080/08841233.2013.828669

Roblyer, M. D., & Wiencke, W. R. (2003). Design and use of a rubric to assess and encourage interactive qualities in distance courses. *The American Journal of Distance Education, 17* (2), 77–98. doi:10.1207/S15389286AJDE1702_2

Shattuck, K. (2015). Focusing research on quality matters. *American Journal of Distance Education, 29*(3), 155–158. doi:10.1080/08923647.2015.1061809

Shelton, K. (2010). A quality scorecard for the administration of online education programs. *Online Learning, 14*(4). doi:10.24059/olj.v14i4.163

Vernon, R., Vakalahi, H., Pierce, D., Pittman-Munke, D., & Frantz-Adkins, L. (2009). Distance education programs in social work. Emerging trends. *Journal of Social Work Education, 45*(2), 263–276. doi:10.5175/JSWE.2009.200700081

Woods, D. (2017, December 17). About the exemplary course program. [Blog post]. Retrieved from https://community.blackboard.com/community/ecp/blog/2017/12/27/about-the-exemplary-course-program

Developing and Supporting Faculty Training for Online Social Work Education: The Columbia University School of Social Work Online Pedagogy Institute

Johanna Creswell Báez, Matthea Marquart, Rebecca Yae-Eun Chung, Delia Ryan, and Kristin Garay

ABSTRACT

With the growth of online and distance education in social work, faculty training and support need to be provided to ensure high-quality online social work education. A model for training social work educators in online teaching is outlined that focuses on pedagogy, technology, and social work values. Columbia University School of Social Work's Online Campus provides a five-week Institute on Pedagogy and Technology for Online Courses for prospective social work instructors. The Institute provides a faculty training model that can be adopted in other social work programs, and seeks to model best practices in online education.

With the rapid growth of online social work education, faculty training and support have become critical. The landscape has shifted from two decades ago when social workers were described as not "high tech" by nature (Gingerich & Green, 1996) now to social workers creating standards for technology in social work education and practice (Beaulaurier & Haffey, 2005; Hitchcock, Sage, & Smyth, 2018; NASW, 2017). Lack of training often has been cited as a reason for social workers being slow to adopt technology, along with social work's historical commitment to face-to-face communication (Berzin, Singer, & Chan, 2015). With the widespread adoption of online programming (CSWE, 2017), social work schools curently need to consider how they are training the next generation of instructors to ensure high-quality online social work education (Levin, Fulginiti, & Moore, 2018). This article provides a tested model for training social work educators in online teaching, with a focus on pedagogy, technology, and social work values.

Background on the Columbia University online campus

Columbia University's School of Social Work (CSSW) dates back to 1898 and is one of the largest and oldest social work programs in the United States, with a rich history of educating generations of social workers (Feldman & Kamerman, 2001). CSSW has continually invested in advancing the profession of social work, including now being at the forefront of online social work education. CSSW launched the Online Campus in 2015, providing access to the Master of Science in Social Work (MSW) program to students around the United States, and it is the only one of the top three schools of social work (U.S. News & World Report, 2019) presently to offer a fully online MSW degree program.

CSSW's model for online education primarily entails synchronous courses, with weekly live online class sessions in the web conferencing platform Adobe Connect, along with weekly asynchronous homework in the learning management system (LMS) Canvas. In order to support online instructors and enable them to focus on teaching, the CSSW online model notably includes three professionals on each instructional team all of whom have an MSW, at minimum: the Instructor, the Associate, and the Live Support Specialist. The Instructor is responsible for designing and teaching the course; the Associate offers academic support in a manner similar to a teaching assistant; and the Live Support Specialist provides technical support for live class sessions in a manner similar to a virtual event producer. This model supports high quality courses and receives positive feedback from students (Marquart & Fleming, 2014; Marquart, Fleming, Rosenthal, & Hibbert, 2016). Currently, CSSW's Online Campus has about 65 Instructors, 90 Associates, and 40 Live Support Specialists providing an average of 100 online classes per year.

As recently as 2015, online education was new to CSSW. From its initiation, the School's Online Campus needed to support instructors in offering the same level of high quality education as on-campus MSW students were receiving. This article outlines the development and current initiative to train social work professionals to become educators for CSSW's Online Campus. The five-week *Institute on Pedagogy and Technology for Online Courses* (Online Pedagogy Institute) provides a prospective training model for online social work educators that can be readily adapted and adopted in other social work programs and was recognized with a 2018 International E-Learning Award (IELA, 2018) and a 2019 United States Distance Learning Association Excellence in Non-Profit Teaching/Training Award (USDLA, 2019).

Faculty development and online social work education

In a comparative analysis of distance education standards, faculty support was one of the six key standards identified as a best practice in online education (Southard & Mooney, 2015). In online education, there are two clear research findings pertaining to such faculty support: (1) effective training influences the quality of the instruction, and (2) online instructional teams need thorough and continued support (Brinkley-Etzkorn, 2018). Higher education institutions are in fact training faculty, but the training activities vary, with the popular format being a one-time, face-to-face workshop and the common training activity being the design of an online course (Meyer & Murrell, 2014). Centers for teaching and learning usually provide this support by retaining instructional design experts (Schwartz & Haynie, 2013); in addition, online resource centers exist, such as the Online Learning Consortium (https://onlinelearningconsortium.org), a collaborative community of higher education leaders dedicated to advancing digital teaching and learning. However, research clearly shows that institutions need to place greater importance on effective faculty development programs along with incentives to support high quality online education (Herman, 2012).

The adoption of distance education requires institutional support and resources, leadership, faculty engagement, and pedagogical clarity in order to uphold social work values and practices (East, LaMendola, & Alter, 2014). Recent studies have identified a clear need and gap in social work programs with regard to developing training for social work educators in online teaching, including enhancement of their comfort and proficiency with technology (Levin et al., 2018). Further, Knowles' (2007) research on implementing online social work education pointed to the importance of the "transformation" (p.20) that instructors must make to provide online instruction, such as moving toward a collaborative teaching model and becoming proficient in technology and "faculty engagement" that will support both a dialog on online pedagogy and an investment in faculty development (Dawson & Fenster, 2015). In preparing future social work instructional teams, both pedagogy and instructional design need to be included in the training in tandem with an integration of the research and theory of instructional technology, cognitive science, and adult education (Reeves & Reeves, 2008).

Online social work pedagogy

In recent years, there has been a growing body of knowledge regarding best practices in online social work education (Beaulaurier & Haffey, 2005; Hitchcock, Sage, & Smyth, 2019; Kurzman & Maiden, 2014). Social work has embraced the pedagogical consensus that online education is a constructivist approach, which includes collaborative learning, reflection, dialog, and the promotion of community (Mayes, 2001). Social work scholars have identified the following best practices for online instruction: the importance of building community and interpersonal relationships between the instructor and students and among students (Secret, Bentley, & Kadolph, 2016); the promotion of small-group mutual aid learning communities where students can learn from each other (Douville, 2013); a focus on social presence and authentic connection with students to support communication (Bentley, Secret, & Cummings, 2015; Rapp-McCall & Anyikwa, 2016); the effective engagement of students, including using a range of technology tools such as webinars, videos, online discussion boards, wikis, blogs, and virtual tools (Farrel et al., 2018; Hibbert, Kerr, Garber, & Marquart, 2016; Levin, Whitsett, & Wood, 2013); promotion of instructor immediacy which requires frequent and purposeful interactions with students to support interactivity (Marquart et al., 2016); and, the use of Universal Design for Learning principles to support accessibility and social justice (Gibson, 2016). Further, social work scholars also have outlined the benefits of building their own learning community to support professional development and continued learning (Hitchcock, 2015; Schwartz, Wiley, & Kaplan, 2016).

Methods to support faculty: the online pedagogy institute

The five-week *Institute on Pedagogy and Technology for Online Courses* evolved at Columbia over the course of several years to address the need to train social work professionals for online teaching. The main objectives of the Institute are to build online instructional skills and confidence in teaching, to learn how to plan engaging live online synchronous classes, to practice how to set up and manage asynchronous homework, and to uphold social work values throughout the content and the engagement with students. [See Figure 1.] Since the summer of 2017, the Institute has graduated four cohorts, representing a total of 152 social work professionals from 31 different states.

The Institute was first developed by Matthea Marquart, MSSW, Director of Administration for the Online Campus at CSSW, and in years 2 and 3, Delia Ryan, LMSW, Live Support Specialist, partnered with Marquart on Institute updates and leadership. The Institute model was influenced by looking at how companies were recruiting and then training employees in their respective fields, such as tax preparation firms that provide free classes and then recruit top students for open positions. This is an approach also adopted recently by Google (Google, 2018), and provides a win-win for the students, receiving valuable free training, and the companies, creating skilled potential employees. Implementation of the Institute was also instructor-driven, with new participants teaching CSSW's pilot online courses openly asking for more support in learning how to teach online, and requesting additional training in online pedagogy. To address these emerging needs, the Institute now includes a complex integration of best practices in learning pedagogy and building skills along with online education technology (Koehler & Mishra, 2005).

The Institute provides opportunities for social work professionals not only to learn best practices in online teaching, but also to develop empathy for what it is like to be a student in an online course. For some participants, the student experience can be a distant memory, and many social work professionals do not have online student experience themselves because distance

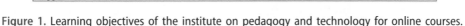

Learning Objectives: Institute on Pedagogy and Technology for Online Courses
1. Plan interactive live online class sessions in the Adobe Connect web conferencing platform, implementing best practices in online pedagogy to successfully engage all students
2. Practice using tools and features in the Canvas learning management system such as assignments, discussion forums, quizzes, and announcements to facilitate learning
3. Recognize that online education benefits from a collaborative approach, and describe the roles and responsibilities for the online Instructor, Associate/TA, and Live Support Specialist at Columbia University School of Social Work (CSSW)
4. Meet web conferencing technology and quality standards required by CSSW's online campus
5. Establish an environment that is welcoming and reflective of social work values, and recognize the importance of tone in communication with students and colleagues
6. Practice new instructional techniques and identify ways to adapt and apply these techniques in the online learning environment
7. Identify ways to motivate students to engage with course material
8. Practice critically reflective teaching
9. Practice using the following educational technology tools as a student: Proctorio for proctoring online quizzes and exams, Quizlet for practicing with digital flashcards, PlayPosit for embedding questions into videos, and BigBlueButton for recording virtual presentations
10. Describe ways to build community and encourage collaboration among participants through discussion during and outside of live class sessions
11. Identify CSSW policies and procedures, including when to contact the appropriate administrative departments as needed and when to contact various options for technical support

Figure 1. Learning objectives of the institute on pedagogy and technology for online courses.

education in social work is a new and emerging trend (Vernon, Vakalahi, Pierce, Pittman-Munke, & Adkins, 2009). The Institute structure mirrors CSSW's online courses, so that instructors have a very realistic student exposure and can quickly come to understand the student side of the online experience. Indeed, the same technology is used for the Institute training as in CSSW's online courses, which helps provide a realistic and relevant program experience for participants.

The model

The Institute is an intensive blend of weekly two-hour live online class sessions in Adobe Connect, taught by an experienced social work online educator, and about three hours of homework each week in Canvas. It is offered twice a year, and the application is open to any master's or doctorate level social work professional that is interested in online social work education. It attracts enough applications that there always is a waiting list. It is a prerequisite for all new online Instructors and Associates to complete the Institute offering before applying to teach with CSSW's Online Campus. The Institute therefore has provided a clear way to recruit, screen, and hire qualified online Instructors and Associates.

The five-week Institute is designed to be both highly engaging and rigorous, with homework that includes relevant readings in online social work education and pedagogy, realistic scenarios, reflection journals, quizzes, small-group and whole-class discussion forums, practice with the LMS tools, and flashcards to reinforce learning. The Institute's weekly live virtual class sessions and discussion forums build a sense of community and enable those enrolled to share their thoughts and expertise. Participants also learn how to establish a virtual classroom environment that is welcoming, and reflective of social work values, and to plan interactive and engaging lessons (for an Adobe Connect virtual classroom) using web conferencing tools.

During the online class sessions, participants practice with actual web conferencing tools, including polls, status icons, webcam, microphone, chat, and breakout groups. The online classes include guest speakers who are experienced online Associates, Instructors, Live Support Specialists, and alumni of the CSSW Online Campus. Further, the Instructor, Associate, and Live Support Specialist roles are modeled for participants, providing a framework for them to develop their own online teaching skills and style. The homework assignments include engaging in critical reflection regarding online education, exploring how to motivate adult learners, and deploying technology to meet instructional goals. Participants learn the basics of using the LMS (Canvas) to create assignments, grade students, and provide feedback. All homework and class participation are graded using rubrics, and an overall grade of 90% is the minimum requirement for graduating from the Institute.

Social justice, diversity, and inclusion themes are interwoven throughout the Institute's curriculum. Social work values require a discussion of the Universal Design for Learning to support accessibility for all learners (Lightfoot & Gibson, 2005; Reeves & Reeves, 2008), and of current events, including those impacting social justice (Adams & Bell, 2016). The Institute includes a focus on teaching and modeling inclusive pedagogy that will support students with diverse backgrounds and needs.

The Institute also seeks to support academic freedom and responsibility for instructional teams by teaching the skills needed to set up and edit assignments in the LMS, as well as create interactive lessons for live class sessions. The curriculum thereby empowers instructional teams to create unique course sections that match their expertise and will ignite their passion for teaching and learning online. Further, the Institute is organized to support self-directed learning; for example, participants can work ahead, at their own pace, to complete their homework by the deadlines. Graduates receive a letter of completion and a digital badge, which can be shared on social media, and includes a printable certificate. Finally, those who are hired with CSSW's Online Campus are provided an array of continuous learning opportunities and support to keep them connected with their Institute colleagues, engage them with the broader Online Campus community, and build upon the knowledge gained during their participation in the Institute. [See Figure 2.]

Quantitative and qualitative findings to date

A feedback survey was deployed, immediately upon completing the training program, as a required final assignment. Qualitative data were recovered in the initial summer 2017 Institute (n = 31). Then numerical scale feedback was collected, in addition to qualitative feedback, for the following Institutes in fall 2017, summer 2018, and fall 2018 (n = 121). The Institute has enjoyed high ratings on these feedback surveys. When asked, "On a scale of one to ten, how would you rate the overall quality of this Institute?" the mean score from the past three cohorts was 9.56. Further, participants provided high scores on "how likely are you to use the skills and information" and "how well did this Institute prepare you to become an online educator." [See Table 1.].

Graduates also provided suggestions for improving the Institute, including providing more time and practice with online teaching, and wanting fewer assignments and ways to better keep track of assignments. Some participants stated that they would like more sessions while others talked about wanting additional training as a "next level version of this course, to continue to enhance the basic skills taught, and continue the dialog around inclusion, community and the other topics taught." Some discussed how dense and fast-paced the course felt and suggested ways to prepare future participants to manage the heavy workload. "While the time commitment of about 5 hours a week is noted upfront," one opined, "I don't think I heard until the end that the Institute tries to partially mimic the workload of what it takes to be an online educator. I think setting that tone more explicitly from the beginning would really help participants."

Continuous Learning Opportunities
1. **Online Faculty Development Series**: A series of online faculty development sessions throughout the academic year, opportunities for guest speaking
2. **Institute on Technical Skills for Online Event Production:** 3-week intensive institute on web conferencing and other skills needed to support live online class sessions
3. **Dedicated Support Team for Each Course:** An Associate and a Live Support Specialist support each online course for the full semester; along with the Instructor, this three-member instructional team meets weekly to plan class sessions and discuss ways to continually improve; the Live Support Specialists provides a written report after every class session that includes feedback and details about student participation
4. **Trainings and One-On-One Mentoring/Coaching:** Provided by the Director of Administration, Program Manager, and Managers of Online Campus Technologies and Course Development
5. **Quality Assurance Reports:** All online course sites are reviewed prior to the start of each semester to provide guidance to the Instructor and Associate on meeting CSSW course standards
6. **Access to Student and Faculty Support Services:** All instructional teams can access CSSW's resources including Advising, Academic Affairs, and the Writing Center, as well as the University's Center for Teaching and Learning and the School's many educational events offered fully online or available via live streaming
7. **Online Support:** Dedicated email helpdesk, 24/7 LMS Support via phone/chat/searchable guides, and a CSSW Online Campus Faculty Site in the LMS with resources

Figure 2. CSSW's online campus: Continuous learning opportunities.

Table 1. CSSW's feedback from participants in the online pedagogy institute (n = 121)*.

	On a scale of 1–10, how would you rate the overall quality of this Institute? M	On a scale of 1–10, how likely are you to use the skills and information you gained from this Institute? M	On a scale of one to ten, how well did this Institute prepare you to become an online educator? M
Summer 2017 (n = 31)	Not Collected	Not Collected	Not Collected
Fall 2017 (n = 26)	9.58	9.81	9.08
Summer 2018 (n = 43)	9.63	9.63	9.28
Fall 2018 (n = 52)	9.46	9.85	9.29
Average (n = 121)	**9.56**	**9.76**	**9.22**

*Note that for the initial Institute in summer 2017 (n = 31), no numerical scale feedback was collected.

Lastly, many participants talked about the empathy they developed for being a student and how it was hard to stay organized and for them keep up with assignment due dates.

Many stated that they did not have any specific feedback and simply stated that the Institute was incredibly valuable. Comments from graduates included, "The Institute set a golden standard for online education. The live sessions, along with the assignments, modeled holistic learning opportunities and effective teaching strategies. It was incredibly well-rounded and of high quality!" and, "Outside of the experiential learning of just knowing what's it like as a student to take a synchronous online course, use of technology was probably most valuable. It pulled us out of our safety zones and showed us how to use the technology as a tool, as opposed to hiding behind it, or setting unnecessary limitations." [See Figure 3 for a list of key themes and sample quotations from participants in the Online Pedagogy Institute.] Further, data are being collected from first-time online CSSW instructors, after each academic year concludes, in order to gather additional feedback on the impact of the Institute on their teaching.

Discussion

The Columbia University Institute provides a training model for online social work educators that may be adapted and then adopted in other social work programs. This training reflects the updated NASW Standards for Technology in Social Work Practice (2017) which mandates that social workers who develop, design, and deliver education using technology engage in appropriate education and training. The Institute may thereby provide a template for how to integrate technology, pedagogy, and social work values when teaching social work online. Some strengths of the model presented here are the Institute's time-limited framework where the curriculum can be taught and completed within five weeks; its peer mentoring paradigm, where prospective faculty and instructional team members learn from social work educators who have been teaching online; and the social work focus on

Themes	Example Quotations
Institute was of high quality	"I found the Institute to be of highest quality…the instructional team and Online Campus department are very informative, supportive, and extremely helpful in the process of learning a monumental skill of teaching online (which can be a bit overwhelming at first as a novice, myself!)."
Learning technology and pedagogy together was helpful	"The instructional team and tech support labored together to ensure that students got the most from the class."
Teaching online is both more engaging and more labor intensive than anticipated	"Before enrolling in this institute, I was skeptical that an online class could be as engaging and rigorous as a residential one, but the past several weeks have taught me that online classes may be even more demanding."
Modeling online teaching was helpful	"I loved how the skills we were learning were also modeled by the teaching team. This was a huge strength of this institute and really speaks to the expertise of the teaching team."
The Institute reflects social work values	"I am also appreciative of the amazing community Matthea and the online instructional team built through their welcoming and supportive presence."
Wanted more time and practice in online teaching	**"My suggestion is to extend the Institute by a couple weeks to build in more practice time using the tools."**
The course requires a significant time commitment	**"If I had to make a suggestion, it would be to be mindful of how dense and fast-paced the course is. I noticed that many of the participants were taking the course in the midst of already busy schedules."**
Wanted fewer assignments or additional ways to keep track of assignments	**"I think the course would be improved if there was a clearer way to access all assignments and their detailed instructions in one place."**

Figure 3. Qualitative themes and quotations from participants in the online pedagogy institute.

empowerment with novice online social work educators who are building the necessary skills to teach synchronous classes in Adobe Connect and create dynamic course elements in the LMS.

For social work educators interested in implementing a similar faculty training program for online teaching, it can be helpful to be aware of challenges and lessons learned. The administration of the Institute takes a significant amount of time, including the following tasks: building an instructional team that can support the live classes and asynchronous homework, offering multiple weekly sections for the live classes to accommodate schedules, and grading several assignments per participant each week which add up to hundreds of weekly submissions for grading. Moreover, enrollment involves a significant time commitment, with the Institute taking five or more hours per week just to complete the online class and homework assignments. For participants who have not been a student for many years, adjusting may involve an emotional impact around the stress of meeting assignment deadlines, or losing points on assignments, or simply functioning as a student once again.

There also may be a steep learning curve for participants who are new to online teaching. Hence, extra support needs to be provided for those who lack comfort and proficiency with technology, or who have questions about expectations and points taken off on assignment grades. The Institute was run by one Instructor (a full-time Administrator of the Online Campus) and a team of Live Support Specialists who managed the multitude of time-sensitive tasks before, during, and after the sessions to create a smooth learning environment.

The Institute did not necessitate a heavy resource allocation because it was run by existing staff. The Instructor was a full-time administrator, so there was no additional cost beyond time, and the support team was composed of existing Live Support Specialists, who were paid at their regular hourly rate. There also was no additional cost for technology, because participants used their own equipment and the Institute used platforms with existing School accounts. The Instructor also oversaw the administration of the Institute and designed and facilitated the live class sessions for three sections of participants each week. Management of the Institute includes recruitment, technology checks, and getting presentation slides from more than 20 guest speakers during the weeks that include such guest speakers as part of the class.

Limitations

Finally, it would be important to note that there are still concerns from some faculty about the effectiveness of online social work education (Levin et al., 2018) and thus there needs to be a keen focus on demonstrating the quality of the online student experience to increase faculty interest in and support for online and distance teaching. As research has shown, institutional support is also critical, as well (East et al., 2014). Overall, this model needs to be evaluated for effectiveness and seeks to add to the scholarly literature on faculty training in online social work education. The Institute is run on a modest budget with one full-time administrator creating and leading the Institute as one small part of an overall administration role. Moreover, only a formative evaluation has been possible given the time and capacity constraints. The Online Campus looks forward to conducting a more formal outcomes oriented evaluation as capacity grows. In addition, the direct experiences of faculty in training programs in the social work field, in general, along with quantitative outcomes, needs to be explored.

Another limitation involves the time and cost investment to create and run an Institute or similar training programs. The initial costs primarily included the considerable time investment from the Instructor (full-time administrator) and the hourly support from the Live Support Specialists.

Further, existing platforms were used for the Institute (e.g., Adobe Connect & Canvas), making the technology cost minimal. Schools starting an online training like this one may want to use their own existing program software to avoid an additional cost. Schools can also consider taking concepts from the model presented here and tailoring them for their institution's needs.

Conclusion

Online social work education has continued to grow exponentially, from approximately 27 different accredited online and distance education Master's programs in 2013 (CSWE, 2013), to 78 programs in 2019 (CSWE, 2019). With the accompanying growth and maturation of technology in the social work field, academic programs need to consider ways to support and enhance the knowledge, preparedness, and comfort level of faculty who will be teaching online courses. The Columbia University Institute provides a prospective training model that can be modified, adapted and adopted by other social work programs, and strives to model best practices in online education. Instructors learn a diverse array of interactive teaching tools including effective engagement and use of technology, best practices in online pedagogy, and how to uphold social work values through content and engagement with students. The Institute also would appear to build skills and confidence in both teaching live synchronous classes, and in setting up asynchronous homework. At a time of ongoing growth in social work education, the authors hope that the Institute offers a constructive model of comprehensive training and professional development for online social work educators to ensure high-quality learning experiences for their students.

Acknowledgments

Dedicated to Steven Schinke and his pivotal role as the Founding Faculty Director of the Online Campus. The authors would like to particularly thank the amazing team of Live Support Specialists who have worked on the Institute: Agata Dera, Ana Quiñones, Chelsea Walus, Elexia Lowe, Erika Wiseberg, Jen So, Jneé Hill, Josh Levine, Kristin Anderson, Krystal Folk, Marianna Da Costa, and Sierra Spriggs.

Disclosure statement

No potential conflict of interest was reported by the authors.

References

Adams, M., & Bell, L. A. (Eds.). (2016). *Teaching for diversity and social justice.* New York, NY: Routledge.

Beaulaurier, R. L., & Haffey, M. F. (Eds.). (2005). *Technology in social work education and curriculum: The high tech, high touch social work educator*. New York, NY: Routledge.

Bentley, K., Secret, M., & Cummings, C. (2015). The centrality of social learning presence in online teaching and learning in social work. *Journal of Social Work Education, 51*, 494–504. doi:10.1080/10437797.2015.1043199

Berzin, S. C., Singer, J., & Chan, C. (2015). *Practice innovation through technology in the digital age: A grand challenge for social work* (Grand Challenges for Social Work Initiative Working Paper No. 12). Cleveland, OH: American Academy of Social Work and Social Welfare.

Brinkley-Etzkorn, K. E. (2018). Learning to teach online: Measuring the influence of faculty development training on teaching effectiveness through a TPACK lens. *The Internet and Higher Education, 38*, 28–35. doi:10.1016/j.iheduc.2018.04.004

Council on Social Work Education. (2013, December 28). *Distance Education*. Retrieved from https://web.archive.org/web/20131228041013/http://www.cswe.org/Accreditation/Information/DistanceEducation.aspx

Council on Social Work Education. (2017). *2017 statistics on social work education in the United States*. Retrieved from https://www.cswe.org/CMSPages/GetFile.aspx?guid=44f2c1de-65bc-41fb-be38-f05a5abae96d

Council on Social Work Education. (2019, January 31). *Online and distance education*. [Website]. Retrieved from https://www.cswe.org/Accreditation/Directory-of-Accredited-Programs/Online-and-Distance-Education

Dawson, B. A., & Fenster, J. (2015). Web-based social work courses: Guidelines for developing and implementing an online environment. *Journal of Teaching in Social Work, 35*(4), 365–377. doi:10.1080/08841233.2015.1068905

Douville, M. L. (2013). The effectiveness of mutual aid learning communities in online MSW practice courses. *Journal of Teaching in Social Work, 33*(1), 15–25. doi:10.1080/08841233.2012.748711

East, J. F., LaMendola, W., & Alter, C. (2014). Distance education and organizational environment. *Journal of Social Work Education, 50*(1), 19–33. doi:10.1080/10437797.2014.856226

Farrel, D., Ray, K., Rich, T., Suarez, Z., Christenson, B., & Jennigs, L. (2018). A meta-analysis of approaches to engage social work students online. *Journal of Teaching in Social Work, 38*(2), 183–197. doi:10.1080/08841233.2018.1431351

Feldman, R. A., & Kamerman, S. B. (Eds.). (2001). *The Columbia university school of social work: A centennial celebration*. New York, NY: Columbia University Press.

Gibson, L. (2016, April). *Challenging social injustice in our own backyard: Using UDL principles to increase access to education*. Workshop presented at the Social Work Distance Education Conference, Indianapolis, IN.

Gingerich, W. J., & Green, R. K. (1996). Information technology: How social work is going digital. In P. R. Raffoul & C. A. McNeece (Eds.), *Future issues for social work practice* (pp. 19–28). Needham Heights, MA: Allyn and Bacon.

Google. (2018). *A new pathway to roles in IT support*. Retrieved from https://www.blog.google/outreach-initiatives/grow-with-google/it-support-professional-certificate/

Herman, J. H. (2012). Faculty development programs: The frequency and variety of professional development programs available to online instructors. *Journal of Asynchronous Learning Networks, 16*(5), 87–106.

Hibbert, M., Kerr, K. R., Garber, A. A., & Marquart, M. (2016). The human element: Fostering instructor presence through online instructional videos. In S. D'Agustino (Ed.), *Creating teacher immediacy in online learning environments* (pp. 91–112). Hershey, PA: IGI Global.

Hitchcock, L. (2015, July 1). *Personal learning networks for social workers.* [Blog post]. Retrieved from https://www.laureliversonhitchcock.org/2015/07/01/personal-learning-networks-for-social-workers/

Hitchcock, L. I., Sage, M., & Smyth, N. J. (Eds.). (2018). *Technology in social work education: Educators' perspectives on the NASW technology standards for social work education and supervision.* Buffalo: University at Buffalo School of Social Work, State University of New York.

Hitchcock, L. I., Sage, M., & Smyth, N. J. (2019). *Teaching social work with digital technology.* Alexandria, VA: CSWE Press.

International E-Learning Association. (2018). *International E-learning awards- past winners.* Retrieved from https://www.ielassoc.org/awards_program/past_winners.html

Knowles, A. J. (2007). Pedagogical and policy challenges in implementing e-learning in social work education. *Journal of Technology in Human Services, 25,* 17–44. doi:10.1300/J017v25n01_02

Koehler, M. J., & Mishra, P. (2005). What happens when teachers design educational technology? The development of technological pedagogical content knowledge. *Journal of Educational Computing Research, 32*(2), 131–152. doi:10.2190/0EW7-01WB-BKHL-QDYV

Kurzman, P. A., & Maiden, R. P. (Eds.). (2014). *Distance learning and online education in social work.* New York, NY: Routledge.

Levin, S., Fulginiti, A., & Moore, B. (2018). The perceived effectiveness of online social work education: Insights from a national survey of social work educators. *Social Work Education, 37*(6), 775–789.

Levin, S., Whitsett, D., & Wood, G. (2013). Teaching MSW social work practice in a blended online learning environment. *Journal of Teaching in Social Work, 33*(4/5), 408–420. doi:10.1080/08841233.2013.829168

Lightfoot, E., & Gibson, P. (2005). Universal instructional design: A new framework for accommodating students in social work courses. *Journal of Social Work Education, 41*(2), 269–277. doi:10.5175/JSWE.2005.200303129

Marquart, M., & Fleming, M. (2014, October 29). *Supporting successful live online classes: Good instructional design is not enough.* Workshop presented at the Online Learning Consortium Conference, Orlando, FL. doi:10.7916/D8HH6HR6

Marquart, M., Fleming, M., Rosenthal, S. A., & Hibbert, M. (2016). Instructional strategies for synchronous components of online courses. In S. D'Agustino (Ed.), *Creating teacher immediacy in online learning environments* (pp. 188–211). Hershey, PA: IGI Global.

Mayes, T. (2001). Learning technology and learning relationships. In J. Stephenson (Ed.), *Teaching & learning online: New pedagogies for new technologies* (pp. 16–26). New York, NY: Routledge.

Meyer, K. A., & Murrell, V. S. (2014). A national study of training content and activities for faculty development for online teaching. *Journal of Asynchronous Learning Networks, 18*(1), 3–18.

National Association of Social Workers. (2017). *NASW, ABSW, CSWE & CSWA standards for technology in social work practice.* Washington, DC: Author. Retrieved from http://www.socialworkers.org/includes/newIncludes/homepage/PRA-BRO-33617.TechStandards_FINAL_POSTING.pdf

Rapp-McCall, L. A., & Anyikwa, V. (2016). Active learning strategies and instructor presence in an online research methods course: Can we decrease anxiety and enhance knowledge? *Advances in Social Work, 17*(1), 1–14. doi:10.18060/20871

Reeves, P. M., & Reeves, T. C. (2008). Design considerations for online learning in health and social work education. *Learning in Health and Social Care, 7*(1), 46–58. doi:10.1111/lhs.2008.7.issue-1

Schwartz, B. M., & Haynie, A. (2013). Faculty development centers and the role of SoTL. *New Directions for Teaching and Learning, 136*, 101–111. Retrieved from https://eric.ed.gov/EJ1029381

Schwartz, S. L., Wiley, J. L., & Kaplan, C. D. (2016). Community building in a virtual teaching environment. *Advances in Social Work, 17*(1), 15–30. doi:10.18060/20875

Secret, M., Bentley, K. J., & Kadolph, J. C. (2016). Student voices speak quality assurance: Continual improvement in online social work education. *Journal of Social Work Education, 52*(1), 30–42. doi:10.1080/10437797.2016.1112630

Southard, S., & Mooney, M. (2015). A comparative analysis of distance education quality assurance standards. *Quarterly Review of Distance Education, 16*(1), 55.

U.S. News & World Report. (2019). *Best schools for social work*. Retrieved from https://www.usnews.com/best-graduate-schools/top-health-schools/social-work-rankings

United States Distance Learning Association Excellence in Teaching/Training Award. (2019). *USDLA awards*. Retrieved from https://usdla.org/awards/

Vernon, R., Vakalahi, H., Pierce, D., Pittman-Munke, P., & Adkins, L. F. (2009). Distance education programs in social work: Current and emerging trends. *Journal of Social Work Education, 45*(2), 263–276. doi:10.5175/JSWE.2009.200700081

The One-minute Paper as a Catalyst for Change in Online Pedagogy

Michael Campbell, Eileen Mazur Abel, and Robert Lucio

ABSTRACT
Online/virtual educators face challenges related not only to tech-nology and pedagogy, but also to student assessment, which remains a critical function to reinforce. Brief assessment tools can be used by the instructor to tailor the learning experience, and where appropriate, to reinforce student-centered learning. In this qualitative study, we explored the use of a one-minute paper as a brief and consistent assessment tool in master's level social work courses in research and advanced clinical practice with individuals courses. The coded segments of qualitative responses (# of coded segments n = 728) from 52 students were examined to explore common themes from the student's experience. Discussion is offered on the use of this tool for brief and consis-tent assessment of knowledge gains in class, as well as the impact these themes may have for the intentional pedagogy for the facilitation of learning.

Introduction

While much has been written about formative approaches for assessing student learning in the traditional classroom, less is known regarding the use of formative assessment in the virtual environment. Effective integra-tion of such assessment in online learning and virtual environments has the potential to offer a mechanism to support meaningful learning and provide feedback to both faculty and students (Baldwin, Ching, & Hsu, 2018; Beebe, Vonderwell, & Boboc, 2010). One of the best established tools for assessing teaching and learning effectiveness is the one-minute paper (OMP) (Lammers & Murphy, 2002; Stead, 2005).

The goal of this paper is to discuss the OMP in light of its role in traditional on ground classes and to assess its utility in the online/virtual environment. Towards this end, the authors review the literature focusing on the rationale, use, and effectiveness of the OMP in traditional classes and then describe how the OMP was used in a virtual teaching environ-ment. The paper highlights the manner in which the OMP was deployed in two first year MSW courses. The authors then delineate the process and outcomes of a qualitative inquiry and provide rich description regarding the use and effectiveness of the OMP in a virtual environment.

Review of the literature

Over the last two decades, there has been a shift in the way teachers and researchers write about student learning in higher education. The discussion of teacher effectiveness has been expanded in recent years to include learner effectiveness (Bloomberg & Grantham, 2015; Vonderwell, Liang, & Alderman, 2007). This shift is compatible with the general move toward student-centered (over teacher-centered) learning (Guerrero-Roldán & Noguera, 2018; McCombs & Whistler, 1997). The phrase *student-centered learning* conceptualizes learning as an iterative process where students and faculty, together, actively contribute to developing knowledge and skill (Lea, Stephenson & Troy, 2003). Within this framework, establishing relationships between students and between students and faculty are critical to the learning process.

The literature indicates that student-centered instruction is most suitable for more autonomous, self-directed learners who can construct their own learning experiences (McCombs & Whistler, 1997; Lea, Stephenson & Troy, 2003). However, though student self-efficacy is important, both Hattie and Temperley (2007), and Nicol and Macfarlane (2006) note the critical role of faculty in providing meaningful feedback. The interplay between student input and faculty feedback is essential for developing effective student learning strategies and enhancing authentic student-centered learning. Similarly, the literature strongly suggests that formative assessment and feedback in higher education should be used to empower students and motivate them to become self-regulated learners (Angelo & Cross, 1993; McCombs, 2015; Pintrich & Zusho, 2002; Weaver & Cotrell, 1985).

Formative assessment is an evaluation process that is employed within the teaching and learning processes in order to support optimal learning (Vonderwell & Boboc, 2013; Zwelijongile, 2015). It enhances faculty ability to identify and utilize ongoing student feedback in order to improve teaching and learning. Using formative assessment strategies faculty can 1) monitor student learning; 2) assess the strengths of their own teaching methods; 3) assess learners' understanding; and 4) accordingly, modify the classroom learning experience (Black & Williams, 1998).

As a formative assessment tool, the OMP is used in the classroom as a means of providing student input into the teaching/learning process. Its origins date back several decades (Weaver & Cotrell, 1985) and its application provides real-time student feedback to the teacher (Chiara and Ostrosky, 1998). The goal of using the OMP is to find out if students have recognized the main points in a class session (Stead, 2005).

The OMP usually is a brief set of no more than three questions assigned at the end of a class session to promote student learning, instructor learning, and assessment of teaching (Almer, Jones, & Moeckel, 1998; Harwood, 1996). Per Stead (2005), typical questions include: 1) identifying the most important learning of the day and 2) additional or unanswered questions that the student might have. Given the nature of the OMP, it is expected that student responses will be brief, spontaneous, and take about a minute to complete (Magnan, 1991). The literature suggests that both teachers and students seem to recognize the value of the OMP (Lucas, 2010). Furthermore, Pintrich and Zusho (2002) have suggested that formative assessment and feedback can enhance student self-regulation. This outcome is particularly relevant in the online environment as self-management of learning often is the key to student success (Vonderwell et al., 2007).

Though the OMP was discussed as an effective assessment tool in the literature as early as the 1980s (Light & Cox, 2001) its effectiveness in the virtual or online teaching environment has not been widely studied. Goffe and Sosin (2010) note that the transition to online learning is not a passing trend which calls for educators to invest energy in efforts to strengthen technology to improve student learning. While it may seem, on the face of it, that this tool would be as useful (Snyder, 2003; Vonderwell, 2004) to the online teacher and student as in the face-to-face environment, little is known about its use in the virtual world. Gikandi, Morrow, and Davis (2011) report that online higher education tends to emphasize summative assessment, with formative assessment receiving relatively little attention (McLaughlin & Yan, 2017; Zwelijongile, 2015).

Sewell, Frith & Colvin (2010) note that an appropriate formative assessment of students' knowledge in online education might be the one-minute paper since it is a recognized tool. Towards this end, Goffe and Sosin (2010) created an active learning activity that combines the convenience of just-in-time email with the one-minute paper (Chizmar & Ostrosky, 1998). This assessment process provides the instructor with timely feedback, and offers students incentives to look back over the material and reevaluate their understanding. Further, in sharing feedback from the OMP with the class, other students can learn from the learning (and lack of learning) of their peers.

Anderson and Burns (2013) investigated student perceptions of the utility of the OMP. Employing a sample of 31 Physical Therapy (PT) and Nurse Anesthesia (NA) students, the authors used an online survey to complete one-minute papers in three separate classes. While study findings indicated that students reported less learning gains from the one-minute paper, as compared to lectures and class discussions, the one-minute paper was found to be useful in enhancing student connections between key ideas and the application of concepts and overall findings, as well as supported the use of the one-minute paper to enhance learning.

Recently, literature has appeared that has contrast the use of the "Muddiest Point" (MP) with the use of OMP (He, 2019; Li & van Lieu, 2018). MP is a format in which faculty ask students to identify one point that they remain confused about. While this technique has been noted to have merit, unlike OMP, it does not ask students to reflect upon material that they have learned. Due to the fact that the MP may inadvertently emphasize the negative, He (2019) notes that it may promote discouragement in both students and instructors.

Educational theory clearly indicates that positive relationships between students and instructors (and among students themselves) enhance the learning experience (Elwood & Klenowski, 2002; McCombs, 2015, Osborne, Byrne, Massey, & Johnston, 2018). While the usefulness of OMP to assess student understanding of course content has been established, the literature has not addressed the utility of the OMP for building connections among students in the online/virtual classroom (Baleni, 2015).

Accordingly, using a grounded method approach (Glaser & Strauss, 1967), this investigation was undertaken to learn more about the use and effectiveness of the OMP in the virtual classroom. The goal of the research was to create a better understanding and richer description of the impact of the OMP as a tool for reinforcing student knowledge, building connections between students and faculty, and enhancing teaching effectiveness in a virtual classroom environment. In this paper, qualitative responses from students' OMP postings were used to explore what themes resonate as key student-centered learning outcomes for a cohort of MSW students in multiple sections of an Advanced Clinical Practice with Individuals and an Introduction to Research Methodology course. The authors' purpose was to explore the utility of the OMP for ongoing process improvement in virtual social work higher education.

Methodology

Study design

A retrospective qualitative review was conducted by reviewing student responses to the session-ending one-minute papers in multiple sections of both a Research Methods and an Advanced Practice with Individuals graduate course. (The University IRB approved the retrospective review of the de-identified OMP responses.) The data were collected from Fall 2016 through Fall, 2017. All classes in which the data were collected met for a sixteen-week term. Students independently completed asynchronous course content and then met weekly in a synchronous virtual classroom environment. The OMP data were collected at the end of each live session.

Data instrumentation and collection

At the close of each class, the instructor directed students to complete a one-minute paper exercise in which they typed into the session chat bar in the online classroom (hosted on Adobe Connect) a response to the following questions:

(1) Identify 1–3 new concepts learned in class today.
(2) Share what you liked about this class session today.
(3) What would you like to see change in future sessions.

The OMP exercise is elective and ungraded, and the student's responses are posted in a virtual chat bar that is visible to the students, their peers, and the instructor. Once the students complete their postings, they are encouraged to review their peer's comments before they exit the virtual class. In this paper, OMP responses were collected from the closing of more than 60 unique sessions embedded in four course sections.

The OMP student responses did not need to be transcribed as they were already in written form, but all data were cut and pasted into a narrative document. All responses to the OMP were de-identified to maintain student anonymity.

Study sample

This purposive sample of students generated data that was reviewed multiple times by the research team. The goal of this iterative process was to better understand the lived experience of the students in the sample and to see what themes rose inductively "from the ground up." Data then were coded into emerging themes.

The sample was drawn across four course sections, with two coming from a research methods course and two coming from a practice course. A total of 52 students provided feedback through the course of the study. All participants were adult students enrolled in an online Master of Social Work program and a majority were enrolled in the two-year MSW program (59.62%), followed by part-time MSW students (21.15%) and advanced standing MSW students (19.23%). A comparison to all students enrolled in the program showed no differences across any of the demographic characteristics. [Complete demographics from the sample are provided in Table 1.]

Data analysis

One-minute paper response transcripts were initially reviewed via an open coding approach and then data were coded independently by two members

Table 1. Demographics.

	N	%
Academic Program		
Two Year	31	59.62%
Part Time	11	21.15%
Advanced Standing	10	19.23%
Race		
White	26	50.00%
Black or African American	11	21.15%
Hispanic/Latino	6	11.54%
Two or More Races	1	1.92%
Unknown	8	15.38%
Gender		
Female	45	86.54%
Male	7	13.46%
Mean Age	52	35.63

of the research team. Identified themes were discussed and consensus was established. A second axial coding process was then initiated. Issues of discrepancy were negotiated by the reviewers to again create consensus. In addition to this hands-on immersion into the data, transcripts also were downloaded from the learning management software and were coded by the research team. The team created a thematic coding tree using MAXQDA (version 12.3.3), which is a qualitative analysis software package. All items were coded separately, and as a team, and each item was discussed until consensus was reached for each code.

In the results section, we will provide details on those themes which accounted for "Primary Themes" and "Other Themes." Primary themes (themes with 50 or more coded segments) will be detailed individually and any themes with fewer than 50 coded segments discussed collectively under the second heading as other themes.

Results

Thematic codes

Students first were asked to provide feedback on important concepts learned in the session and then to provide process improvement feedback on aspects of the session that were positive, and conversely, which they wish would change for future lessons. The analysis of the student comments from the one-minute papers revealed ten major themes [see Table 2]. These included activity-based learning, course content, connection with asynchronous content, critical thinking, relationship building, technical issues, the flow of the course, negative feedback, programmatic discussions, and professionalism. Each of these areas will be described below in greater detail.

Table 2. Thematic Code Distribution.

Primary Themes (50 or more coded segments)	N Segments	% of total
Activity Based Learning	208	28.57%
Course Content	208	28.57%
Connection with Asynchronous Content	92	12.64%
Critical Thinking	85	11.68%
Relationship Building	67	9.20%
Other Themes (Less than 50 coded segments)	N Segments	% of total
Technical Issues	26	3.57%
Flow of class	23	3.16%
DELTA – negative feedback	11	1.51%
Programmatic Discussion	7	0.96%
Professionalism	1	0.14%
TOTAL of all Themes/Coded Segments	728	100.00%

Primary themes

Primary themes include all themes with over 50 coded segments. These include activity-based learning, course content, connection with asynchronous learning, critical thinking, and relationship building. Each of these will be described in detail throughout this section.

Activity based learning (*# of coded segments* = 208)

Overall, 28.3% of all coded sections were related to the theme of activity-based learning. Within this area, students referred to the course content and activities in four primary areas: the actual content covered, the information that was provided through the activities, the impact of the activities on student learning, and suggestions for improvements.

Content (*# of coded segments* = 144): Students mentioned the content or activities they participating in during their live online class sessions. A majority of these comments simply noted they found helpful or liked a specific activity within the course session. These included practice activities, role plays, handouts, small discussions, group activities, polls, and breakout groups.

Impact (*# of coded segments* = 35): Some students specifically mentioned the impact that the activity-based learning had on their performance or perspective. These comments consistently noted the change in their perspective or skills that came from the activities. In some cases, students remarked that they had learned a new skill that they had not known before or which helped them see the problem from a client's view in a way they had never done before. Students appreciated the ability to put what they were learning into action.

Information (*# of coded segments* = 27): Students also mentioned the information they were provided in terms of feedback from the instructor and other students during their activity-based learning. This outcome was seen through feedback on activities by peers or the instructor, clarification of expectations about class activities, additional questions that were asked to clarify the activity, or detailed expectations about the activity.

Suggestions (# *of coded segments* = 2): Several students mentioned specific ways the activities could be improved upon moving forward. These were simply provided as ways to enhance these activities in the future.

The overall sentiment of the theme of activity-based learning can be illustrated by one student who noted:

> *I like the interactive parts of our class where we get to really discuss something with our peers as it really helps with seeing things in a new or different way and helps me to understand things in a way that just reading a textbook does not.*

Course content (# *of coded segments* = 208)

Comments related to course content were tied for the highest number of coded segments (28.3%). When it comes to course content, students generally mentioned either some social work practice technique or specific content knowledge they gained in the course session. The student comments did not cluster into sub-themes for course content, but instead often simply mentioned specific items from their classes. For students, this might be something completely new, or it might clarify what they had already been learning. For instance, one noted the ideas were reinforced when "emphasizing the vocabulary, which is also a great help. The examples, such as the tables that we dissect, make the reading more understandable." On the other hand, they might cite something new, as illustrated by a student comment that she was "aware of the miracle question, however, I did know that it was a therapeutic technique of Solution Focused Therapy."

Connection with asynchronous content (# *of coded segments* = 92)

Connection with asynchronous content accounted for 12.64% of all coded segments. The four primary areas that emerged related to connection with asynchronous content were (1) that the live sessions assisted learning processes,(2) students learned additional content, (3) the material they read was reinforced, and (4) they were able to practice and apply what they had read or learned.

Assisted Learning as a Process (# *of coded segments* = 60): A majority of the students' comments in relation to asynchronous content centered around the idea that the synchronous session was useful as a process to learn the information that they had read about or learned elsewhere. This meant that the flow of the course, the feedback on what they were learning, and being able to talk through the materials in a live session helped clarify and provide further insight into the asynchronous materials.

Learned Additional Content (# *of coded segments* = 18): Students also noted that the asynchronous content was a starting point, but they were able to learn additional content in the synchronous sessions. They commented that they were able to learn more about the assignments and that applying the content allowed them to gain a deeper understanding than just reading the textbook. This was a consistent message – whether they were discussing research, the application of theories, or direct practice skills.

Reinforced Readings (# *of coded segments* = 8): Throughout their written comments, students again noted that the synchronous content reinforced what was learned via the other materials. They frequently were able to refresh their knowledge of topics they had previously learned about in other courses or had read in their current course materials.

Applied Content (# *of coded segments* = 6): The ability to practice the content that was covered both in the course readings and in class was helpful to students. They observed that reading about an idea or concept was one thing, but to be able to practice that skill helped reinforce their learning. A student commented, "the book taught me what an evaluation was, but I liked that the activity helped me see how an evaluation is really applied," and "breaking down this report in different sections was an excellent example to assist in understanding what our work should look like."

Critical thinking (# *of coded segments* = 85)

Students expressed some notion of critical thinking in 11.68% of all coded segments. The concept of critical thinking was displayed by how they looked at course materials and assignments, self-reflection, client's perspective, and the actions of others in the readings or role plays.

Course Materials and Assignments (# *of coded segments* = 52): A majority of the comments written around critical thinking were focused on taking a deeper look at the course materials and assignments. Students were able to look at how to apply what they learned to social work practice, but also how to look more deeply at what they were reading and learning. For instance, students reported being able to better understand how to apply research scales and to differentiate between research and non-research articles.

Self-Reflection (# *of coded segments* = 18): Throughout the comments, it was apparent that students were able to apply self-reflection as part of their critical thinking skills. This included examining what therapy style would suit them, and how to ask and rephrase questions in order to be most effective. Some of the skills students mentioned they still needed to work on covered different therapeutic techniques, how to respond to specifically difficult questions, and the need to learn and grow as a social worker before deciding on which style to use.

Clients Perspective (*# of coded segments* = 8): Students wrote about how they were able to see the client's perspective on different situations. The students acknowledged that this is helping them develop empathy towards clients' situations, which is essential in social work practice.

Actions of Others (*# of coded segments* = 7): In this area, students wrote about how they viewed the actions of others in the context of critical thinking. This was seen when thinking about what they read or when they watched others role play. When discussing what they read, students remarked about the impact of ethics in both research and practice.

Students were able to apply what they are learning to their own lives, and start to think deeply about the impact of social work in their own lives. This was exemplified by a student who is trying to separate personal helping skills from the needs of families:

> *I liked when we discussed how to deal with counseling our family members. I currently am dealing with personal issues at home and I try to tell them that I would rather not, but I will help them find help.*

> *The practice of single-subject design research is interesting to me. Being able to design the questions on a scale that's understandable and easy for the client to relate to helps you to connect better with the client and the subject.*

Relationship building (*# of coded segments* = 67)

Students discussed relationships in terms of general support for each other, help or support on specific class activities, and the interactional support they received from their peers.

General Support (*# of coded segments* = 28): Students noted that they enjoyed the interaction with classmates and expressed a sense of support overall. This feeling might be due to tough circumstances going on or just general encouragement to keep a positive outlook in the course. Additionally, some students noted the support the instructor provided throughout the course by caring about their success and providing overall help.

Specific Support for Class Activities (*# of coded segments* = 20): Some students expressed gratitude for being supported in specific class activities. They also noted specific activities which facilitated in-class discussions that were helpful.

Interaction with Peers (*# of coded segments* = 19): Through their one-minute paper comments, students also conceptualized relationship building as interaction with their peers. This came in the form of specific help on activities or with technical difficulties, to the interactive nature of the class. The idea of sharing thoughts back and forth was helpful to learning. Relationship building was best exemplified through a student who commented:

> *Everyone in this class is so supportive and provides helpful feedback. This is definitely a plus! I didn't feel great about my session tonight, but I think it helped me learn a lot about different types of clients I may assist.*
>
> *They help me understand what I need to focus on, Love interacting with my classmates.*

Other themes

This section discusses all of the other thematic codes which had fewer than 50 coded segments each. These include technical issues (# of coded segments = 26), flow of class (# = 23), negative feedback (# = 11), programmatic discussion (# = 7) and professionalism (# = 1). Technical issue themed responses comprised three general areas (general technical difficulties, trouble with the internet, and issues with other users/peers). Overall, the general technical issues appeared to be the largest area of concern for students. This included issues with figuring out how to navigate the technology to not being able to download course materials that were loaded by the instructor.

The second most frequently mentioned area of technical issues revolved around the Internet. Some students reported having trouble with their internet connection due to company or weather issues and others reported missing some of the lectures due to only intermittent connection or being "kicked off" the system. Students also complained when other students did not mute their microphones, causing distractions and background noise which interfered with their learning.

When it came to the flow of the class, students noted the process and structure of the class which referred to using a timer to keep things moving on track, the flow of moving from one activity to another, the interactivity of each activity, and the ability to exchange ideas with each other. Students also mentioned programmatic issues about the courses including having a clearer understanding of how the course fits into the overall sequence of the program and course policies. They also provided some "negative feedback," or areas that could be improved, by noting that the set-up of the course could be improved, how class time was spent, and the need for providing clearer instructions for activities. Finally, one noted that other students were not always professional when giving feedback on role plays.

Discussion

The student's responses to the one-minute paper (OMP) constituted several primary themes: *Activity-based learning, Course content, Connection with asynchronous material, Critical thinking, and Relationship building.* These themes are reflective of the utility of the OMP as a tool for helping graduate students to actively identify learning outcomes across asynchronous and synchronous content domains. Additionally, these topics seem to support the notion (Vonderwell, 2004) that student-centered learners actively participate in ongoing meaningful feedback to improve the learning experience/environment when given a consistent platform for sharing feedback.

The themes, gleaned from the student's responses, also seem to support the findings of Lea, Stephenson, & Troy (2003) given that the impact of the OMP can be used as a tool for assessing student-centered learning and reinforcing student knowledge. It also helped to discern which concepts resonated for the students at the time. The OMP, as well, offers the instructor the opportunity to use this information to extend learning on the subject and to bolster other key aspects of learning that did not get recorded by students. In a similar way, the OMP was effective in building connections between students and faculty through a transparent feedback loop. This increased communication, extending Harwood's (1996) findings, enhances teaching effectiveness in the virtual classroom environment.

The results of this study indicate that students took an active stance in both the presentation of knowledge acquired and with respect to ways to promote student-centered learning. This action-oriented approach, in keeping with the work of Goffe and Sosin (2010), models active learning and appears to be a good tool for both assessment and reinforcement (Chizmar & Ostrosky, 1998).

It is of interest to this study that student comments in the OMP seem to indicate a synergistic connection between content items presented in a synchronous virtual session (Course Content) and the learning that took place outside of the classroom (Connection with Asynchronous Content). An argument can be made that the OMP could be a tool to help bridge the gap that Gikandi et al. (2011) identified wherein online learning settings tend to excel at summative assessment but lag behind with effective formative assessment and also can help to bridge the synchronous and asynchronous learning platforms.

Another key finding of this research is that MSW students demonstrated an active application of learned concepts (Critical Thinking) in OMP responses. Much like the findings of Anderson and Burns (2013), this study found that the OMP is useful in enhancing student integration of central ideas and offers a forum for information exchange among peers and with faculty. These data serve to support the generally accepted theme that engaged students take a more active role in their learning. They also reinforce the notion that when students are offered a forum to state their preferences for the flow and delivery of their classroom experience they will leverage that opportunity to highlight appreciative feedback, for the aspects of course delivery that they like, as well as constructive feedback, for aspects they wish to have changed. Finally, this data strongly supports the role that one-minute papers can play as a micro assessment tool in an online environment. In these settings, where time management is critical and student engagement is complicated by issues of distance and time, technology (such as the chat bar in the online class setting) can quickly and easily offer a functioning forum for routine student feedback to promote, and facilitate engagement in the process.

This qualitative study offers a breadth of knowledge regarding themes generated through the use of the OMP. While this provides a unique context for student perceptions and feedback on their courses, content, and relationships, it should be noted that the findings are specific to this sample of students. Since the goal of the investigation, per qualitative methods, is not generalizability, this outcome is not a design flaw. Rather, the goal of this inquiry is for educators to gain a deeper understanding of the utility of the OMP as a formative assessment tool in the virtual classroom.

We recommend that future research on the role of the OMP in virtual and online social work education focus on the interplay between the qualitative findings in the student responses and their relationship with student achievement in learning and self-efficacy (Hattie & Temperley, 2007). Later, in mixed method designs, research might involve predictive analytics regarding the connection of the OMP responses to self-directed learning (Lea, Stephenson & Troy, 2003).

Disclosure statement

No potential conflict of interest was reported by the authors.

References

Almer, E. D., Jones, K., & Moeckel, C. L. (1998). The impact of one-minute papers on learning in an introductory accounting course. *Issues in Accounting Education, 13*(3), 485–497.

Anderson, D., & Burns, S. (2013). One-minute paper: Student perception of learning gains. *College Student Journal, 47*(1), 219–227.

Angelo, T. A., & Cross, K. P. (1993). *Classroom assessment techniques: A handbook for college teachers* (2nd ed.). San Francisco, United States: Jossey-Bass.

Baldwin, S., Ching, Y. H., & Hsu, Y. C. (2018). Online course design in higher education: A review of national and statewide evaluation instruments. *Technology Trends, 62*, 46. doi:10.1007/s11528-017-0215-z

Baleni, Z. (2015). Online formative assessment in higher education: Its pros and cons. *The Electronic Journal of e-Learning, 13*(4), 228–236. Retrieved from http://files.eric.ed. gov/fulltext/EJ1062122.pdf

Beebe, R., Vonderwell, S., & Boboc, M. (2010). Emerging patterns in transferring assessment practices from face-to-face to online environments. *Electronic Journal of E-Learning, 8*, 1.

Black, P., & Williams, D. (1998). Inside the white box: Raising standards through classroom assessment. *Phi Delta Kappan, 80*(2), 139–148.

Bloomberg, L. D., & Grantham, G. (2015). Teaching in graduate distance education: Perspectives on evaluating faculty engagement strategies. *International Journal of Online Education, 29*, 56–66.

Chiara, J. F., & Ostrosky, A. L. (1998). The one-minute paper: Some empirical findings. *Journal of Economic Education, 29*(1), 3–10. doi:10.1080/00220489809596436

Chizmar, J. F., & Ostrosky, A. L. (1998). The one-minute paper: Some empirical findings. *The Journal of Economic Education, 29*(1), 3–10. doi:10.1080/00220489809596436

Elwood, J., & Klenowski, V. (2002). Creating communities of shared practice: The challenges of assessment use in learning and teaching. *Assessment & Evaluation in Higher Education, 27*(3), 243–256. doi:10.1080/02602930220138606

Gikandi, J. W., Morrow, J., & Davis, L. (2011). Online formative assessment in higher education: Review of the literature. *Computers & Education, 57*(1), 2333–2351. doi:10.1016/j.compedu.2011.06.004

Glaser, B. G., & Strauss, A. L. (1967). *The discovery of grounded theory.* Chicago, IL: Aldine.

Goffe, W. L., & Sosin, K. (2010). Teaching with technology: May you live in interesting times. *The Journal of Economic Education, 36*(3), 278–291. doi:10.3200/JECE.36.3.278-291

Guerrero-Roldán, A., & Noguera, I. (2018). A model for aligning assessment with competences and learning activities in online courses. *The Internet and Higher Education, 38*, 36–46. doi:10.1016/j.iheduc.2018.04.005

Harwood, W. S. (1996). The one-minute paper: A communication tool for large lecture classes. *Journal of Chemical Education, 73*(3), 229–230. doi:10.1021/ed073p229

Hattie, J., & Temperley, H. (2007). The power of feedback. *Review of Educational Research, 77* (1), 81–112. doi:10.3102/003465430298487

He, Y. (2019). Traffic light cards: A cross and modification between the minute paper and muddiest point. *College Teaching, 67*(1), 70–72. doi:10.1080/87567555.2018.1522612

Lammers, W. J., & Murphy, J. J. (2002). A profile of teaching techniques used in the university classroom: A descriptive profile of a US public university. *Active Learning in Higher Education, 3*(1), 54–67. doi:10.1177/1469787402003001005

Lea, S. J, Stephenson, D, & Troy, J. (2003). Higher education students' attitudes to student-centred learning: beyond 'educational bulimia'?. *Studies in Higher Education, 28*(3), 321–334. doi:10.1080/03075070309293

Li, M., & van Lieu, S. (2018). Traditional and online faculty members' use of Classroom Assessment Technique (CATs): A mixed-method study. *Journal of Instructional Research, 7*, 90–99. doi:10.9743/JIR

Light, G., & Cox, R. (2001). Assessing: Student assessment. In *Learning and teaching in higher education: The reflective practitioner.* London, UK: Paul Chapman Publishing.

Lucas, G. M. (2010). Initiating student-teacher contact via personalized responses to one-minute papers. *College Teaching, 58*(2), 39–42. doi:10.1080/87567550903245631

Magnan, B. (1991, January) Teaching idea: The one-minute paper'. *Teaching Concerns* [University of Virginia Newsletter]. Retrieved from http://cte.virginia.edu/resources/teaching-idea-the-one-minute-paper-3/

McCombs, B. (2015). Learner-centered online instruction. *New Directions for Teaching and Learning, 144*, 57–71. doi:10.1002/tl.20163

McCombs, B., & Whistler, J. (1997). *The learner-centered classroom and school: Strategies for increasing student motivation and achievement.* San Francisco, United States: Jossey-Bass.

McLaughlin, T., & Yan, Z. (2017). Diverse delivery methods and strong psychological benefits: A review of online formative assessment. *Journal of Computer Assisted Learning, 33*(6), 562–574. doi:10.1111/jcal.v33.6

Nicol, D. J., & Macfarlane, D. (2006). Formative assessment and self-regulated learning: A model and seven principles of good feedback practice. *Studies in Higher Education, 31* (2), 199–218. doi:10.1080/03075070600572090

Osborne, D.M, Byrne, J.H, Massey, D.L, & Johnston, Amy N.B. (2018). Use of online asynchronous discussion boards to engage students, enhance critical thinking, and foster staff-student/student-student collaboration: a mixed method study. *Nurse Education Today, 70*, 40-46. doi:10.1016/j.nedt.2018.08.014

Pintrich, P. R., & Zusho, A. (2002). The development of academic self-regulation: The role of cognitive and motivational factors. In A. Wigfield & J. S. Eccles (Eds.), *A Vol. in the educational psychology series. Development of achievement motivation* (pp. 249–284). San Diego, CA: Academic Press.

Sewell, J. P., Frith, K. H., & Colvin, M. M. (2010). Online assessment strategies: A primer. *MERLOT Journal of Online Learning and Teaching, 6*(1), 297–305.

Snyder, K. D. (2003). Ropes, poles, and space: Active learning in business education. *Active Learning in Higher Education, 4*(2), 159–167. doi:10.1177/1469787403004002004

Stead, D. R. (2005). A review of the one-minute paper. *Active Learning in Higher Education., 6*(2), 118–132. doi:10.1177/1469787405054237

Vonderwell, S. (2004). Assessing online learning and teaching: Adapting the minute paper. *TechTrends, 48*(4), 29–31. doi:10.1007/BF02763442

Vonderwell, S., Liang, X., & Alderman, K. (2007). Asynchronous discussions and assessment in online learning. *Journal of Research on Technology in Education, 39*(3), 309–328. doi:10.1080/15391523.2007.10782485

Vonderwell, S. K., & Boboc, M. (2013). Promoting formative assessment in online teaching and learning. *Tech Trends, 57*(4), 22–27. doi:10.1007/s11528-013-0673-x

Weaver, R. L., & Cotrell, H. W. (1985). Mental aerobics: The half-sheet response. *Innovative Higher Education, 10*(1), 23–31. doi:10.1007/BF00893466

Zwelijongile, G. B. (2015). Online formative assessment in higher education: Its pros and cons. *The American Journal of Distance Education, 29*, 56–66.

Cutting the Distance in Distance Education: Reflections on the Use of E-Technologies in a New Zealand Social Work Program

Nicky Stanley-Clarke, Awhina English, and Polly Yeung

ABSTRACT

The development of new e-technologies and an increased focus on developing distance social work education programs has created the impetus for social work educators to consider the tools they can employ in delivering distance courses. This article reflects on an action learning research project involving the development of an online toolbox of e-technologies to support social work educators in the delivery of distance courses. It highlights the opportunities and challenges when considering the integration of e-technologies as part of social work education.

Introduction

The growth of new technologies, student demand, and institutional pressures to develop online platforms for teaching social work are profoundly changing the nature of social work education (Pelech et al., 2013; Vernon, Vakalahi, Pierce, Pittman-Minke, & Frantz Adkins, 2009). Social work educators are putting aside their reluctance to embrace e-learning and considering how to use the emerging technology in a way that will support the interpersonal nature of social work engagement (Coe Regan & Youn, 2008; Wilson, Brown, Wood, & Farkas, 2013). This article reports and reflects on an action learning research project that involved the process of developing an online toolbox of e-technologies for social work educators. The goal of the research was to trial the new tools and consider both their appropriateness and effectiveness within a distance learning social work program in New Zealand.

E-learning is the emerging paradigm of modern education (Sun, Tsai, Finger, Chen, & Yeh, 2008) involving the use of online tools and networking mechanisms to engage with students to "create, foster, deliver and facilitate learning, anytime and anywhere" (Liaw, 2008, p. 864). Utilizing e-learning can occur in a number of ways including synchronous, asynchronous, or hybrid (blended) learning. Synchronous e-learning involves both the faculty and students being online at the same time and engaging with one another through the use of webconferencing tools such as virtual classrooms and discussion forums. Asynchronous learning involves students being able to engage with material via an online platform at a time that best suits them. A hybrid or blended learning approach involves a combination of both synchronous and asynchronous learning tools, thereby providing a varied learning experience.

Social work education and E-learning

A lack of technology to support role-plays, home visits, and simulated counseling sessions historically has created barriers to the development of e-learning within social work education (Wilson et al., 2013). The essence of the struggle is, How can social work educators feel confident that their students embody social work values and are able to effectively engage and practice clinically with clients if they have not actually been able to assess the student in a physical classroom? In addition, questions have been raised regarding how social work students can be socialized into the profession through an online learning environment (Coe Regan & Youn, 2008). Despite these concerns, there have been several comparative studies confirming equivalence in grades and outcomes for distance versus classroom-based social work programs (McAllister, 2013; Pelech et al., 2013). In addition, the development of new e-technologies such as Adobe Connect, Skype, virtual classrooms, and social media tools (such as Facebook and Twitter) has created new possibilities and opportunities (Coe Regan & Youn, 2008; Iverson Hitchcock & Young, 2016; Vernon et al., 2009).

Nevertheless, in considering using e-technologies, social work educators struggle with creating equality of opportunities for social work students, minimizing structural barriers, and ensuring that the learning environment works congruently with the reality of students' lives (Reamer, 2013).Therefore, educators have to balance the inclusion of new e-learning technologies with the ability of students to have access to and the resources to engage with this method of learning (Maidment, 2005; Parker-Oliver & Demiris, 2006). To address the disparity in student access to a good Internet connection, lack of technological support, and the cost of technological upgrades, distance programs traditionally have opted for the banking method of learning (Desai, Hart, & Richards, 2008; Maidment, 2005). This asynchronous form of teaching involves placing course material online that students can then access at a time and place convenient to them. The use of an online platform and similar technologies removes the physical constraints of the traditional classroom, providing a 24-hour-a-day, 7-days-a-week learning environment and often more realistically respond to the learning requirements of students in the 21st century (Desai et al., 2008; Parker-Oliver & Demiris, 2006; Sun et al., 2008). However, increased access to the Internet and a wider array of devises for rapidly accessing online materials means that social work students may become frustrated with courses that are not regularly updated to reflect students' changing needs, such as more hybrid approaches to learning (Maidment, 2005; Pelech et al., 2013).

The integration of e-technologies and resources in the delivery of social work programs has created some unexpected alignments with social work values, such as equality and social action, as well as the development of skills, including reflexivity and critical engagement. In addition to the flexibility of the learning environment there are opportunities to improve student decision making, reflection, and critical thinking (Iverson Hitchcock & Young, 2016; Vernon et al., 2009). Iverson Hitchcock and Young (2016) found that students using Twitter, a microblogging social media platform, could engage and follow current social work and social policy issues. This raised students' awareness of social work issues, encouraged them to participate in social action, and supported both reflective thinking and collaboration with others beyond the classroom—meaning that students could contribute to conversations about the profession from their role as students. This process of connected learning, which is informed by and empowered through the use of e-technologies, allows students to network beyond the bounds of the traditional learning domain (Iverson Hitchcock & Young, 2016; Maidment, 2005).

Another persuasive reason for integrating more e-learning experiences into social work education is to keep pace with the changing nature of social work and to equip students to practice within the current social work context and culture (Maidment, 2005; Parker-Oliver & Demiris, 2006). There is a growing need for social workers to engage with technology in working with clients—from using social media to connect, to the delivery of online programs, support groups, and social work interviews using Skype (Iverson Hitchcock & Young, 2016). In response, social work practitioners, as well as educators, need become literate with these tools and come to understand the benefits of using them.

Despite the growing body of evidence supporting the use of e-technologies in the delivery of social work education, there still is resistance from many educators as they continue to debate the effectiveness of teaching clinical skills through this modality (Cappiccie & Desrosiers, 2011; Coe Regan & Youn, 2008; Levin, Witsett, & Wood, 2013; Parker-Oliver & Demiris, 2006; Pelech et al., 2013). This is the point at which this research project commenced as the authors—all social work educators—struggled to balance the competing demands of the university, students, and a belief in social work pedagogy, on one hand, with the need to learn about and develop skills in the use of e-technologies to deliver social work programs, on the other.

The project

The project was undertaken at a university in New Zealand. The university taught both undergraduate programs (including a BSW) and postgraduate or postqualifying social work programs (including MSW, Master of Applied Social Work, Doctor of Social Work, and the PhD). Students in all programs were a mix of high school graduates as well as more mature adult students.

Initially established as an internal or in-person teaching program, the university had delivered distance-based social work programs since the mid-1990s. The distance programs were offered as hybrid courses. Course content was delivered online as well as in-person on contact days. A number of the courses also provided supplemental printed materials. The university utilized a Moodle e-learning platform as the primary management system for delivery and engagements. To support the project, the authors applied for and were awarded an academic fellowship grant from the university, which enabled them to purchase teaching and grading release time, which in turn provided them with dedicated time to learn, trial, and reflect on the effectiveness of the e-technologies being deployed.

The project was a qualitative action learning research project utilizing the cyclical approach of planning, inquiry, intervention, and reflection (Baum, MacDougall, & Smith, 2006; Silver, 2009). Action learning is an applied form of social research that aims to produce useful knowledge through a process of generating experiential learning that creates knowledge through praxis (Baum et al., 2006; Marlow, 2011; Silver, 2009). It is exploratory in nature and evolutionary, as the research evolves through the process of critically reflecting on the prior action and then altering the approach accordingly (Castro Garcés & Martínez Granada, 2016; Coghlan, Shani, & Roth, 2016; Silver, 2009). This reflexive process generates learning from experience and in doing so creates new opportunities for action.

As noted earlier, the three authors were social work educators involved in teaching both undergraduate and postgraduate social work. They all had worked for the university in combined research and teaching positions for a period of more than 4 years. Castro Garcés and Martínez Granada (2016) explained that undertaking action research within an educational setting enables faculty to explore issues they come across in their teaching in order to understand and improve educational practices. Such was the case in this study, with the idea for the research stemming from the authors collectively evaluating their existing methods of teaching delivery, considering ways in which to further develop their teaching, and to be able to engage more effectively with distance students and then create a toolbox for other social work educators wishing to use these e-technologies in their teaching.

The project occurred over a semester of teaching. At the start, the authors identified some e-technologies they wished to trial within the courses they were teaching at the time, which were social policy and clinical social work in the 1st, 2nd, and 3rd years of the BSW, an advanced clinical practice in the MSW and a social policy course in the Master of Applied Social Work degree program. They met with a teaching and learning consultant regularly to learn more about e-technologies and to reflect on the usefulness of the tools that had been employed in the intervening period. The creation of a Moodle demonstration platform (known as a sandbox) complemented the face-to-face meetings and further facilitated the sharing of ideas, knowledge, and reflection. The process of working collectively created a mechanism for sharing and cogenerating knowledge, linking well to the core values of action research (Castro Garcés & Martínez Granada, 2016; Coghlan et al., 2016; Marlow, 2011). Following the completion of the project, the sandbox would prospectively be transformed into a toolbox for all social work staff to be able to access information about how to develop and use the e-technologies.

Over the course of the semester the authors tried a range of e-technologies within the Moodle sites to create a hybrid or blended learning environment. Among the tools were a few of the built-in technologies within Moodle, including a dynamic glossary module related to the content of a course, which could be updated on a regular basis; a polling tool, known as Choice; and asynchronous discussion forums. As the authors' confidence in using e-technologies increased, they tried other tools including Adobe Connect for synchronous, interactive lectures and tutorials as well as for creating a platform for students to practice role plays. The authors also tried other asyncronous tools including inserting Twitter feeds into their Moodle platforms, using Mediasite to edit and record podcasts, and an online polling tool known as Mentimeter (https://www.mentimeter.com/app).

Results

The research project's process of reflection and collaboration highlighted the authors' different responses to using the same tools, with each preferring to utilize a slightly different approach to the e-technologies related in part to the nature of the course but also their own confidence and personal teaching preference. The following section provides the results from the authors' experience in using the e-technologies.

Using podcasts or prerecorded lectures

As noted, Adobe Connect was one of the main technologies the authors used across the project with varied success. Students in the program had expressed a desire for podcasts or prerecorded lectures related to course content, and the authors were keen to try the technology and to reflect on its effectiveness as a teaching tool. Adobe Connect was initially used by the authors to provide podcasts to students introducing their papers for the semester. Adobe Connect, as well as Mediasite, were further employed to make podcasts more related to course content and to provide explanations related to course assessment.

The first author used Adobe Connect to provide explanations related to assessment and supported this practice with a weekly blog to students providing learning goals, clarifying key terms, and highlighting core tasks that needed completion. Student feedback found the inclusion of these tools to be positive and supported their learning, with one commenting, "The online learning environment was really useful and the weekly posts from the lecturer were helpful." Another student said, "The videos from the lecturer were excellent and made a big difference for me. They make the content of the paper much more accessible."

The second author used Adobe Connect on a fortnightly basis to provide tutorial sessions to students and creating an opportunity for "open discussion." Weekly lectures were also recorded using Mediasite, an asyncronous tool that enables digital recording and editing of lectures and other course material, which students then can view in their own time. The second author found that the use of Mediasite was particularly successful for 1st-year students. Course evaluations noted that students thrived off the regular interaction with their educator and from the opportunity to ask detailed questions about the course. The following comments were reflective of the general student experience:

> Loved the lectures, and the live tutorials with the lecturer were extremely helpful, no question was a stupid question, she was so good and clear. Her lectures were not just straight from the text either; she related personal stories and examples and I find this way of learning really helpful, putting it into realistic scenarios.

The second author found that student engagement improved through the use of weekly online lectures. Students reported that they enjoyed the ability to pause and rewind these lectures and were highly motivated by having the slides, alongside the author's reflections, as part of the lecture. In the past, students often would be given weekly PowerPoint slides, but without the author's input they appeared to struggle to align the slides with the reading material. Students frequently listened to the recorded lectures more than once and often used the Mediasite lectures as a weekly starting point, where ideas would blossom and they then would research and read more on their ideas after the lectures. As one student commented,

> Weekly lectures have been great. Great delivery, heaps of resources. [The author] is an amazing lecturer that appears to have put a lot of time and effort into developing the resources she has made available to students. I found this paper [course] really interesting and informative.

The second author identified several challenges involved in using Mediasite lectures including the slow process of "video making," having to be an "actor," and needing to keep material up-to-date. The first challenge involved the slow process of preparing, recording, and processing the lecture before it could be accessed by the students. In the early stages, when the second author was still learning how to use Mediasite, it often would take a whole day to record, process, and upload the lecture. Sometimes the challenge would be getting the content right, other times the Internet speed would mean that it might take a whole afternoon for the file to process. This reality led to the second challenge—the author being prepared and able to become an "actor." The authors each found that there is a certain type of confidence needed to be able to record a lecture to a computer screen and it is, for some, more intimidating than for others. The second author struggled and found that students commented on the use of "ums" throughout the lectures: "Lectures were rather distracting with the amount of 'Ums' mentioned in the lecture which took away my interest from the actual messages." However, given the new teaching tool and their ability to "act" the second author felt that presenting an "um-free" video lecture would be near impossible. The final challenge was that often the information in the lectures quickly became outdated, and therefore much material could not be reused in following years.

Live connect sessions

The first and second authors both used Adobe Connect meeting rooms to host orientations, tutorials, or question and answer (Q&A) sessions with students. (Students were provided with instructions about how to use Adobe Connect prior to the session.) In this scenario, they created a meeting room and inserted a brief PowerPoint overview, which was spoken to at the start of the session. In addition, a chat module was created where students could type any questions they had about the presentation or course material. The session was recorded, with the consent of students, and made available to those who could not attend. Both authors A and B liked the use of the synchronous Adobe Q&A or tutorial sessions and felt that they generated student engagement and participation in ways that were not facilitated as easily by the prerecorded podcasts. Student evaluations captured their comments about the Q&A sessions: "The exam Q&A session was valuable and supported me a lot to know what to study for the exam" and "The Adobe Q&A sessions explained the assignments in detail; without these I would have found completing assignments through distance much more difficult."

Role-plays online

A central concern of distance students in clinical social work programs at this university was related to the lack of a platform in which to practice their clinical skills. The first author attempted to address this concern in the distance offering of their 2nd-year social work skills course. Students enrolled in the internal offering of the course were required to attend weekly laboratories where they learned clinical skills and could develop expertise in applying social work models. Although the distance students were required to attend a compulsory contact course, which included a laboratory component, this did not provide for the same weekly progression of skills across the semester. The first author decided to create a virtual platform for the distance students to practice their role-plays. To do this, the author created an Adobe Connect meeting room that the students could access and use as a platform for practicing their interview skills. They, of course, needed to have access to a camera and microphone to be able to participate. The author provided the students with a lab book with examples of role-plays and the core skills to be explored in each session. She also offered instruction to students on how to use the forum and allocated students to the role of meeting host so they could access the room at a time that was convenient to them without the author needing to be in attendance. Students then were able to book a time in the lab room, through the paper's Moodle site, and could meet in groups of three (social worker, client, and observer) to practice the skills.

The first author found the process of setting up and orientating the students to the room to be straightforward, and initially they were very enthusiastic about using the room. However, upon completion of the course, the author noted that the room was rarely used. Students commented in the course evaluation that they liked the idea but found that creating time, and coordinating with other students to participate, was problematic, adding an extra workload burden on top of the required coursework. One commented, "Being a full time student I also found it very hard to find any extra time to do these on top of all my other paper requirements." Students also commented that they lacked sufficient confidence to use the facility on their own and felt that they would have liked the educator present to support the process: "I feel like at this stage we need proper supervision from a tutor to be able to get the best out of it." It was the first author's reflection that, despite the ease in setting up the room and the success students had when they engaged with it, the facility would be better used with Year 3 or Year 4 students who have greater levels of confidence in undertaking role-plays. The additional workload burden for students in participating in the role-plays through the online platform also needed to be factored in to overall course planning.

Twitter

Inserting a Twitter feed into the Moodle site was found to be an easy and effective way to keep students engaged in recent events in social policy. Both the first and third authors inserted a feed from their Twitter accounts into a HTML block within the Moodle sites for their social policy papers. The HTML block worked by simply displaying anything the authors retweeted. The first author also experimented with creating Twitter lists and inserting these into a master's-level clinical issues paper. In the Twitter list, all tweets made by people allocated to the lists automatically showed in the paper's Twitter feed. She felt that this worked best at a postgraduate level, where the students had the academic maturity to discern between tweets. The first author felt that this would not work as well for undergraduate students, and that having the author selecting and retweeting relevant tweets was more appropriate.

The use of a Twitter feed for the third author stemmed from a 2nd-year social policy assignment in the BSW program that required students to choose a social policy area (e.g., health, income support, social welfare, housing, disability). The assignment asked students to locate and analyze five news articles from their selected area in relation to social policy theories (e.g., neoliberalism, feminism) and goals of well-being (e.g., justice, equality). Given that social policy entails the study of the social relations necessary for promoting human well-being, social media was deemed an appropriate tool to influence students' information-seeking trends. Consequently, news stories on social issues were tweeted daily by the author. An advantage of engaging social work students with social and political issues via Twitter was that more government and social services organizations are using social media platforms to engage, recruit, and educate the public. Students therefore benefited by learning how to deploy these networks as a means of information-seeking and professional communication. Linking students with local and national social and welfare issues opened discussion opportunities related to global events, international social work, and social policy practices. For example, during the 2nd-year social policy class, students located information and discussion about the Vulnerable Children Act 2014, a policy that made significant changes to child protection in New Zealand, which they then circulated on Twitter.

Student feedback about the use of Twitter as a teaching tool, was that it provided them with a quick and easy way to remain engaged and connected with current affairs. One student commented, "I think keeping connected and abreast of conversations really helped enhance my learning."

Online polling tools

The depth and breadth of social policy content makes the topic well suited for traditional lecture delivery. However, such a lecture format, although widely accepted, has been criticized for lack of effectiveness as a teaching method, due to a lack of student centeredness (Isseks, 2011). Use of questions during lectures is an effective strategy to break up the content and gives students opportunities to immediately assess their understanding. Historically, students have been reluctant to participate using traditional approaches (such as hand-raising or the use of response paddles) because they do not want people to know if they got an answer wrong (Stowell & Nelson, 2007). The third author therefore trialed two e-technologies to engage students: Choice and Mentimeter.

Choice is a tool embedded in Moodle that allows the educator to create Q&A options to gauge feedback from students; however, the answers are not anonymous to the educator. The third author experimented with Choice across both in-person and distance classes to explore students' progress and confidence in completing an assignment. Disappointingly, less than 10% of the students participated. The polling app Mentimeter was also employed to develop true/false, multiple-choice, Likert-scale questions and to produce short written comments. Mentimeter enables tracking of the live result, while students are voting, with the web-based mobile polling app using their mobile phones, tablets, or laptops. This app was used during an in-class lecture to gauge students' stances on certain social and welfare issues. Although distance students were not able to vote "live," questions embedded into the PowerPoint and online podcasts encouraged them to participate within a specified period. Results then were collated and presented back to all students via Moodle. Given that the polling feature in Mentimeter provided results only from those who voted, it helped to ensure anonymity among those who participated, thereby minimizing direct judgment related to student progress or ability. Mentimeter was trialled three times during the semester, and more than 30% of distance students participated.

Discussion and implications

As discussed in the introduction, the purpose of this project was to test a range of e-technologies and consider their appropriateness and effectiveness for inclusion within a distance learning social work program. The key findings from the project were as follows:

- The use of e-technologies, in particular synchronous classrooms, provided opportunities to engage and build relationships with distance students that are not offered in traditional asynchronous programmes.
- Social work schools should consider developing a digital strategy or online toolbox when evaluating the integration of e-technologies into their teaching program. This should consider staff and student workload, the management of student expectations, and the different needs of students in relationship to their learning journey.

Key to using e-technologies successfully is finding new ways to engage students (Desai et al., 2008; Jeffrey, Milne, Suddaby, & Higgins, 2012; Sun et al., 2008). Hence, educators need to think about how to redefine their communication to facilitate a process of engagement and relationship building (Desai et al., 2008). In addition, they need to identify the relevant student characteristics (Liaw, 2008). The nature of the course is the most important concern, with e-technologies needing to support rather than dominate the learning experience (Sun et al., 2008). The authors in this study observed that there is a risk of overwhelming students, leading some to opt out of using the tools (such as the online role-plays used by the first author) and becoming disengaged from the program. This reality requires that faculty be selective in the tools they employ, always considering the workload, and the different technological abilities of students.

Nevertheless, e-technologies do provide benefit in engaging with distance students. One of our deepest fears was that the experience of teaching online would be impersonal. After all, many of us got in to teaching because of the opportunity to build relationships that might make a difference. Although this project helped the authors facilitate learning in a mechanical way, it also assisted in building the relationships that are so critical to effective instruction. The use of online synchronous classrooms (such as Adobe Connect) provided a vehicle for students to build a relationship with their instructors, potentially leading to increased openness and communication across the degree. However, in agreement with Cappiccie and Desrosiers (2011), we found that it was important to keep online sessions short because most students struggled to find focused time without interruptions. Also, students preferred the synchronous Adobe Connect sessions to asynchronous discussion boards and taped lectures because the latter did not provide the level of interpersonal engagement they preferred. Students also often did not engage with e-technologies if this required a commitment over and above what was prescribed for the course.

The authors also discovered that the use of e-technologies created expectations from students that there would be a one-size-fits-all approach to course delivery across the programme. There is value in the diversity of tools and approaches used to engage with students in offerings on clinical social work and social policy, reflecting the reality of clinical practice, and being able to engage with difference. We found that these expectations needed careful management so that students did not become dissatisfied or wholly reliant on e-technologies for their learning.

Although Twitter was only a component of the third author's social policy courses, the potential of this social media tool created the opportunity for students to engage and participate dynamically in real-world issues. Confirming the findings of Iverson Hitchcock and Young (2016), our use of Twitter highlighted the benefits of deploying social media to engage students in their own learning so that they can teach themselves, or one another, by contributing to a knowledge base of professional conversation. In this project, it was found that once students grasped the potential for Twitter as a nexus of information, they seemed to take a newfound sense of agency over their own learning, following other people's tweets, retweeting news and information to others. This provided some indication that the educator does not always have to be the one facilitating student learning.

Realistically, online learning can take at least twice the time needed when compared with face-to-face teaching. A review of the literature on this topic by Pelech and colleagues (2013) revealed reports of up to 40% more time being required, involving multiple factors such as educator experience, extent of interaction desired, and class type and size. It was concluded that the online experience for students may be comparable to face-to-face courses if it is strategically and rigorously developed and monitored. The experiences of the authors in this project support that e-learning and online courses do require intensive educator presence and frequent, consistent, and highly responsive interaction with students within a variety of structured and well-facilitated opportunities. When these criteria are present, with adequate infrastructure and resources, the quantity and quality of interaction may well extend beyond the traditional format of face-to-face teaching.

For online curriculum and e-learning delivery to be effective, the university, educator, and student all need to make a substantial investment of resources. A grant was received to undertake this endeavor enabling the authors to buy out teaching and marking in order to have focused time for the project. Further, the university provided additional expert assistance from a teaching and learning consultant who had experience in the use of e-learning technologies. The project could not have occurred without this financial and in-kind support. Jones (2015) claimed that the availability of university infrastructure to support e-learning is crucial to ensure quality, and we would agree. Although online courses offer more flexibility than on-campus courses, instructors need additional equipment, skills, training, and time to successfully teach in this format because providing quality online education for social work students is a time and resource intensive task.

Conclusion

In conclusion, the purpose of the article was to provide a reflection on the process of trialing e-technologies within a distance social work program. The outcomes of this action learning project do in fact affirm existing research that e-technologies can be used effectively to support the delivery of social work education. The findings also confirm the need for social work educators to carefully consider how they choose to use and adopt e-technologies and to formalize their selections through the creation of a digital strategy or online toolbox.

Funding

This work was funded by an academic fellowship grant provided by Massey University in New Zealand.

References

Baum, F., MacDougall, C., & Smith, D. (2006). Participatory action research. *Journal of Epidemiology Community Health*, 60(10), 854–857. doi:10.1136/jech.2004.028662

Cappiccie, A., & Desrosiers, P. (2011). Lessons learned from using adobe connect in the social work classroom. *Journal of Technology in Human Services*, 29(4), 296–302. doi:10.1080/15228835.2011.638239

Castro Garcés, A. Y., & Martínez Granada, L. (2016). The role of collaborative action research in teachers' professional development. *Profile Issues in Teachers' Professional Development*, 18(1), 39–54. doi:10.15446/profile.v18n1.49148

Coe Regan, J. A. R., & Youn, E. J. (2008). Past, present, and future trends in teaching clinical skills through web-based learning environments. *Journal of Social Work Education*, 44(2), 95–116. doi:10.5175/JSWE.2008.200600592

Coghlan, D., Shani, A. B., & Roth, J. (2016). institutionalizing insider action research initiatives in organizations: The role of learning mechanisms. *Systemic Practice and Action Research*, 29(2), 83–95. doi:10.1007/s11213-015-9358-z

Desai, M. S., Hart, J., & Richards, T. C. (2008). E-learning: Paradigm shift in education. *Education*, 129(2), 327–334.

Isseks, M. (2011). How Powerpoint is killing education. *Educational Leadership*, 68(5), 74–76.

Iverson Hitchcock, L., & Young, J. A. (2016). Tweet, tweet! using live twitter chats in social work education. *Social Work Education*, 35(4), 457–469. doi:10.1080/02615479.2015.1136273

Jeffrey, L. M., Milne, J., Suddaby, G., & Higgins, A. (2012). *Help or hindrance: Blended approaches and student engagement*. Wellington, New Zealand: Ako Aotearoa National Centre for Tertiary Teaching Excellence.

Jones, S. H. (2015). Benefits and challenges of online education for clinical social work: Three examples. *Clinical Social Work Journal*, 43(2), 225–235. doi:10.1007/s10615-014-0508-z

Levin, S., Witsett, D., & Wood, G. (2013). Teaching social work practice in a blended online environment. *Journal of Teaching in Social Work*, 33(4–5), 408–420. doi:10.1080/08841233.2013.829168

Liaw, S. (2008). Investigating students' perceived satisfaction, behavioural intention, and effectiveness of e-learning: A case study of the Blackboard system. *Computers & Education*, 51(2), 864–873. doi:10.1016/j.compedu.2007.09.005

Maidment, J. (2005). Teaching social work online: Dilemmas and debates. *Social Work Education*, 24(2), 185–195. doi:10.1080/0261547052000333126

Marlow, C. R. (2011). *Research methods for generalist social work* (5th ed.). Belmont, CA: Cengage.

McAllister, C. (2013). A process evaluation of an online BSW program: Getting the student perspective. *Journal of Teaching in Social Work*, 33(4–5), 514–530. doi:10.1080/08841233.2013.838200

Parker-Oliver, D., & Demiris, G. (2006). Social work informatics: A new speciality. *Social Work, 51*(2), 127–137. doi:10.1093/sw/51.2.127

Pelech, W., Wulff, D., Perrault, E., Ayala, J., Baynton, M., Williams, M., … Shanker, J. (2013). Current challenges in social work distance education: Responses from the Illuminati. *Journal of Teaching in Social Work, 33*(4–5), 393–407. doi:10.1080/08841233.2013.834863

Reamer, F. G. (2013). Distance and online social work education: Novel ethical challenges. *Journal of Teaching in Social Work, 33*(4–5), 369–384. doi:10.1080/08841233.2013.828669

Silver, C. (2009). Participatory approaches to social research. In N. Gilbert (ed.), *Researching social life* (3rd ed., pp. 101–124). London, UK: Sage.

Stowell, J. R., & Nelson, J. M. (2007). Benefits of electronic audience response systems on student participation, learning, and emotion. *Teaching of Psychology, 34*(4), 253–258. doi:10.1080/00986280701700391

Sun, P. C., Tsai, R. J., Finger, G., Chen, Y. Y., & Yeh, D. (2008). What drives a successful e-Learning? An empirical investigation of the critical factors influencing learner satisfaction. *Computers & Education, 50*(4), 1183–1202. doi:10.1016/j.compedu.2006.11.007

Vernon, R., Vakalahi, H., Pierce, D., Pittman-Minke, P., & Frantz Adkins, L. (2009). Distance education programmes in social work: Current and emerging trends. *Journal of Social Work Education, 45*(2), 263–276. doi:10.5175/JSWE.2009.200700081

Wilson, A. B., Brown, S., Wood, Z. B., & Farkas, K. J. (2013). Teaching direct practice skills using web-based simulations: Home visiting in the virtual world. *Journal of Teaching in Social Work, 33*(4–5), 421–437. doi:10.1080/08841233.2013.833578

Human Service Administrator Perceptions of Online MSW Degree Programs

Laura Curran, Ray Sanchez Mayers, and Fontaine Fulghum

ABSTRACT

Online programs have proliferated rapidly in higher education, and this reality holds true for social work education as well. Employing a mixed methods design, this study looked at employer perceptions of online degrees compared to traditional degrees. Data was collected through an online survey that included Likert type and open-ended questions assessing employer attitudes and hiring practices regarding individuals who possess online MSW degrees. Results suggest that a majority of social service administrators believe traditional MSW degrees are preferable to those attained online, especially with respect to clinical training. These findings have significant implications for online MSW programs and graduates with online degrees.

Online courses and degree programs have proliferated rapidly in higher education since the advent of web-based technologies in the 1990s. An oft-cited national survey, conducted by the Babson Group and using data from the National Center for Education Statistics' Integrated Postsecondary Education Data System, found that over one fourth (28%) of all students enrolled in 2- and 4-year degree-granting higher education institutions took at least one of their courses fully online or in a hybrid format (combining face-to-face instruction with online learning). Another 14% of all higher education students were exclusively enrolled in distance education courses (Allen, Seaman, Poulin, & Straut, 2016). Despite the popular equation of distance education with for-profit educational institutions, the overwhelming majority of students taking some distance education courses (79%), and those completing their degree entirely in an online/hybrid format (70%), were enrolled at public or private nonprofit institutions. Moreover, distance enrollments continued to grow at such public and nonprofit institutions between 2012 and 2014, despite a decline in overall enrollment (Allen et al., 2016).

This shift holds true for social work education as well. In a recent study of deans and directors of schools of social work, 66 of 121 respondents reported that their schools provided one or more web-based courses (East, LaMendola, & Alter, 2014). According to the Council on Social Work Education (CSWE), the accrediting body for social work programs, in 2014 there were nine BASW programs (1.8%) and 27 MSW programs (11.8%) that reported having fully online programs. Another 162 (32.9%) bachelor's programs and 106 (46.5.%) master's programs reported that parts of their programs were online. In addition, 51 bachelor's programs and 28 master's programs said that they were developing online/distance education courses (CSWE, 2015).

Despite this rapid growth and student interest in online programs, few studies have looked at employer hiring practices and perceptions of online graduates. This is particularly true in social work, where studies of employer attitudes toward online degree holders appear nonexistent in the literature. This absence is of concern given that graduates from online MSW programs will proliferate in the labor market in the coming years, assuming that current trends continue. As more and more MSW programs are delivered online, schools of social work have an ethical obligation to examine employer attitudes and track employment outcomes for these graduates. As Kurzman (2013) noted, research has yet to examine the post-MSW career achievement of online versus traditional graduates. This study begins to fill this research gap by examining employer attitudes toward online MSW degree holders in the Northeast.

Background

Employer Attitudes toward Online Degree Holders

A small body of literature examining employer and/or hiring manager attitudes toward online degree holders has recently emerged. This literature is in its infancy despite the fact that in a national survey approximately 40% of chief academic leaders identified the "potential lack of acceptance of online education by potential employers" as a barrier to the growth of online degree programs (Allen & Seaman, 2015, p. 27). Other extant studies primarily rely on relatively small-scale survey data that query potential employer and hiring managers' attitudes toward online degree holders in comparison to traditional degree holders. Although mixed, findings from these studies generally indicate employers' or gatekeepers' preference for employees with traditional on-the-ground (OTG) degrees across a variety of fields (Adams, DeFleur, & Heald, 2007; Adams, Lee, & Cortese, 2012; Fogle & Elliott, 2013; Grossman & Johnson, 2016; Metrejean & Noland, 2011; Richardson, McLeod, & Dikkers, 2011).

For instance, Kinneer's (2014) recent study of healthcare recruiters found that participants reported being significantly more likely to hire registered nurses with traditional degrees than those with online degrees.

This literature further suggests that these negative perceptions stem from employers' beliefs that online programs are generally either of lower quality or unable to teach critical skills within their virtual delivery format (Richardson et al., 2011). For example, in their study of administrators in the healthcare sector, Adams and colleagues (2007) found that employers perceive online degree programs as lacking the face-to-face interaction, field work components, and close mentoring deemed necessary for practice in the healthcare sector. Similarly, Adams and colleagues' national survey of high school principals revealed that respondents perceive online coursework as unable to provide students with the interpersonal skills and values orientation necessary for employment in an educational setting. This body of research also indicates that employer experience with online education (Fogle & Elliott, 2013), the reputation of the degree-granting institution (Adams et al., 2007), grade point average, licensure, and communications skills (Metrejean & Noland, 2011) may moderate employer attitudes. Although they stem from somewhat disparate professions, some of these findings may pose issues relevant to social work.

Findings concerning negative employer attitudes toward online degrees may partially mirror some academics' attitudes toward online coursework. Skepticism about online education lingers among educators, academic gatekeepers, and the general public despite its rapid growth (Allen & Seaman, 2015; Straumsheim, Jaschik, & Lederman, 2015). For instance, the Babson Survey Research Group of Babson College reports that fewer than 30% of academic leaders believe their faculty "accept the value and legitimacy of online education" (Allen et al., 2016, p. 26). The leaders reported more faculty support in institutions with higher numbers of distance enrollments (Allen et al., 2016). According to the national *2015 Inside Higher Ed Survey of Faculty Attitudes on Technology*, only 17% of faculty agreed or strongly agreed with the statement "For-credit online courses can achieve student learning outcomes that are at least equivalent to those of in-person courses" at any institution (Straumsheim et al., 2015, p. 14). However, agreement was higher (28%) among faculty who had taught online (Straumsheim et al., 2015).

There is evidence of ongoing skepticism among faculty within social work. While CSWE and the National Association of Social Workers, the largest professional social work organization, are generally supportive of current developments in online education (Kurzman, 2013), and outcomes literature (discussed next) is generally positive, the academic community continues to question the effectiveness of teaching and assessing clinical skills via web-based means (Levin, Whitsett, & Wood, 2013; Moore, 2005; Reamer, 2013; Regan & Youn, 2008). Moore's (albeit somewhat dated) 2005 survey concerning social work faculty perception of online courses found that the majority believed face-to-face instruction to be more effective across the curriculum, with the largest perceived difference in clinical content areas. Other social work educators caution about the lack of spontaneous dialogue and nonverbal communication that may delimit learning in the online classroom (Sawrikar, Lenette, McDonald, & Fowler, 2015) and raise ethical concerns, including issues of proper gatekeeping (Reamer, 2013). Moreover, discussion within the social work clinical community suggests that disfavor toward online degrees may exist among human services agencies (Clinical Social Work Association, 2013). Such concerns seem to center around the ability to convey helping and humanistic-oriented skills and values via an online modality.

Learning Outcomes in Online Education

Despite considerable caution, a significant amount of empirical evidence points to equivalent learning outcomes in online and face-to-face classes. The oft-cited meta-analysis of 50 study effects conducted by the U.S. Department of Education (2010) found that, across a variety of academic disciplines, online students performed modestly better in comparison to students learning the same material in face-to-face settings. Research examining online coursework in social work education has generally reached similar conclusions. A number of small studies, some quasi-experimental in design, have found equivalent learning outcomes when measured by skills acquisition, grades, and student satisfaction in traditional and online social work courses (Ouellette, Westhuis, Marshall, & Chang, 2006; Siebert, Spaulding-Givens, & Siebert, 2006; Woehle & Quinn, 2009). Extant studies also suggest that clinical skill development of online students is comparable to that of traditional learners (Wilke & Vinton, 2006). For instance, Ouellette and colleagues (2006) reported no significant difference between interviewing skills acquired by online and OTG learners. Interestingly, Cummings, Chaffin, and Cockerham's (2015) recent study comparing online and traditional MSW students found no significant differences in the majority of educational outcomes between the student populations, although field instructor ratings were higher for online students in an extended study program.

Employer Attitudes and Online MSW Degrees

Despite the significant growth of online MSW degrees, we found only one published study to date concerning employment outcomes for online degree holders in social work. This study found that employment outcomes were similar between OTG students and online degree holders, although OTG students were more likely to be employed in full-time positions and working toward licensure than online graduates (Potts & Kleinpeter, 2001). Given the small sample size ($N = 72$) and the geographical concentration of the graduates, the generalizability of these findings is limited. In sum, the current literature concerning online learning in social work generally overlooks labor market considerations, including employer attitudes, and this study seeks to fill this gap.

Methods

This study posed the following research questions:

RQ1: Is there a difference in employer attitudes toward online MSW and traditional OTG degree holders?

RQ2: What factors may influence differences in employer attitudes toward online and traditional MSW degree holders?

RQ3: What factors might account for employer preference toward OTG graduates with MSW degrees?

Procedure and Sample

The study utilized an exploratory, cross-sectional, mixed method design. A purposeful sample was used to capture the population of interest, that is, social service agencies employing MSWs. Online surveys were sent to 934 social service agencies in three neighboring states affiliated with a mid-Atlantic social work school and identified through field affiliation contracts. Project staff called the agencies to ascertain the name and e-mail for the person in charge of staff hiring at each agency. The introductory letter of invitation, consent form, and survey instrument were sent via e-mail inviting these individuals to participate in the survey via Qualtrics survey software. A reminder e-mail was sent 2–3 weeks after the initial mailing. Only one staff person per agency in charge of hiring decisions was sent the survey. Three hundred seventy administrators responded, and 332 surveys were completed in their entirety (90%). Of those, 100 also responded in some format to open-ended qualitative questions. The study was approved by the Institutional Review Board of the university.

Instrument

The survey consisted of three parts: demographic and descriptive information about the respondents and their agency settings, questions regarding respondent views of online programs, and two open-ended questions addressing attitudes toward hiring MSW graduates and regarding online social work education. The questions regarding views of online programs were closed ended using a Likert scale from *strongly disagree* to *strongly agree* (and *don't know*) and included questions regarding perceptions of quality, clinical and macro course outcomes, and student self-discipline. Survey items development was informed by the extant literature. The two open-ended qualitative questions asked (a) "Do you have any concerns in hiring someone with an online degree? If so, can you tell us what they are?" and (b) "Is there anything else you want to tell us about this topic?" The dependent variable in the study was based on a question that asked, "Do you think that online programs are 'not as good,' 'just as good,' or 'better than' traditional programs?" In this survey, the term "online degree" refers to 60-credit MSW programs in which all coursework was completed in an online format.

Quantitative Analysis

Quantitative data analysis was done using SPSS 23.0 after the recoding of some variables. As noted, the dependent variable was perception of online programs. Only two respondents said they were "better than traditional," and those were not included in the analysis. Therefore, a dichotomous variable was created with the two responses "not as good" and "just as good." Bivariate chi-square analyses were done to identify associations between perception and potential predictors. Logistic regression was conducted to model the relationship between perception and explanatory variables using backward stepwise regression. In this approach, we start with all independent variables of interest in the model and proceed backward, removing one insignificant variable at a time until we are left with the variables that have a significant relationship to the dependent variable. Our qualitative data analysis entailed a conventional content analysis (described below) and was conducted using Microsoft Excel.

Results

Quantitative Findings

Sample Characteristics

The majority of sample respondents was female (68.6%) and White (81.7%). Of those sampled, 68.4% were older than 46, whereas only

7.1% were younger than 35. The majority of the respondents had such job titles as Executive Director, or Chief Executive Officer, or similar administrative titles (81.4%). Although one respondent had an A.A. degree, the educational level of the rest of the respondents ranged from B.A./B.S. degrees (12%) to doctoral degrees (11.4%). Forty-four percent were MSWs, with job experience ranging from zero to 40-plus years. Of those surveyed, 42.7% reported that they had taken an online class. Only 9.1% of the respondents had ever hired social work staff with an online degree, whereas 17.4% were unsure whether those hired had an online degree. The majority (73.5%) said that they had never hired anyone with an online degree (see Table 1).

Table 1. Demographic and Organizational Profile of Sample.

	No.	%
Individual characteristics		
Gender[a]		
Male	101	31.4
Female	221	68.6
Age[b]		
35 and younger	23	7.1
36–45	79	24.5
46–55	76	23.5
Older than 55	145	44.9
Race/Ethnicity[c]		
White	254	81.7
African American	29	9.3
Hispanic/Latino	13	4.2
Other	15	4.8
Education[d]		
BA/BS/BSW	40	12.0
MSW	147	44.0
Other master's	86	25.7
PhD/PsyD/EdD	38	11.4
Other	23	6.9
Job title[e]		
Exec. Dir/CEO	285	81.4
Supervisor, Case manager	24	6.9
Other	41	11.7
Organizational characteristics		
Type of agency[f]		
Public	50	14.8
Private nonprofit	235	69.5
Private for profit	53	15.7
Location of agency[g]		
New York area	16	4.7
Northern New Jersey	115	34.0
Central New Jersey	116	34.3
Southern New Jersey	54	16.0
Philadelphia area	10	3.0
Other	27	8.0

Note. Approximate number of employees ($n = 314$). Range = 1–3,700, $M = 218.55$, $SD = 454.37$. Numbers in the sample vary, as not every question was answered; no imputation of data was conducted.
[a]$n = 322$. [b]$n = 323$. [c]$n = 311$. [d]$n = 334$. [e]$n = 350$. [f]$n = 338$. [g]$n = 338$.

A majority of the agencies were private nonprofits (69.5%), with about an equal number of public and private for-profit agencies as well (see Table 1). Most were located in New Jersey (84.3%), and others were in the New York City area and the Philadelphia area; a few were affiliated with statewide or national organizations. The number of employees in these agencies ranged from just one to 3,700 ($M = 218$, $SD = 454$).

Perceptions of Online Degree Programs

When asked their perception of online degree programs, 57.4% of respondents said they were not as good as traditional programs. Yet a majority either agreed or strongly agreed that "some of the best colleges and universities offer online courses" (65.9%; see Table 2). Conversely, a large number disagreed or strongly disagreed that "most online programs are offered by lower-quality schools" (51.9%), although 20.4% of them said they "didn't know." A large percentage of the respondents disagreed or strongly disagreed that "students can develop effective clinical skills through online coursework" (57.5%). On the other hand, 54.5% agreed or strongly agreed that "students can develop effective macro practice skills though online coursework." Respondents were also divided on whether "students who take online courses are more self-directed and disciplined," and 24.8% said they "didn't know."

In the bivariate chi-square analysis, we found that female participants were significantly more likely than male to view the quality of online programs "as good as traditional programs" (48.5%). MSWs and doctoral administrators were significantly less likely to view them "as good". Those who agreed that online programs were offered by better schools were significantly more likely to view online programs positively, as were those who agreed that clinical skills and macro skills could be taught online. Respondents who had hired staff with online degrees were significantly more likely to report that online degrees were "just as good" as

Table 2. Perceptions of Online Programs (%).

	Strongly disagree	Disagree	Agree	Strongly agree	Don't know
Some of the best colleges and universities offer online courses[a]	3.1	14.5	48.1	17.9	16.4
Most online degrees are offered by lower quality schools[b]	10.2	41.8	24.2	3.7	20.1
Students can develop effective clinical skills through online coursework[c]	16.4	40.9	22.9	4.6	15.2
Students can develop effective macro practice skills through online coursework[d]	6.8	23.8	46.6	8.0	14.8
Students who take online courses are more self-directed and disciplined[e]	4.4	31.4	27.3	12.1	24.8

[a]$n = 325$. [b]$n = 324$. [c]$n = 324$. [d]$n = 325$. [e]$n = 323$.

Table 3. Bivariate associations between perceptions of the quality of online programs "as good as traditional programs" and respondents' characteristics/attitudes.

	As good (%)	p
Gender		.006**
Male	31.5	
Female	48.5	
Education		.011*
BA/BS	60.0	
MSW	34.6	
Other master's	50.0	
PhD/PsyD/EdD	34.3	
Other	61.1	
Ever hired staff with online degree		.013*
Yes	57.1	
Not sure	57.1	
No	37.8	
Better schools offer online programs		< .001***
Strongly disagree	10.0	
Disagree	11.4	
Agree	45.4	
Strongly agree	74.6	
Don't know	37.5	
Lower quality schools offer online programs		< .001***
Strongly disagree	85.7	
Disagree	59.3	
Agree	13.2	
Strongly agree	10.0	
Don't know	33.3	
Students can develop clinical skills online		< .001***
Strongly disagree	12.2	
Disagree	30.8	
Agree	71.0	
Strongly agree	92.9	
Don't know	51.1	
Students can develop macro skills online		< .001***
Strongly disagree	15.0	
Disagree	15.5	
Agree	53.6	
Strongly agree	72.0	
Don't know	52.4	
Online students more self-directed and disciplined		< .001***
Strongly disagree	7.1	
Disagree	21.5	
Agree	56.6	
Strongly agree	80.6	
Don't know	44.4	

traditional ones than those who had never hired someone with an online degree. Finally, those who saw online students as more self-directed viewed online programs being "as good as traditional" ones (see Table 3) The bivariate analysis also revealed no statistical difference by age, race/ethnicity, or having themselves taken an online course.

Observed variations on gender remained in the multivariate analyses: The odds of viewing online courses positively were higher for female participants. This result was true for gender differences once all other covariates were controlled for. The findings related to degree type did not remain. The findings on age, race/ethnicity, and having taken an online course also remained the same, that is, they were not significant. The most significant predictor of positive attitudes toward online education was the question as to whether clinical skills could be learned online. Those who agreed or strongly agreed that clinical skills could be learned online were more likely to view online courses positively, whereas those who disagreed were much less likely to do so (see Table 4). Another important factor was the perception of online students as having more self-discipline. Those who agreed or strongly agreed with this statement were also more likely to view online programs as "just as good as" traditional ones.

Table 4. Multivariate predictors of perceiving online courses as "just as good as traditional programs".

	Odds ratio	95% CI
Gender: Female	3.08***	[1.43, 6.63]
Some of the best colleges and universities offer online degrees		
Disagree	1.75	[0.07, 46.02]
Agree	3.31	[0.16, 66.80]
Strongly agree	10.88	[0.48, 248.95]
Don't know	6.03	[0.25, 144.79]
Most online degrees are offered by lower quality schools		
Disagree	1.58	[0.35, 7.27]
Agree	0.35	[0.06, 1.92]
Strongly agree	0.12	[0.00, 13.87]
Don't know	0.53	[0.09, 3.04]
Students can develop effective clinical skills through online coursework		
Disagree	8.94***	[1.94, 41.28]
Agree	24.62****	[4.93, 122.94]
Strongly agree	98.30***	[4.80, 2012.63]
Don't know	7.16**	[1.09, 47.00]
Students can develop effective macro practice skills through online coursework		
Disagree	0.09**	[0.01, 0.82]
Agree	0.28	[0.03, 2.43]
Strongly agree	0.17	[0.01, 2.00]
Don't know	0.23	[0.02, 2.88]
Students who take online courses are more self-directed and disciplined		
Disagree	4.11	[0.15, 112.86]
Agree	15.87*	[0.60, 423.12]
Strongly agree	25.65*	[0.91, 725.81]
Don't know	10.86	[0.41, 289.16]

Note. $n = 281$. Reference categories are as follows: male, strongly disagree that clinical skills can be taught online, strongly disagree that macro skills can be taught online, strongly disagree that online students are more self-disciplined. Overall model fit: $\chi^2(20) = 149.229$, $p < .000$, -2 Log Likelihood $= 235.433$, Nagelkerke $R^2 = .553$. CI $=$ confidence interval.
*$p < .10$. **$p < .05$. ***$p < .01$. ****$p < .001$.

Qualitative Findings

Analysis

As described earlier, the survey contained two open-ended qualitative questions: (a) "Do you have any concerns in hiring someone with an online degree? If so, can you tell us what they are?" and (b) "Is there anything else you want to tell us about this topic?" The questions were designed to elicit in-depth information about respondents' attitudes, including potentially negative perceptions. The qualitative data were analyzed according to principles of conventional qualitative content analysis with codes derived inductively from the textual data. Conventional/classical content analysis seeks to understand the phenomenon under study through the categorization of text, and may quantify or count qualitative themes, but does not generate theory (Hsieh & Shannon, 2005). This classical approach to data analysis is appropriate to the exploratory and descriptive aims of this study. Data analysis here commenced with multiple readings of the data and proceeded with the development of codes, and the eventual sorting of codes into categories, once the relationships between codes were established (Miles & Huberman, 1994). Rereading and refinement of the coding and thematic categories occurred throughout the analysis process. The analysis concluded with the establishment of categories. To strengthen the rigor and trustworthiness of the analysis, a second member of the study team applied the coding scheme to the data. The final categories included lack of interpersonal interactions; interpersonal interaction impacts clinical skill development; most concerned about field; reputation of university most important; rigor/quality of the courses; students most important; and other.

Concerns Hiring Someone with an Online Degree

Of the 100 participants who responded to the first question ("Do you have any concerns in hiring someone with an online degree"), 35 said they had no such concerns and another five indicated that the question wasn't applicable. The most common reservation concerning the hiring of individuals with online degrees involved the perceived lack of interpersonal interactions in a virtual classroom. Thirty-three respondents suggested that online courses did not provide sufficient opportunities for interpersonal interactions between faculty and students or between classmates. Many suggested that this lack of interactivity potentially undermined the educational experience and hindered learning outcomes.

Responses suggested that social interaction in the classroom was perceived as particularly critical for social work education, given the relational aspects of the profession. One participant wrote,

> Social work is an interactive skill. Learning to listen and "hear" are critical and I don't believe these are skills that can be taught or learned "online". The collaborative nature of group learning—sharing with colleagues in a live setting—is an integral component of social work education.

Another respondent similarly opined, "[My concern is for] ... the interpersonal experience ... the colleague/peer interaction before, during and after session. Many key social work skills involve the ability to interact in person with other people—this is lost in an online school."

Ten participants suggested that traditional pedagogical strategies for teaching clinical skills, such as role-plays, could not readily translate to a virtual environment, hence compromising the clinical education of online students. According to one respondent,

> I am concerned that they do not have the interpersonal skills necessary to work with clients. The use of role playing and other similar activities teaches students how to respond clinically in the moment. ... in traditional programs professors can detect who does not possess the interpersonal skills that are paramount in developing a therapeutic relationship, and work with students to develop these critical skills, or coach them out of the social work profession.

Another respondent echoed this sentiment: "Staff should have experience learning and providing in vivo counseling. Qualities such as tone and body language cannot be accurately assessed or displayed through a computer." Interestingly, several of these same respondents nevertheless thought that macro practice skills could be learned online.

Outcomes also indicated that the perceived quality of the field education experience may moderate attitudes toward online MSW degrees. Sixteen respondents noted that the field education experience would be central to their evaluation of an online degree. One participant expressed this sentiment by writing, "I am more concerned about the quality of the field placement if the candidate has an online degree." Notably, there was evidence that some mistakenly believed that online programs did not contain a field education component. For instance, one respondent wrote that a "lack of field experience" was a concern in hiring an individual with an online degree. Another alluded to a similar deficit in field education, stating,

> Preparation for certain skills is limited, particularly in the area of interpersonal skills. Client contact is required to build assessment skills, case management skills, and counseling skills. This cannot be acquired on-line without additional learning experiences.

Finally, a smaller group of respondents (seven) suggested that the reputation of the university or the vigor of coursework (two) was more important than the delivery mechanism of the degree, or mitigated the negative connotations sometimes associated with online degrees. One participant wrote,

"The field is changing and as better schools offer this, we would be more likely to consider hiring someone." Another similarly noted, "It would depend on the university, as we've had social work interns that were taking mostly online courses through [institutional name omitted] and were great candidates. However, there are some online universities that do not have good reputations."

Participant responses to the second question ("Is there anything else you want to tell us?") largely mirrored findings from the first question. There were 100 qualitative responses, and a majority responded to this follow-up query with a "no" (44) or a "NA" (six). Of interest, nine respondents expressed positive attitudes toward online education. For instance, one noted the flexibility of online degrees and the ways in which online education allowed students to fulfill multiple responsibilities in a demanding economy: "You need to make people's lives easier. They need to work to support themselves and online learning can help so they can do both." Another respondent indicated that a growing familiarity with online education contributed to an attitude shift: "The more I learn about how online programs work, I am more open to considering applicants who hold online degrees." One noted the growing import of online education and advocated for greater university investment: "High quality online education is important. I would like universities to invest in making their online learning experiences as good, if not better, than the in class experience."

Discussion and Implications for Social Work Education

Although this study looked at human service administrator perceptions of online social work programs, there are some limitations. First, a higher participation rate would have been desirable. Yet our 36% response rate is within the norm for online surveys, which tend to yield lower response rates than traditional paper surveys (Fan & Yan, 2009). Shih and Fan's (2009) meta-analysis of 29 published studies, for example, found the average response rate for online surveys to be 34%. Moreover, our response rate may reflect population characteristics, as some suggest that survey response rates for nonprofit organizations (Hager, Wilson, Pollak, & Rooney, 2003) and high-level executives (Cycyota & Harrison, 2002) tend to be lower. In considering nonresponse bias, it may be that respondents who were more familiar with (or more opinionated about) online education were more likely to respond, although we are unable to confirm this conjecture. The agencies sampled are affiliated (through field work agreements) with a school of social work that runs an online program. However, very few of these agencies host online students, and it is highly likely that many of the respondents are unaware of the school's online program. It is also possible that small human service agencies, which do not have technology resources, might have been excluded.

Furthermore, we used a purposive sample drawn from a social work program's database of affiliated human service agencies located in three Eastern states. There were 934 agencies included in the initial mailing, but we have no way of knowing how representative these agencies (or our respondents) are of the larger, national universe of human service agencies, and the results of this localized study naturally are not generalizable. The survey also focused fully on online degrees, without a nuanced articulation of various permutations, such as hybrid programs and synchronous versus asynchronous learning. Had we asked about other forms of online learning, the results may have been different. Finally, we requested that the individual who is primarily in charge of hiring be the person to complete the survey. This decision poses a potential limitation, given that hiring often involves multiple staff members. Nevertheless, we believed this individual would best represent organizational and leadership perspectives regarding hiring criteria. Despite these limitations, we believe that the 370 administrators who responded to the survey do reflect some prevailing attitudes about online social work programs that we previously had heard only anecdotally. Since there has been very little research in this area, we hope to have contributed to a further understanding of this question.

In sum, this study finds that a majority of surveyed social work administrators believe that traditional MSW degrees are preferable to those attained online. It supports anecdotal evidence about social work's somewhat negative perception of online clinical education, despite empirical evidence supporting equivalent learning outcomes. Our results also suggest that social work administrators may have limited or even mistaken understandings of online MSW program content and expectations. For instance, some respondents incorrectly suggested that field education is not an online MSW program requirement. Hence, administrators' lack of knowledge about online education may contribute in part to negative perceptions. In fact, there is some initial evidence to suggest that greater familiarity with online education may correlate with more positive attitudes toward online degrees. For instance, respondents who have hired staff with online degrees are more likely to feel that online programs are as good as traditional ones. However, simply having taken an online course was not associated with a more positive attitude toward online degrees.

Our results, of course, must be interpreted with caution given the study's limitations, but they do raise concerns that students with degrees obtained from online programs could face challenges when seeking employment. Assuming that student demand for this degree option continues, it is incumbent upon social work programs to assess, ensure, and communicate the quality, rigor, interactivity, and innovation of online MSW degrees to various stakeholders, including field agencies, the broader social service community, and other educational partners.

As noted, initial research suggests that clinical learning outcomes and field education performance are equivalent for online and traditional MSW students. Additional evidence that compares larger cohorts of students naturally is needed to confirm or refine these early findings. Helpfully, CSWE's 2015 Educational Policy and Accreditation Standards call for assessment of learning outcomes and the achievement of social work competencies by program option. This requisite should facilitate larger scale data collection and a comparative analysis of outcomes between traditional and online programs.

In addition to conducting ongoing educational research, schools of social work offering online programs have an obligation to closely monitor the employment outcomes of their online graduates. Future research also should examine comparative data, including employment rates, salaries, licensure, and areas of practice. Finally, social work program administrators should use a variety of communication strategies to showcase the content and rigor embedded in their online programs, including innovations in clinical pedagogical strategies, to the profession at large.

References

Adams, J., DeFleur, M., & Heald, G. (2007). The acceptability of a doctoral degree earned online as a credential for health professionals. *Communication Education, 56*(3), 292–307. doi:10.1080/03634520701344959

Adams, J., Lee, S., & Cortese, J. (2012). The acceptability of online degrees: Principles and hiring practices in secondary schools. *Contemporary Issues in Technology and Teacher Education, 12*(4), 408–422.

Allen, I., & Seaman, J. (2015). *Grade level: Tracking online education in the United States, 2015.* Babson Park, MA: Babson Survey Research Group and Quahog Research Group. Retrieved from http://www.onlinelearningsurvey.com/reports/gradelevel.pdf

Allen, I., Seaman, J., Poulin, R., & Straut, T. (2016). *Online report card: Tracking online education in the United States.* Babson Park, MA: Babson Survey Research Group and Quahog Research Group. Retrieved from http://onlinelearningsurvey.com/reports/onliner eportcard.pdf

Clinical Social Work Association. (2013, September). *Position paper: Online master's of social work programs.* Garrisonville, VA: Author. Retrieved from http://www.clinicalsocialworkas sociation.org/Resources/Documents/CSWA%20-%20Position%20Paper%20-%20Online% 20MSW%20Programs%20-%209-13-1.pdf

Council on Social Work Education. (2015). *2014 Statistics on social work education in the United States.* Alexandria, VA: Author.

Cummings, S., Chaffin, K., & Cockerham, C. (2015). Comparative analysis of an online and a traditional MSW program: Educational outcomes. *Journal of Social Work Education, 51*(1), 109–120. doi:10.1080/10437797.2015.977170

Cycyota, C., & Harrison, D. (2002). Enhancing survey response rates at the executive level: Are employee- or consumer-level techniques effective? *Journal of Management, 28*(2), 151–176. doi:10.1177/014920630202800202

East, J. F., LaMendola, W., & Alter, C. (2014). Distance education and organizational environment. *Journal of Social Work Education, 50*, 19–33.

Fan, W., & Yan, Z. (2009). Factors affecting response rates of the web survey. *A Systematic Review Computers in Human Behavior, 26*, 132–139. doi:10.1016/j.chb.2009.10.01

Fogle, C. D., & Elliott, D. (2013). The market value of online degrees as a credible credential. *Global Education Journal, 2013*(3), 67–95.

Grossman, A., & Johnson, L. (2016). Employer perceptions of online accounting degrees. *Issues in Accounting Education, 31*(1), 91–109. doi:10.2308/iace-51229-2016

Hager, M., Wilson, S., Pollak, T., & Rooney, P. M. (2003). Response rates for mail surveys of nonprofit organizations: A review and empirical test. *Nonprofit and Voluntary Sector Quarterly, 32*(2), 252–267. doi:10.1177/0899764003251617

Hsieh, H., & Shannon, S. (2005). Three approaches to qualitative content analysis. *Qualitative Health Research, 15*(9), 1277–1288. doi:10.1177/1049732305276687

Kinneer, J. W. (2014). The acceptability of online and for-profit nursing degrees: A study of hiring gatekeeper perceptions. *Online Journal of Distance Learning Administration, 17*(2). Retrieved from http://www.westga.edu/~distance/ojdla/summer172/Kinneer172.html

Kurzman, P. A. (2013). The evolution of distance learning and online education. *Journal of Teaching in Social Work, 33*(4–5), 331–338. doi:10.1080/08841233.2013.843346

Levin, S., Whitsett, D., & Wood, G. (2013). Teaching MSW social work practice in a blended online learning environment. *Journal of Teaching in Social Work, 33*(4–5), 408–420. doi:10.1080/08841233.2013.829168

Metrejean, E., & Noland, T. (2011). An analysis of CPA firm recruiters' perceptions of online masters of accounting degrees. *Journal of Education for Business, 86*(1), 25–30. doi:10.1080/08832321003713754

Miles, M. B., & Huberman, A. M. (1994). *Qualitative data analysis: An expanded sourcebook.* Thousand Oaks, CA: Sage.

Moore, B. (2005). Faculty perceptions of the effectiveness of web-based instruction in social work education: A national study. *Journal of Technology in Human Services, 23*(1–2), 53–66. doi:10.1300/J017v23n01_04

Ouellette, P. M., Westhuis, D., Marshall, E., & Chang, V. (2006). The acquisition of social work interviewing skills in a web-based and classroom instructional environment: Results of a study. *Journal of Technology in Human Services, 24*(4), 53–75. doi:10.1300/J017v24n04_04

Potts, M., & Kleinpeter, C. (2001). Distance education alumni: How far have they gone? *Journal of Technology in Human Services, 18*(3/4), 85–99. doi:10.1300/J017v18n03_06

Reamer, F. (2013). Distance and online social work education: Novel ethical challenges. *Journal of Teaching in Social Work, 33*(4–5), 369–384. doi:10.1080/08841233.2013.828669

Regan, J. A. C., & Youn, E. J. (2008). Past, present, and future trends in teaching clinical skills through web-based learning environments. *Journal of Social Work Education, 44*(2), 95–115. doi:10.5175/JSWE.2008.200600592

Richardson, J. W., McLeod, S., & Dikkers, A. G. (2011). Perceptions of online credentials for school principals. *Journal of Educational Administration, 49*(4), 378–395. doi:10.1108/09578231111146461

Sawrikar, P., Lenette, C., McDonald, D., & Fowler, J. (2015). Don't silence "the dinosaurs": Keeping caution alive with regard to social work distance education. *Journal of Teaching in Social Work, 35*(4), 343–364. doi:10.1080/08841233.2015.1068262

Shih, T. H., & Fan, X. (2009). Comparing response rates in e-mail and paper surveys: A meta-analysis. *Educational Research Review, 4*, 26–40. doi:10.1016/j.edurev.2008.01.003

Siebert, D. C., Spaulding-Givens, J., & Siebert, C. (2006). Teaching clinical social work skills primarily online: An evaluation. *Journal of Social Work Education, 42*(2), 325–336. doi:10.5175/JSWE.2006.200404103

Straumsheim, C., Jaschik, S., & Lederman, D. (2015). *The 2015 Inside Higher Ed survey of faculty attitudes on technology: A study by Gallup and Inside Higher Ed.* Washington, DC: Gallup. Retrieved from https://www.insidehighered.com/system/files/media/Faculty%20Attitudes%20on%20Technology%202015.pdf

U.S. Department of Education, Office of Planning, Evaluation, and Policy Development. (2010). *Evaluation of evidence-based practices in online learning: A meta-analysis and review of online learning studies.* Washington, DC: Author.

Wilke, D., & Vinton, L. (2006). Evaluation of the first web-based advanced standing MSW program. *Journal of Social Work Education, 42*(3), 607–620. doi:10.5175/JSWE.2006.200500501

Woehle, R., & Quinn, A. (2009). An experiment comparing HBSE graduate social work classes: Face-to-face and at a distance. *Journal of Teaching in Social Work, 29*, 418–430. doi:10.1080/08841230903249745

Index

Note: **Bold** page numbers refer to tables and *italic* page numbers refer to figures.

Printed and bound by CPI Group (UK) Ltd, Croydon, CR0 4YY

21/10/2024

01777183-0001